PSYCHOLOGICAL TORTURE

D1556226

Sadly, it is highly likely that psychological torture is committed by governments worldwide and yet, notwithstanding the serious moral questions that this disturbing and elusive concept raises, and limited research in the area, there is no operational or legal definition. This pioneering new book provides the first scientific definition and instrument to measure what it means to be tortured psychologically, as well as how allegations of psychological torture can be judged.

Ground in cross–disciplinary research across psychology, anthropology, ethics, philosophy, law and medicine, the book is a tour de force which analyses the legal framework in which psychological torture can exist, the harrowing effects it can have on those who have experienced it, and the motivations and identities of those who perpetrate it.

Integrating the voices both of those who have experienced torture as well as those who have committed it, the book defines what we mean by psychological torture, its aims and effects, as well as the moral and ethical debates in which it operates. Finally, the book builds on the Istanbul Protocol to provide a comprehensive new framework, including practical scales, that enables us to accurately measure psychological torture for the first time.

This is an important and much–needed overview and analysis of an issue that many governments have sought to sweep under the carpet. Its accessibility and range of coverage make it essential reading not only for psychologists and psychiatrists interested in this field, but also human rights organisations, lawyers and the wider international community.

Pau Pérez-Sales is Chair of the World Psychiatric Association Section of Psychological Consequences of Persecution and Torture, Editor-in-Chief of *Torture Journal*, a practicing psychiatrist in Hospital La Paz (Madrid) and Director of the SiRa-GAC Center.

PSYCHOLOGICAL TORTURE

Definition, evaluation and measurement

Pau Pérez-Sales

WITHDRAWN
UTSA LIBRARIES

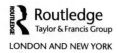 Routledge
Taylor & Francis Group

LONDON AND NEW YORK

First published 2017
by Routledge
2 Park Square, Milton Park, Abingdon, Oxon OX14 4RN

and by Routledge
711 Third Avenue, New York, NY 10017

Routledge is an imprint of the Taylor & Francis Group, an informa business

© 2017 Pau Pérez-Sales

The right of Pau Pérez-Sales to be identified as author of this work
has been asserted by him in accordance with sections 77 and 78 of the
Copyright, Designs and Patents Act 1988.

All rights reserved. The purchase of this copyright material confers the
right on the purchasing institution to photocopy pages which bear the
photocopy icon and copyright line at the bottom of the page. No other
parts of this book may be reprinted or reproduced or utilised in any form
or by any electronic, mechanical, or other means, now known or hereafter
invented, including photocopying and recording, or in any information
storage or retrieval system, without permission in writing from the
publishers.

Trademark notice: Product or corporate names may be trademarks or
registered trademarks, and are used only for identification and explanation
without intent to infringe.

British Library Cataloguing in Publication Data
A catalogue record for this book is available from the British Library

Library of Congress Cataloging in Publication Data
Names: Pâerez-Sales, Pau, author.
Title: Psychological torture : definition, evaluation and measurement /
Pau Pâerez-Sales.
Description: New York : Routledge, 2017. | Includes bibliographical
references.
Identifiers: LCCN 2016013433| ISBN 9781138671546 (hbk : alk. paper) |
ISBN 9781138671553 (pbk : alk. paper) | ISBN 9781315616940 (e-book)
Subjects: LCSH: Psychological torture.
Classification: LCC HV8593 .P457 2017 | DDC 364.6/7019—dc23
LC record available at https://lccn.loc.gov/2016013433

ISBN: 978-1-138-67154-6 (hbk)
ISBN: 978-1-138-67155-3 (pbk)
ISBN: 978-1-315-61694-0 (ebk)

Typeset in Bembo
by diacriTech, Chennai

Printed and bound in the United States of America by Publishers Graphics,
LLC on sustainably sourced paper.

Library
University of Texas
at San Antonio

ACKNOWLEDGEMENTS

agrade**CIMIENTOS**

To

```
                          h
              M           É
        m     A     r     C     o     S
              r           t
              I           O
              N           r
              a
```

Marcelo Viñar and Alberto Fernández, friends and psychiatrists, contributed by sharing and discussing personal memories. Sara López, colleague, lawyer and human rights activist, reviewed legal concepts. Carmelo Vazquez, always enthusiastic and supportive, provided insightful suggestions to the text. Genevieve Roudané and Beth Gelb have been more than style editors, and felt personally involved in the project. Thanks to all of them.

TABLE OF CONTENTS

EXTENDED TABLE OF CONTENTS

TABLES

FIGURES

WHY THIS BOOK: THE NEED TO DEFINE AND OPERATIONALISE TORTURE IN THE PRESENT CENTURY

Much has been written about torture from philosophical, ethical, legal and medical points of view since the early writings of Beccaria in the 17th century. However, defining torture remains a challenge: even after over 50 years of considerable efforts by academic researchers, a 2010 review based on 209 peer-reviewed research papers concluded: 'there is no consensus about how to define and operationalize torture. Only a quarter of published studies presented an explicit definition of torture leaves the impression that few in the field believe that defining their primary construct is even a worthwhile endeavor' (Green, Rasmussen and Rosenfeld, 2010b). As the authors stated: 'Obtaining a definition of "torture" is a critical starting point for understanding the impact of its primary construct and its operationalization'.

Torture methods are quickly evolving, faster than the understanding of both society and judges (who are, ultimately, part of society). It is a fact that torture is widespread in our times, even in parliamentary democratic societies. We face an era of change in which old methods based on the production of insurmountable pain coexist with techniques that operate mainly psychologically. Contemporary torture is increasingly the result of sophisticated methods aimed to make torture 'cleaner' for the torturer, widely acceptable to society, hidden from the media, and outside the legal protection available to the average citizen.

This book has several objectives:

1. To define torture in general and psychological torture specifically, while understanding that although pain and brute physical torture is still the main avenue through which torture currently occurs, it is increasingly being replaced by methods centred on the mind and self. Even when torture is purely physical, pain is merely the main but not the only door to access free will and influence the mind. Psychological torture exerting mild and controlled pain is plausibly the main avenue through which torture will occur in the future.
2. To build a theoretical framework for understanding contemporary torture as a necessary step towards redefining torture in legal and medical terms.

3. To propose operational criteria of torture enabling the advancement of academic research in the field.
4. To propose working criteria that would assist legal agents (judges, attorneys, lawyers and others) in deciding when a case could qualify as torture from a medical point of view.
5. To propose adjustments in the Istanbul Protocol (the main tool used worldwide for the documentation of torture) according to the aforementioned objectives.

SECTION 1
Premises

1

WHERE THINGS STAND: THE CONCEPT OF TORTURE AND PSYCHOLOGICAL TORTURE

The definition of torture in the legal arena

Torture is an ill-defined concept. Although many assume they understand it based on the influence of media and films, the fact is that the concept of torture (especially psychological torture) is elusive and blurred. This is not an accident. The UN definition of torture is concrete in certain aspects, but intentionally ambiguous in others, due to a belief that a narrow and overly operational definition of torture would allow governments to dodge the definition easily. Thus, this ambiguity served both a logical and political end.

Legislators seek a broad, qualitative definition of torture while leaving judges the discretion to interpret this definition in specific cases. While this approach may be legitimate, such general definitions undermine researchers' need for a measurable definition of torture. It is undoubtedly difficult to build a common framework for understanding the anthropological, ethical, psychological and legal aspects of torture. The lack of a measurable definition has made the advancement of a comprehensive theory of torture mechanisms extremely difficult, while depriving courts of the medical and psychiatric tools needed to improve decision-making.

In a review Green et al. (2010) found that only thirty per cent of academic research on torture included a definition, and of those studies, two out of three sources cited the 1984 United Nations Convention against Torture (CAT), which is the uncontested legal reference point. Article 1 of the Convention defines torture as:

> Any act by which (1) severe pain or suffering, (2) whether physical or mental, (3) is intentionally inflicted on a person (4) for such purposes as obtaining from him or a third person information or a confession, punishing him for an act he or a third person has committed or is suspected of having committed, or intimidating or coercing him or a third person, or for any reason based on discrimination of any kind, (5) when such pain or suffering is inflicted by or at the instigation of or with the consent or acquiescence of a public official or other person acting in an official capacity. It does not include pain or suffering arising only from, inherent in or incidental to lawful sanctions. *(Numbers added for clarity)*

The remaining sources use the definition of the World Medical Association.[1] Although most countries are signatories of the UNCAT, national legislation varies and sometimes includes a definition of torture that is not always compliant with the United Nations standard.[2]

The UNCAT definition has important operational problems, and the two main difficulties are defining severity of suffering and the motivational criteria (Table 1.1).

The fact that these criteria cannot be easily defined impedes the development of an operational definition of torture that could foster human rights research. This difficulty is reflected in the fact that half of the studies reviewed by Green et al. (2010) used broad categories that included torture victims among other victims of different kind of abuses, or made a single category of victims of torture 'and other ill-treatment' (Green et al., 2010).

The severity of suffering criteria is a problem specific to the UN definition; the World Medical Association avoided it. It is also excluded in the definition of the Inter-American Convention to Prevent and Punish Torture, which, drawing from the experience of its predecessor (the UNCAT definition), provided what may well be the best contemporary legal definition of torture. The definition agreed upon by the Inter-American Commission of Human Rights, though limited in its application to the Latin American countries that signed it, deserves special consideration because it goes much further than that of the UN:

> For the purposes of this Convention, torture shall be understood to be any act intentionally performed whereby physical or mental pain or suffering is inflicted on a person for purposes of criminal investigation, as a means of intimidation, as personal punishment, as a preventive measure, as a penalty, or for any other purpose. Torture shall also be understood to be the use of methods upon a person intended to obliterate the personality of the victim or to diminish his physical or mental capacities, even if they do not cause physical pain or mental anguish. (Article 2 of the convention)[3]

The definition explicitly recognises that (1) *physical pain* is not necessarily a requirement for torture; (2) the 'severity' of suffering is not a criterion because the emphasis must be on the *methods* used and not the consequences; and (3) the purpose of torture can be 'to obliterate the personality of the victim', or to 'diminish his mental capacities'. In other words, it specifically recognises psychological torture *even in absence of mental suffering*, if there is an attack to the psychological integrity of the person. The Inter-American Court has affirmed that when the state is clearly involved, there is no need to know the 'intentionality' of the perpetrator, as this is sometimes impossible to elucidate (see discussion in Chapter 6). The Rome Statute of

TABLE 1.1 Key problems in the UNCAT definition of torture

Criteria	Problems with the criteria
Severity of Suffering: Torture is an act that inflicts severe pain or suffering whether physical or mental.	• What is 'severe'? How is severity defined? • How is 'mental suffering' defined? • When is 'mental suffering' so severe as to amount to torture?
Motivational Criteria: Torture is intentionally inflicted to obtain a confession, intimidation, coercion.	• How can we ascertain the alleged perpetrator's 'intentionality'? • How can the alleged perpetrator's motives and purposes of be ascertained?

the International Criminal Court and, in the 1990s, the International Criminal Tribunals in the former Yugoslavia and Rwanda are also reference points that have established additional criteria for defining torture.

With few exceptions, torture is measured using questionnaires that typically include a checklist of torture methods, and then the total 'number' of torture methods suffered is calculated, as if all the methods were comparable.[4] Thus, torture is often measured based only on the quantity and types of acts. A more refined tool would consider key variables of the torturing environment and the subjective experience of the survivor. For instance: (1) the relationship pattern between torturer and tortured; (2) circumstances of the torturing system (political persecution, ethnic cleansing, law enforcement procedure, etc.); (3) whether techniques target identity; and (4) the severity of each experience from both an objective and subjective point of view.

The boundaries of torture: the concept of Cruel, Inhuman and Degrading Treatment (CIDT)

There are excellent, up-to-date reviews on the concept of torture and Cruel, Inhuman and Degrading treatment (CIDT) in international human rights law and international criminal law (Nowak and McArthur, 2008; Rodley and Pollard, 2009; Vos, 2007). Here we will briefly review the most essential topics; Chapter 4 will focus on aspects directly related to the consideration of mental and psychological suffering as factors in the determination of torture allegations in the context of international law.

The definition of torture is closely linked to the legal debate about its boundaries. In 1969 the European Commission of Human Rights (ECHR) introduced the distinction between 'torture' and 'ill-treatment' and in different sentences established a progressive criterion, considering torture an 'aggravated and deliberate form of cruel, inhuman or degrading treatment or punishment', a formula also adopted in 1975 by the General Assembly of the United Nations in their first Declaration against Torture. This distinction disappeared in 1984 when the UN finally approved the Convention against Torture (CAT) and other Cruel, Inhuman or Degrading Treatment or Punishment in which no distinction is explicitly made between 'torture' and 'ill-treatment' (see Article 1, above). Article 16 of the Convention equates torture and CIDT by stating that any state party is obligated to 'prevent' CIDT. However, the level of obligation by the signatory states is not the same. Although the Convention unequivocally prohibits both torture and CIDT under international law (even in times of exception or war), the obligation to criminalise torture and to bring the perpetrators to justice (Articles 4 to 9), the principle of *non-refoulement* (Article 3) and the prohibition of using evidence extracted by torture (Article 15) apply exclusively to torture and not to CIDT. It is, therefore, of the utmost importance to draw a legal distinction between torture and other forms of CIDT in the application of the CAT (Nowak, 2009).

The European Court (1969), when considering allegations of torture by the State of Greece against political opponents, set an historical precedent and established three levels of treatment (Table 1.2).

The Court established that:

- In Level 1 the key point is dignity and the act does not necessarily need to be intentional.
- Level 2 and 3 are indistinguishable with the only difference that 3 (torture) would be an aggravated form of 2 (inhuman treatment).

TABLE 1.2 Classical distinction between torture and cruel, inhuman and degrading treatment

Level 1. Degrading treatment	'Treatment that grossly *humiliates* a person or drives him to act against his will or conscience.'
Level 2. Cruel or inhuman treatment	'Treatment that *deliberately* causes *severe* suffering, mental or physical, which in the particular situation is unjustifiable.'
Level 3. Torture	'Inhuman treatment which has a purpose of obtaining information or confessions, or the infliction of punishment, and it is generally an *aggravated* form of inhuman treatment.'

The concept of 'unjustifiable' disappeared in all future definitions and has no application under current international law, although it was at the centre of the recent debate in the United States within the context of the so-called 'war against terrorism', where some scholars apply the principle of 'necessity' and 'proportionality' to advocate for the legalisation of torture under certain conditions (Allhoff, 2005; Dershowitz, 2008; Sussman, 2005)

This distinction was the basis of the well-known sentence *Ireland v. United Kingdom* that established the boundaries of torture for the European Court of Human Rights (ECHR) in the 1970s and the beginning of the 1980s (ECHR, 1978a). The tribunal considered a complaint by the Irish government regarding the case of a group of 228 Irish citizens detained and interrogated by the British Army between 1971 and 1974 and systematically subjected to five techniques[5] (wall-standing, hooding, subjection to noise, sleep deprivation and deprivation of food and drink). The European Commission found that the combined use of the five techniques 'did not occasion suffering of the particular intensity and cruelty implied by the word torture . . . [but] amounted to a practice of inhuman and degrading treatment' (Weissbrodt, Aolain, Fitzpatrick and Newman, 2009).

The tribunal was asserting that there was a particular stigma attached to the term 'torture', and therefore it should be used selectively and cautiously (Nowak, 2009). For some authors (e.g. Spjut, 1979) this meant that, in practice, treatment should only be declared *torture* when 'there were acts of extreme barbarity' and excluded from torture 'the systematically researched and applied subtle techniques of psychological manipulation which nullify the human will'. This reasoning criminalised the types of crude torture more commonly performed in 'third world' countries, while providing legal protection to the more subtle non-pain based forms of ill-treatment practiced in European democracies (Nowak, 2006).

After facing criticism, the court reconsidered their position in subsequent sentences. In the case of *Ahmed Selmouni v. France* (ECHR, 1999), the Court clearly changed its doctrine.[6] It ruled that sustained beatings and humiliation leaving evidence of physical injury (acts that it would have previously categorised as only 'inhuman') *did* constitute torture. The Court also supported the qualification of torture based on psychological suffering (in the form of humiliation, debasement and instilling fear or anguish), noting 'the regrettable failure to order a psychological report'. The Court stated that: 'Having regard to the fact that the Convention is a living instrument which must be interpreted in the light of present-day conditions . . . the Court considers that certain acts which were classified in the past as "inhuman and degrading treatment" as opposed to "torture" could be classified differently in the future.' The Court took the view that greater firmness was needed to defend the fundamental values of contemporary democratic societies.

Two years later, in *Keenan v. United Kingdom* (ECHR, 2001a) the Court moved even further towards disavowing severity of suffering as the defining factor. The sentence explained that: 'While it is true that the severity of suffering, physical or mental, attributable to a particular measure has been a significant consideration in many of the cases decided (. . .) under Article 3, there are circumstances where proof of the actual effect on the person may not be a major factor. For example, in respect of a person deprived of his liberty, recourse to physical force which has not been made strictly necessary by his own conduct diminishes human dignity and is in principle an infringement of the right set forth in Article 3.' For some authors (e.g. Rodley and Pollard, 2009), the idea implicit in this sentence was that the five techniques once considered 'inhuman and degrading treatment' would be qualified as torture and that the Court was moving away from the concept of 'severity of suffering' (Vos, 2007).

The UN Human Rights Committee adhered to this doctrine from the beginning, and in 1997, they explicitly challenged the Israeli Government's claim that the use of the 'five' techniques did not cause severe suffering and therefore did not violate Article 1 of the Convention (Ginbar, 2009; Imseis, 2001). The Committee rejected this argument, noting that other criteria, 'such as intent and purpose of extracting information, were met'.[7] The underlying idea was that purpose and motivation, not severity of suffering, were the core criteria for deciding if torture had occurred.

Under the administration of President George W. Bush, the US tried to bring back the distinction based on the severity of suffering assuming that only torture, not CIDT, would be subjected to prosecution under international law (Greenberg, 2006; Jaffer and Singh, 2006; Nordgren, McDonnell and Loewenstein, 2011). CIDT would therefore be permissible during the interrogation of Guantanamo detainees, and those responsible would not be liable to international prosecution (Rumsfeld, 2003). International human rights groups unanimously rejected this position[8] (because the Convention prohibits both).[9]

There is growing consensus in international law to establish a common threshold of 'severe pain and suffering' for both torture and cruel or inhuman treatment, and to shift emphasis from the intensity of suffering to its 'purpose' and motivation (Rodley and Pollard, 2009). This approach has been adopted by the ECHR, the UN Committee, and the Inter-American Court. It is also compatible with the Rome Statute of the International Criminal Court (ICC), which does not require aggravation of pain or suffering in order to identify torture in war crimes. Most experts consider this to be the simplest and most practical position (Nowak, 2009; Rodley and Pollard, 2009; Vos, 2007). Thus, if 'purpose' is established as the defining criteria which distinguishes torture from cruel or inhuman treatment, it is no longer necessary to define the minimum threshold of pain or suffering. Moreover, this definition reflects the reality of contemporary torture (as well as torture in the foreseeable future), in which interrogators use more subtle mechanisms that are not necessarily based on pain or suffering. This definition prevents attempts by governments to distinguish between subjective gradations of pain and erode the mandate of the Convention while escaping full responsibility for ill-treatment of prisoners (Luban et al., 2012). The resulting gradation would resemble Table 1.3.

In all cases, the above only applies when such pain or suffering is inflicted by (or at the instigation of, or with the consent or acquiescence of) a public official or other person acting in an official capacity. It does not include pain or suffering arising only from, inherent in, or incidental to lawful sanctions.

In a personal interpretation, former United Nations Special Rapporteur Manfred Nowak proposed that in addition to purpose, *powerlessness* is an additional key factor for distinguishing torture from CIDT (Nowak and McArthur, 2006). Nowak argues that when a person is rendered

TABLE 1.3 Contemporary distinction between torture, cruel, inhuman and degrading treatment

Level 1. Degrading treatment	Treatment that grossly *humiliates* a person or drives him to act against his will or conscience.
Level 2. Cruel or inhuman treatment	Treatment that *deliberately* causes [severe] *mental or physical* suffering.
Level 3. Torture	Treatment that *deliberately* causes [severe] *mental or physical* suffering with the purpose of obtaining information or confessions, or the infliction of punishment, or any other reason based on discrimination (Cunniffe, 2013).

completely helpless and cannot defend him or herself from the aggressor, such powerlessness should be included as an element in identifying torture. For instance, even though legal force used against protestors would not be considered torture under the UNCAT definition because the aggression was exercised legally, Nowak's principle of proportionality and powerlessness could apply. Beating a person lying on the ground, whether unconscious or defenseless, for the purpose of humiliation or punishment could be considered CIDT or even amount to torture.

Psychological torture: early definitions

There is not an official definition of or consensus on the meaning of **psychological torture** (PT). Some definitions emphasise the *results* and define PT as the methods 'used to break down a detainee psychologically' (Kramer, 2010), or to 'disrupt profoundly the senses or the personality' (PHR, 2005, citing a US law[10]). The Inter-American Convention specifies, as mentioned above, that PT is 'the use of methods upon a person intended to obliterate the personality of the victim or to diminish his physical or mental capacities, even if they do not cause physical pain or mental anguish'.[11]

Others emphasise the *method* of torture. In such cases, PT is defined as methods which cause aversive stimuli not *based on producing physical pain or that do not physically attack the body* (Quiroga and Jaranson, 2008; Reyes, 2008). Cunniffe (2013) argues that because all torture methods affect the mind, the term psychological torture should be reserved for no-touch torture. In their report on torture methods used in Guantanamo, the Center for Constitutional Rights (Center for Human Rights and Humanitarian Law, 2006) classified the following as psychological torture methods: 'Solitary confinement, light and sound manipulation, exposure to the elements and to extreme temperature, . . . sleep deprivation, and threats of transfer for torture in another country.' The report found that 'physical methods' included 'beatings, short-shackling (being tied in painful positions for hours) and stress positions'.

Another point of view sees PT as a set of practices to inflict pain or suffering *without resorting to direct physical violence*, thus including in the definition of PT those techniques in which there is no 'aggression' but there is physical pain (like being held in stress positions for hours) (CSHRA, 2005).

Finally, some authors distinguish PT from **brain torture**, defined as *physical torture that targets the brain*.[12] Examples include: mild but repeated head contusions with a newspaper, a book, or an open hand, as well as dry anoxia through hooding. These torture techniques leave no external marks, and they directly affect brain functioning, and, if repeated, can cause permanent damage as detected by fMRi or SPECT (Panayiotou, Jackson and Crowe, 2010).

White torture, no-touch torture and clean torture

Although some authors use it interchangeably with the concept of psychological torture (Mausfeld, 2009), the concept of **white torture** refers specifically to torture based on the use of sensory deprivation techniques (Suedfeld, 1990). White torture is named after studies performed by Donald Hebb and others in the 1950s (McCoy, 2012). They showed that a person who was blindfolded, isolated from noise and placed in a closed water tank or wearing special clothes designed to block sensory inputs presented symptoms of confusion after just a few hours, signs of disintegration of personality after twenty-four hours, and hallucinations and psychotic symptoms after about two days. The effects were long lasting: some subjects of these experiments even suffered permanent mental damage. These studies formed the basis for the design of maximum security experimental prisons (like F-Prisons in Turkey for Kurdish prisoners, which are now closed, or the special security modules in Evin prison in Iran). The design of the cells precluded any human contact and the environment was comprised entirely of white tones, with minimal stimulus.

McCoy (2006, 2012) has coined the term **no-touch torture** to specifically describe techniques developed since 1950 by the Central Intelligence Agency (CIA) in different psychology research programs (of which MK Ultra is the most famous). The KUBARK Manual (Central Intelligence Agency, 1963), later refined and updated in the Human Resource Exploitation Manual (Central Intelligence Agency, 1983), describes and explains techniques designed 'to induce psychological regression in the subject by bringing a superior outside force to bear on his will to resist' (p. 89). McCoy groups these techniques into two categories: 'sensory disorientation'[13] and 'self-inflicted pain'.[14]

In his exhaustive review of torture methods throughout history, Rejali (2007) introduces two new terms: **coercion torture** and **clean torture**. He points out that many painful physical techniques of interrogation or control leave few marks. Such practices are referred to as 'clean techniques' in contrast to the scarring techniques of torture; Rejali does not consider them to be psychological techniques. He says that most torture techniques in democracies are clean torture because although they may involve intense physical pain, they leave almost no marks: a fist punching the body leaves few lasting physical traces.

Ojeda (2008), in a seminal review on psychological torture methods, assumes that it is difficult to formulate a satisfying definition because it is impossible to define 'psychological pain' or how much suffering qualifies as enough to reach the level of 'torture'. His solution is to opt for an alternative **extensional definition** of PT, that is, to enumerate a list of categories of techniques that could be considered 'psychological torture' according to the CIA training manuals, scientific knowledge, and other sources.

In this text we will consider psychological torture to be *the use of techniques of cognitive, emotional or sensory attacks that target the conscious mind and cause psychological suffering, damage and/or identity breakdown in most subjects subjected to them; such techniques may be used alone or together with other techniques to produce a cumulative effect.* Thus, PT involves manipulating the input received by the conscious mind, input that allows the person to stay oriented in the surrounding world, retain control and have the adequate conditions to judge, understand and freely make decisions – in effect, the essential constitutive ingredients of an unharmed self.

Most torture techniques are in fact both physical and psychological because the distinction between body and mind is artificial: the two are inseparably interconnected. Sensory deprivation, deprivation of food and inundation with white noise are all techniques that attack basic functions of the body, weakening the person and finally attacking the mind. Hunger, in theory a 'no-touch' technique, can produce unbearable physical pain.

Thus, we can distinguish:

- Pure psychological techniques (such as humiliation)
- Attacks on the self through attacks on bodily functions (such as sleep deprivation)

The range of views on torture presented so far reveal the complexity and lack of consensus in the field. How can psychological torture be understood from a multidisciplinary point of view? Can psychological research produce an operational definition based on objective scientific criteria to improve clinical and epidemiological studies, while facilitating the forensic assessment of cases? Is it possible to reach a consensus on the criteria that could help refine a legal framework to protect against torture? These are the challenges we will address in this book.

Notes

1   The Tokyo declaration of the World Medical Association (1975) is often cited as a precedent. 'Torture is defined as the deliberate, systematic or wanton infliction of physical or mental suffering by one or more persons acting alone or on the orders of any authority, to force another person to yield information, to make a confession, or for any other reason.'

2   In the United States, torture is defined as 'an act committed by a person acting illegally, specifically intended to inflict severe physical or mental pain or suffering (other than pain or suffering incidental to lawful sanctions) upon another person within his custody or lawful control' (18 U.S.C. 23490(1) 1998). 'Severe physical or mental pain or suffering' is defined as follows: '(A) the intentional infliction or threatened infliction of severe physical pain or suffering; (B) the administration or application, or threatened administration or application, of mind-altering substances or other procedures calculated to disrupt profoundly the senses or the personality; (C) the threat of imminent death; or (D) the threat that another person will imminently be subjected to death, severe physical pain or suffering, or the administration or application of mind-altering substances or other procedures calculated to disrupt profoundly the senses or personality.'

3   www.oas.org/juridico/english/treaties/a-51.html

4   See Başoğlu, Livanou and Crnobarić, 2007. The Semi-Structured Interview for Survivors of Torture (Başoğlu et al., 2007) for instance, operationalises torture severity by calculating a combined index. The index includes the total number of types of torture (from a list of 44 events), frequency of exposure to torture, duration of detention and perceived severity of each type of experienced torture (i.e. distress) rated along a 5-point Likert scale.

5   (1) Wall-standing: forcing the detainees to remain for periods of some hours in a 'stress position', described by those who underwent it as being 'spread-eagled against the wall, with their fingers put high above the head against the wall, the legs spread apart and the feet back, causing them to stand on their toes with the weight of the body mainly on the fingers'; (2) hooding: putting a black or navy colored bag over the detainees' heads and, at least initially, keeping it there all the time except during interrogation; (3) subjection to noise: pending their interrogations, holding the detainees in a room where there was a continuous loud and hissing noise; (4) deprivation of sleep: pending their interrogations, depriving the detainees of sleep; (5) deprivation of food and drink: subjecting the detainees to a reduced diet during their stay at the centre and pending interrogations (*Ireland v. United Kingdom*, paragraph 96).

6   The full text states: 'The Court found that . . . he had been subjected while in police custody [to] physical and—undoubtedly (notwithstanding the regrettable failure to order a psychological report on Mr. Selmouni after the events complained of)—mental pain and suffering. The course of the events also showed that pain and suffering had been inflicted on the applicant intentionally for the purpose of, inter alia, making him confess to the offense which he had been suspected of having committed. (. . .) The acts complained of had been such as to arouse in the applicant feelings of fear,

anguish, and inferiority, capable of humiliating and debasing him and possibly breaking his physical and moral resistance. (. . .) It remained to establish in the present case whether the "pain or suffering" inflicted on Mr. Selmouni could be defined as "severe" within the meaning of Article 1 of the United Nations Convention against Torture (. . .). The Court considered that this "severity" was, like the "minimum severity" required for the application of Article 3, in the nature of things, relative; it depended on all the circumstances of the case, such as the duration of the treatment, its physical or mental effects and, in some cases, the sex, age, and state of health of the victim, etc. The Court was satisfied that a large number of blows had been inflicted on Mr. Selmouni. (. . .) The Court also observed that the applicant had been subjected to a certain number of acts which would have been heinous and humiliating for anyone, irrespective of their condition. (. . .) Under these circumstances, the Court was satisfied that the physical and mental violence, considered as a whole, committed against the applicant's person had caused "severe" pain and suffering and had been particularly serious and cruel. Such conduct had to be regarded as acts of torture for the purposes of Article 3 of the Convention' (Summary, paragraph 4).

7 Report of the Committee Against Torture, GAOR, 52nd Session. Supplement n. 44 (1997), paras 24–5.

8 For a review see http://en.wikisource.org/wiki/Working_Group_Report_on_Detainee_Interro gations (last consulted May 2014).

9 Secretary of Defense Donald Rumsfeld authorised the use of thirty-five techniques. Seventeen were already in use and described in intelligence army manual FM 34–52. Techniques 20–21, 27–29 and 31–35 were explicitly recognised as involving physical contact that can produce pain or harm, or threats of pain or harm. They included: the prolonged use of stress positions for up to four hours; continuous interrogations for up to twenty hours; solitary detention for up to thirty days; forced grooming; hooding; removal of clothing; auditory/environmental manipulation; and other methods. Rumsfeld stated in 2005, prior to the army's internal investigation, 'My impression is that what has been charged thus far is abuse, which I believe technically is different from torture . . . I don't know if . . . it is correct to say . . . that torture has taken place, or that there's been a conviction for torture. And therefore I'm not going to address the torture word' (cited in Vos, 2007, p. 6).

10 18 U.S.C. §2340(2)(B)

11 www.oas.org/juridico/english/treaties/a-51.html

12 Another similar category is physical torture when the target is the senses. Again, hearing or sight can be a target for aggression, leaving no external marks.

13 A mix of sensory overload and sensory deprivation via isolation then intense interrogation, heat and cold, light and dark, noise and silence, for a systematic attack on all human stimuli.

14 Fighting against an external source of pain (like in beatings or shocks) is substituted by fighting against an internal source of pain (such as endless hours of the stress of forced positions) so that there is no aggression and the detainee becomes his or her own enemy.

SECTION 2
The voices

2

INTANGIBLE ELEMENTS OF PSYCHOLOGICAL TORTURE: LEARNING FROM THE VOICES OF SURVIVORS

'Usually, the testimonies denouncing torture that are delivered to agencies working on Human Rights – detailed as they are – merely recount what happened from beginning to end as a chronological narrative. When they mention certain kinds of torture, they are almost always referring to techniques: "they used the bathtub on me," [or] "the bag"; "they put electrodes on me." (. . .). Sometimes the reports are very detailed. And yet, when you ask torture victims privately about the testimony, they usually end up confessing that the testimony does not satisfy them, that it pales before all that was actually done to them, that it barely touches on everything they experienced. "I say: They put electrodes on my testicles, but can anyone imagine what that means? Or the theater and the madness that surrounded me? What I felt? Only someone who has been through that can understand." (. . .). For the readers of the testimonies that regularly circulate, it is very important to know that they are only outlines, small sketches of a skeleton that lacks meat; they give data, list techniques, collect specific phrases. (. . .) Years ago, another victim of torture told me, "If you haven't been there, you can't understand anything." And it's true.' (Eva Forest, On Torture, 2006)

Torture is a widespread phenomenon. Testimony is one of the elements that helps give meaning to the torture experience, though it often presents challenges and feelings of hopelessness, pain and skepticism. There are many autobiographical accounts of torture survivors from all over the world and ample documentation from rehabilitation centres offering descriptions of the subjective experience of survivors. It is possible to access testimonies from almost all conditions and contexts. In this chapter, we offer an overview of the key elements of torture *from the perspective of survivors*. We include a selection of published texts from survivors with especially revealing insights into the psychology of torture.

We will limit ourselves to the question, *What are the core elements of a torture survivor's experience that can help create a definition of psychological torture?* We will only analyse torture (and not other, connected, forms of exerting strength or coercion linked to politically motivated violence that could be included under a broader spectrum of 'torture experiences'); we focus on the emotional and psychological components in the description of the experience (not the description of actions or methods).

Out of a great number of testimonies, we have chosen a group of survivors with especially enlightening ways of putting words to feelings and experiences that are usually unspeakable and indescribable. Testimonies from survivors from Uruguay (Carlos Liscano, Jacqueline Gurruchuga and Beatriz Brenzano, Henry Engler, and Marcelo Viñar) and Argentina (Mario Villani), as well as Cambodia (Vann Nath), Austria (Jean Améry), Spain (Javier Larreta) and the former Soviet Union (Alexander Solzhenitsyn) are represented below.

Vann Nath – *A Cambodian Prison Portrait*

Vann Nath is one of seven people who survived imprisonment and torture in the S-21 detention centre in Phnom Penh, during the Pol Pot regime in Cambodia.[1] His memoir (Nath, 1998) describes the routines in the prison and mass killing by starvation and hunger.

'I lay exhausted on the floor, without one grain of rice in my belly. I fell asleep. (. . .). I woke up early the next day, my body aching. I was famished and I wondered what kind of food they would give me when they let me eat (. . .). Then a man carrying porridge in a bucket on a shoulder pole came in the room (. . .). Everyone got four small spoonfuls of porridge and some watery soup with banana leaves floating in it. It tasted delicious to me because I was so hungry. But after a couple of spoonfuls, the food was all gone and the guards ordered [us] to go to sleep. I lay down on the floor and realized that they were not going to give me water. I turned to the prisoner nearby, named Chath. His eyelids were drooping. "Two or three spoons of rice – is that enough?" I asked. "I'm so hungry . . ." (. . .). "Keep quiet, be careful," he said. Eventually I fell asleep.'

An estimated 12,000 people were killed in the centre through torture and extrajudicial killings.

'When I woke up, I wanted badly (. . .) to drink some water. (. . .). I began to feel hungry. (. . .). The sky began to darken. The electric power came on in the room, [and] it was bright as daylight. I lay back and looked at a small gecko on the ceiling that was catching insects around the electric light. The gecko was luckier than me, I thought, because it had plenty of insects to eat!'

Hunger and thirst become an obsession.

'My belly felt like it was almost touching my backbone. When will they give us another plate of rice porridge? Maybe they only gave one a day. We would starve to death in less than half a month (. . .). Then, I heard the guards ordering us to wake up. I sat up quickly and saw the rice porridge had come. I swallowed my spit because I was so hungry. They were passing the plates out, the same as in the morning. I wanted to save some but I was too hungry. The others were the same and in a blink of an eye, everything was gone and the bowls were licked clean.'

'After living that kind of life for several days my body began to deteriorate. My ribs were poking out and my body was like an old man of 70. My hair had overgrown like bamboo roots and had become a nest for lice. I had scabies all over my body. My mind and spirit had flown away. I only knew one thing clearly: Hunger.'

'Each night if any crickets or grasshoppers fell down from the electric lights above, we would scramble for them and toss them into our mouths as if they were delicious. When the guard caught us, he would smack our heads as hard as he could with his thick sandal made of rubber auto tire, giving us black eyes or bloody noses.'

'I lived that way for more than 30 days. I was never released from the shackles (. . .) If I needed to defecate, I asked the guards to bring the bucket over.'

'One day I felt unusually weak and exhausted. I could not hear anything clearly – it felt like my ears were filled with cotton. (. . .). I whispered to Chath, the man next to me: "Brother, I don't think I can make it another ten days. I'm so hungry and I can hardly hear or see." "I feel the same – we have

no hope now." Maybe they were going to kill me, maybe not. It did not matter. Wisdom and spirit had *flown from me. All I thought about was my stomach . . .'* (p. 42–50).

The text also describes the environment of absolute terror and the permanent state of fear and panic, just waiting for the final moment of torture and killing, while watching trucks arriving with new detainees and hearing how the newcomers are also tortured and disappeared. Nath later explains that even the guards ultimately disappeared.

In a meeting between survivors and torturers, over fifteen years later, in the context of filming a documentary (Panh, 2003), Nath said:

'I have two types of wounds. One is bodily injury. They have electrocuted me to look for a supposed betrayal, facts about enemies whom I did not know. (. . .). The other one is an injury to the emotions, a psychological wound. I live in fear. They have taken from me everything that is human; they have removed the right to be a human being. I have been tied up and abandoned in a corner, hungry, undignified, humiliated. . . . When you go through all that suffering, you will never be able to forget. (. . .). I would like to live like a father, with the same rights as others. But when humans are tortured so deeply, they will never be able to forget. Even today, I am afraid of everything, without reason or logic. I'm scared and I can never find the causes.'

'Forget? Forget? Although I want to forget, I cannot forget. Tonight, for example [before the encounter], I've only slept one hour. Every time I wake up, the images of the prison come to me again and again. I do not want them, but they come. I see you now, and I will see you tonight in my dreams, in front of me as you were at the time. How you walked and talked, your gestures. . . . Your voice will come back to me again. Everything returns again and again. . . . (. . .) If I want to sleep, I have to take medication. I do not want to think about the past, but the past haunts me . . .' (pp. 39–40).

Elements for a definition of psychological torture based on Vann Nath's testimony

Torturing System. S–21 is described as a place of extermination in the context of a country where large parts of the population were annihilated. The communication between guards and detainees, the absolute and unquestionable submission and the extreme terror experienced are only understandable in this context. A person could be tortured to death for any spurious reason, in this context of constant psychological pressure often combined with illogical actions, contradictory messages, arbitrary decisions, cruelty and nonsense.

Torture cannot be separated from the context in which it occurs. Torture and its effects are not isolated events, but part of a larger context that gives birth to torture and keeps it alive. This is what Montagut (2012) and others refer to as *the torturing system*.

Hunger as an extremely painful, slow death of the body, as a method for breaking the psyche. Nath's testimony shows the interplay between physical and psychological factors. Food and water restriction, as examples of manipulation of bodily functions, are elements not usually associated with physical pain. They are considered part of the 'softening' process that makes detention uncomfortable and facilitates cooperation. But Nath describes how hunger can come to break the spirit and the mind. Starving, physical pain and emotional and cognitive breakdown go together. He remembers starving as a devastating experience and defines hunger as worse than any other torture method.

Endless time, no hope. Time is endless, torture could go on forever, but one thing is for sure: everyone dies, without exception. Even guards, eventually, will die. Suffering is prolonged when one is subjected to a slow death.

Permanent changes in worldviews. Nath describes how torture changes the way the person sees others and the world; this change is irreversible. After torture, nothing can be the same again.

Introjection of fear. Permanent fear remains years after release, even in minor situations. The persons lives as if he was waiting for (delayed and unexpected) death at any moment.

Carlos Liscano – *The Truck of Fools*

The Truck of Fools is Carlos Liscano's detailed account of nine months of daily torture suffered in Uruguay, followed by thirteen years in various maximum-security prisons and, finally, exile in Sweden (Liscano, 2004). Through a detailed and introspective narrative, the author creates a portrait of the main psychological dilemmas that a prisoner faces, the complex relationship with his torturer, and the intricate, strange and ambivalent relationship with his own body. It is a text unlike any other we know.

The two of us: my body and me. '*They have just brought me from the room where they torture; that's on the floor below, down the stairs to the left. You can hear screams, one person tortured, then another and another, all night. I don't think about anything. Or I think about my body. I don't think about it; I feel my body. It's dirty, beaten up, tired, smelly, sleepy, and hungry. Just now, the world consists of my body and me. I don't say it to myself like that, but I know there is no one else but the two of us. It will be many years, almost thirty, before I can tell myself what it is I feel. Not tell myself "what I feel," but what it and I felt*' (p. 17).

Make the prisoner fight against him or herself. '*The prisoner's other unequal struggle is with himself. Talk or not talk. In either case he loses, as there is no way to win at this game. If he does not talk, torture and the suffering continue, the prisoner does not know for how long. If he believes he can stay firm on his feet to the end, but can't, and breaks down, it could be disastrous, could lead to his giving out all the information he has without resistance, without making the torturer pull it out. If the tortured prisoner talks, he will be faced with his worst enemy, be left alone with himself, for weeks, months, years, thinking he is shit, asking himself why, telling himself he should and could have stood more, a little more, one more night, another session, another dunking of his head in the tank*' (p. 54).

Wanting to stop the pain, but fearing guilt. '*The first thing one wants is for pain to stop, all the rest is secondary. The sick person can do no more than wait for the results of medical treatment. But for the person tortured, relief depends on himself or herself. Only talk, and torture will stop. (. . .). But the pain, when will it stop? It depends on the torturers, they will decide the moment when not to interrogate a prisoner – man or woman – any longer. But the pain also depends on the prisoner: all he has to do is turn over the information wanted for the pain to stop. But then conscience returns: this pain will pass, eventually it will pass. He begs a little more of the body, another bit, another night. Because one day the body will get over the pain. The other pain is forever, to be lived with.*'

Torture is unique for each person. '*The details have to do with intimate knowledge of the body, not the human body in general, but one's own. Torture is like an illness, not everyone hurts the same, and only those who have gone through it know what it feels like (. . .). No matter what you know, what you have heard, what you have read about torture. Experience in torment is unlike anything one imagined, and it is unique for everyone*' (pp. 48–49).

Wishing for death as an escape. '*Later torture will make me think my age and good health are disadvantages. If my heart gave out in the middle of torture, I'd die, and that would be the end of it. But my heart does not fail me; it is the heart of a strong young man active in sports all his life*' (p. 49).

Adaptation even to the horror. '*At night you hear men and women screaming, dogs barking to terrify prisoners. The officers also shout, threaten, yell insults. After a while in the cells one can sleep even with the desperate cries of the tortured (. . .). The torture room smells of mildew and tobacco*' (p. 49).

Scenery of horror and fear. '*As a workplace it is inhospitable and insalubrious. There is a two-hundred-liter metal tank, cut in half, full of water. The prisoner, male or female, enters the room, led in with shoves and blows. Torture has not begun yet; this is only to frighten, the "loosening up" process*' (pp. 49–50).

Alone with the pain: the work of 'softening'. '*After torture sessions, handcuffed behind his back, the prisoner is placed "de plantón" facing the wall, legs far apart, in the cell or in the corridor. The toes swell, legs swell, the back can barely remain upright. Wrists hurt from the tight handcuffs, lose feeling, first the thumbs, then other fingers, the whole hand. The handcuffs are designed to squeeze on their own accord (. . .). Best leave them the way they are. But in the struggle during torture, the handcuffs tighten of their own accord (. . .). That hurts permanently and so [it] works at softening up [the prisoner]*' (p. 55).

Manipulation and deceit. '*There is a good torturer and a bad one. The good torturer [informs] the prisoner that he does not like to torture, but that his partner is a very tough, violent guy, of few words, able and willing to do the worst. To demonstrate, the bad torturer makes himself understood. If it were left to him, the prisoner would soon learn how things work around here (. . .). But the good one has not yet given up on his [friendly] method, and continues arguing*' (p. 50). '*The dialogue, or whatever you want to call this, ends at last when the prisoner repeats that he knows nothing. The good torturer gets annoyed, or acts annoyed, and gives his place to the bad one. The bad one hits him, gives him a kick. The prisoner does not know whether it is the good [one] or the bad [one] who is beating . . . him, but supposes it is both. The torturers – there are always four or five – bring the prisoner up to the edge of the tank of water. One sticks his hand in and removes it. Does the prisoner hear the water? (. . .). After a while, long or short, the torturer gets bored and tries to put the prisoner in the tank. It's not an easy task. The prisoner resists. Then . . . the softening up of the stomach muscles [begins]. From the blows, the prisoner doubles over with pain and then is plunged head-first into the tank. This lasts, how long? Impossible to tell. For the prisoner it is an eternity*' (pp. 50–51).

The unbearable anguish of suffocation: skirting the edge of death. '*Thanks to blows to the stomach, when the prisoner is ducked in the tank he has no air in his lungs. He is hooded and handcuffed behind. He swallows water, feels he's drowning. That is what it feels like, choking to death. When they take him out of the tank, the cloth hood is full of water. So a hand closes the hood around his neck, and the water takes time to drain out. The drowning sensation goes on for seconds longer. The prisoner yells and yells. They are not normal cries of pain, but bestial, like a desperate animal. His nose and mouth cannot get enough air. The sound comes out in gasps, a succession of explosions. It's a bellow more than a shout. The body moves, jerks. There is no air anywhere*' (p. 52).

'*When he is in the water, the prisoner exerts strength he does not normally have, kicks his legs, moves his torso and bangs his head against the side of the tank. The officers, two of them, have to hold him while he is in the water (. . .). If he does go down to the bottom, a heavy body is hard to lift out, and the pris-oner may drown. It's a matter of seconds. An instant of distraction and a corpse is removed from the water. When they do take him out, the prisoner lashes out desperately, hitting whoever is holding him without meaning to. Tough job, torturing – takes strength, resolution, self-forgetfulness*' (pp. 54–55).

'*The body has infinite capacity for resistance*' (p. 65).

The battle for time and the possibility of hope. '*[The interrogator] does not approve of torture (. . .). If the prisoner chooses, [everything could] be worked out without violence. All he has to do is answer what he's asked (. . .). Because, the prisoner should know, they have all the time in the world to* *extract information (. . .). [But] The torturer, however, does not have everything in his favor. Even though he shouts repeatedly, "We have all the time in the world to get information out of you," the prisoner knows, that is not so. (. . .). Facts the prisoner might give tonight that would lead to the arrests of others, won't be any good by dawn. The torturer is in a hurry, that is his disadvantage'* (p. 53).

Dependency and hatred towards the torturer and the 'owner' of the prisoner. *'Each prisoner is assigned a "responsable," a person who is responsible or in charge of him, usually a captain if the prisoner is "important." Lieutenants and second lieutenants take charge of prisoners of "minor importance." (. . .). The "responsable" is the prisoner's owner: perhaps not of his life, because to kill intentionally he is supposed to get permission, but he is the owner of everything else. (. . .). The prisoner is the property of his "responsable." (. . .). In my case, I am the property of a captain who arrested me. My captain has illusions of being just. "If you give me the information I want, I shall treat you well." (. . .). It is up to me for the captain to be able to demonstrate his [sense of] justice. (. . .). He's not original; they all say the same [things]. My captain is a little older than I am, perhaps thirty. He's a little heavy, shorter than I am, taciturn, with a thick voice. Smokes all the time. Sometimes gives me a cigarette. The ownership of the prisoner by the "responsable" is absolute. The prisoner sleeps the hours the "responsable" decides, eats if the "responsable" wishes, is handcuffed in front or behind as the "responsable" decides, will have a blanket if the "responsable" orders it (. . .). The "responsable" is "his" owner, but both belong to each other'* (p. 58).

'As the "responsable" directs the torture of his prisoner, he gets to know him intimately. He sees him at his worst, which is when you know a human being to his depths. He sees him suffer, hears him scream, feels his useless resistance [like that] of a trapped animal. When the prisoner begs to breathe, [begs] that they not beat him, asks to go to the bathroom, lies, invents, humbles himself, the "responsable" is there. When the prisoner is wounded flesh, wet with urine, smelling bad, a soaking rag on a filthy [mattress], the "responsable" is there. To the "responsable" nothing about the prisoner is unfamiliar.'

'A good "responsable" looks after his prisoner. He does not let others torture him, or a soldier on guard hit him for no reason. A good "responsable" is a little paternalistic with his prisoner; he never tortures beyond what is necessary. He is [possessive], does not allow anyone of the same or lesser rank to interfere with his prisoner. Sometimes, in the early morning, the "responsable" takes a little time to converse with his prisoner in his cell (. . .). He asks after the family, who they are, how many there are, what they do. He also lets the prisoner in on his own feelings, his social and political concerns. The "responsable" might speak of his origins, say he too belongs to the people. He might even let the prisoner know he is not totally in agreement with the form of interrogation, but is not the boss. From which the prisoner should understand that from a certain point of view, the two are victims of the same mistaken decisions of his superiors (. . .). The fact of the "responsable" lends an order to things, to the barracks and also to the prisoner' (pp. 60–61).

"The "responsable" is the prisoner's reference point, a mixture of authoritarian and punishing father, slave-owner, and minor god, who doles out pain, food, water, air, clothing, personal hygiene, trips to the bathroom. The "responsable" is a necessary person to this world of pain (. . .). After a time in the barracks, the prisoner and his "responsable" have developed a relationship in which the "responsable" is treating the prisoner with certain condescension – or maybe not condescension so much as that the "responsable" [is no longer] seeing the prisoner objectively. He thinks he knows everything about his prisoner, but suspects the prisoner is hiding an important part of his life, of his activities. So for a night the rules are changed, and prisoners under suspicion are separated from their "responsable" and interrogated by someone else. (. . .) If the special session gives no result, the "responsable" is assured he can trust his prisoner. But if under brief and intense torture the prisoner gives information his boss does not know, the relationship deteriorates. The "responsable" feels betrayed (. . .). The "responsable" gets irritated, scolds his prisoner for not having given him the information, for making him look bad in front of his colleagues and superiors' (pp. 58–63).

Battles of the body, and dignity. *'To defecate is a more complicated objective. It must be done hooded, into an invisible hole in the floor. Handcuffs are switched to the front. Then the soldier takes off the handcuffs when the prisoner finishes so he can wipe himself. Then puts them on again, at the back. Many operations. Although it hardly matters because the hood does not let him see, the prisoner knows the toilet has no door and that the soldier is there, leaning against the doorframe, watching him or conversing with another soldier. (. . .). As the difficulties are so many, prisoners would rather not defecate. Then they get diarrhea or become constipated. The last is my trouble; I go four weeks, five, six, without being able to defecate'* (pp. 64–65).

'But [something] stronger and more necessary than the body's ability to endure pain, something else sustains the prisoner. It is not ideology, not even ideas, nor does it affect all the same or equally. The prisoner holds onto something beyond the rational, the definable. Dignity sustains him. (. . .). He buries himself in his misery and gathers his forces, yells, lies, wants to die to lessen the pain, and wants to live to remember one day that even in torment he held onto the dignity he was taught, remember that he never trusted the torturer, hated him, was capable of killing him with his bare hands, bathing in his blood, and destroying him until not even the dust of his bones remained. Because loathing, pure loathing, also sustains, helps pass the night, another night, endure successive deaths in the tank, the cries of other prisoners' (pp. 65–66).

Shifting worldviews, confronting tangible evil and horror. *'Although sometimes I may doubt, I'll never stop believing in a human being's shining capacity for indescribable acts of loyalty and sacrifice. But I also know human beings are capable of absolute evil, of hurting others for sport, of allowing a person to die in torment. Before I became a prisoner I did not know that such infinite degradation, such a descent [into] the abyss, was possible. It is scary to look at oneself in the mirror. Those things I learned in solitary prison cells'* (p. 72).

Could I ever be like them.? *'And I wake up and am afraid. Not afraid of them, but of me, of my feelings, this hatred, so old, so deep that still lives somewhere inside me. And I think: Is this me? Am I like this? Able to do this? I ask my body if it is he who has not been able to forget'* (p. 66).

Disgust as bodily experience. Nausea and the struggle for identity and dignity. *'Bad smells, urine on clothing, spit and [leftover] food stuck to the beard, hair stiff from not being washed for weeks, skin beginning to shed for lack of sun and washing, all this brings on loathing. No one would put up with someone in such a state next to him. But one has to put up with his own self. This body, dirty, smelling bad, in pain from beatings and from lack of rest, sleepy, that can't so much as move a foot without asking permission, provokes disgust. It's one thing to think, "This is disgusting." It's different to feel, "Now I am disgusting." (. . .). But one can't ask the body to bear pain and at the same time tell [the body that] it is disgusting. You feel for this animal. It's disgusting but one wants to love it, because it is all one has, because dignity depends on its resistance, some dignity. Because what the torturer wants is for the prisoner to feel disgust toward himself. That he is so defenseless that he thinks he's worth nothing, and therefore keeping his mouth shut, lying, resisting, will cease to make sense. If one is not worth anything, if one is disgusting, what has he got to defend in the torment? Not even future memories. I don't know how to explain [the extent to which] disgust toward one's own body [makes] one see himself differently, and that that knowledge is for life'* (pp. 69–70).

Torturers envy prisoners. *'Then other times, some nights, torturers show a curious aspect: envy of the prisoners. Because deep down the torturer knows that never will what he does have any dignity, any human, cultural, moral, or ethical value. Suppose they get the information they want, then what? They may succeed in having every man and woman in the country afraid of them – in the street, in factories, in the university – who until they lock up the house and go to bed at night, will fear the torturer.*

Then what? Will that make the torturer feel proud? Never, not in a thousand years will he be proud to say to his children, "There was a man, or a woman, with information he did not want to give me. He was hooded, handcuffed behind his back. He refused. But I took him to the limit, smashed him, broke him down. Made him feel he was garbage. Made he feel what death was like under water, once, many times, and in the end he gave me the information"' (pp. 74–75).

The particular method of torture does not matter: it is merely the transactional space built by the torturer to subjugate the tortured. *'I think every torturer develops his own skills and techniques. He learns to use common instruments – water, electricity, [the] "garrote" – as one learns to use any tool, on the material, which in his case is the body of tortured prisoners. (. . .) My "responsable" has specialized in the tank. (. . .) I don't think he beats me. (. . .) I am sure his thing is the tank. In fact, years later I learn that every arrest center had its own specialized method of torture. (. . .) Where I am there are no electric prods; the tank dominates. Once, as a threat, an officer said he'd bring a prod, and then I'd see what was what. That the tank was nothing compared to the prod'* (p. 81).

Elements for a definition of psychological torture based on Liscano's testimony

Liscano explains that in torture there is always a double struggle: the relationship with the torturer, and the fight against oneself and against one's own body.

1. **The struggle against the torturer**
   a. Torture is a **psychological struggle** against the torturer. Liscano describes physical pain as the space in which that struggle is waged. Understanding the torturer's personality is essential to survival. Liscano describes this as a macabre game of chess in which the torturer seeks the breaking point of the detainee and the detainee seeks to understand and adapt to the demands and peculiar crazes of his torturer in order to stay one step ahead of him, save time, and minimise pain.
   b. There is the obvious relationship based on **domination** and **submission** (involving the 'owner' or 'responsable' of the prisoner), but Liscano also describes a **mutual dependence**. The interrogator needs information and has less time than it may seem. Liscano even goes so far as to suggest that it is unclear whether the torturer always dominates. A link, a type of special relationship definable as a sadistic paternalism, is established.
   c. This means that there are constant attacks on, and questioning of, the detainee's identity by the torturing system and his or her 'responsable'. Knowing how to bend the 'identity', the 'inner self' of the prisoner is the ultimate goal. Torture is then structured around the creation of a sadistic, paternalistic, and manipulative relationship.
2. **The prisoner's relationship with his or her body**
   Torture is a painful process of becoming aware of one's own body as something unknown and strange.
   a. Liscano describes pain as an extreme form of knowledge that pushes the mind to its limit. Over the course of hours, pressure from a clothing seam or a shackle can cause excruciating pain, and the person needs to put all of their mental energy into turning that pain into a kind of anesthesia.
   b. The prisoner establishes an ambivalent relationship with his or her body: an abject, painful body that is nevertheless the only thing he or she has left. The prisoner has no other option but to love it in spite of the aversion and hate that it provokes.

Nausea and disgust are basic emotions that exemplify the struggle of the prisoner to preserve his or her dignity and identity.

c.   Liscano shows the psychological nature of physical torture even in the apparently banal event of using the toilet. Defecating or urinating can dominate a prisoner's thoughts, as could other simple things like drinking water, hearing a deafening noise or other psychophysical elements. The system establishes seemingly minor situations that foster a situation of dependence on the torturer and cause a battle for dignity in the face of degradation, humiliation and self-rejection; the final point is to break down resistance and make the detainee give up.

3.   The torturing system creates a **deceptive trick**: it is not a struggle between the torturer and the tortured, but a battle of **the tortured against himself**.

This causes devastating physical and psychological exhaustion, especially because (in Liscano's description), the system creates a situation in which the enemy is internal: one has the power to stop the torture simply by saying something, but must face the possibility of later suffering permanent guilt. The system designs a situation in which the detainee must rethink everything all the time as they are faced with stressful, exhausting dilemmas.

4.   **Torture is a process** with a perfectly defined way of operating. It is 'professional work' carried out by 'professionally trained' interrogators.

Liscano explains how the torture environment includes various routines:

a.   'Softening': hitting, yelling, chaos, loneliness. Scenarios of terror.

b.   Initial 'talk'. 'We have all the time in the world.' Instilling hopelessness. The sooner you talk, the less you will suffer.

c.   Manipulation: different pre-established roles of the interrogators.

d.   Pain so strong that the victim wants to die in order to end it.

5.   Detainees will learn:

a.   Another way to view and understand their own bodies. What their limits are, and how far they are willing to go.

b.   To hate other human beings as a way to protect themselves and to resist. Trying to remember who they are, where they are and why they are there. They will learn that this hatred will last forever.

In short, Liscano's book describes torture based on the use of physical pain as a transactional space which establishes a relationship of 'trust/submission' between the prisoner and their 'responsable', in which the prisoner is pushed progressively into a state of submission and surrender, but also identification with the aggressor in an attempt to break down the prisoner's identity.

Jacqueline Gurruchaga and Beatriz Brenzano – *Memories of Sexual Torture*

In 2009, Gurruchaga (JG) and Brenzano (BB), together with a group of 30 other women from Uruguay, collectively chose to report the sexual torture they suffered as political prisoners during the Uruguayan dictatorship (Grupo de denuncia de la violencia sexual sufrida durante el terrorismo de Estado, 2014). They had remained silent for over 30 years.

Message: absolute dominance – we can do anything we want. *'We were in places where the neglect and filth was intentional. The inadequate ventilation, the amount of light, ramps, hooks,* *hangers, cattle prods, hoods, handcuffs, toilets, everything was designed for the task at hand. (. . .). The combination of actions was calculated to make us feel extremely vulnerable, denigrated, completely at their mercy. (. . .). In a context of extreme violence, sexual abuse operated as part of the 'varied menu' of abuses seeking to break us. They made us feel like they could do anything they wanted to us, even stripping us, groping us, forcing us to touch them, penetrating us with different objects, etc., etc.' (JG)*

Torture: finding the detainee's limits. *'They combined different types of torture, separated by "softening period" in which they tested more subtle methods, but always with a purpose: to find our limits. The helplessness, the chaos, remaining tied up, hooded, without food, drink, or rest, ragged and filthy, surrounded by loud music and screaming for days on end (. . .).' (JG)*

'Feeling dirty, soiling ourselves and still wearing the same clothes, menstruating, [and] smelling our smells and their smells made our torture worse, worked against us.' (JG)

'We never spoke of torture in general, let alone sexual abuse. It was like a learned behavior. Perhaps it was a matter of decency and dignity. As if it was not okay to feel bad about something that we knew would happen more or less like it finally did. (. . .) In retrospect, it is a bit odd that we have not sought to reflect collectively or in small groups about what torture meant to us, at least in the various places where I went.' (JG)

Embodied memory of pain. *'The recollection persists as a permanent mark on the memory of the body – the blood, the tears are still there – and to this day it harms us and also affects many of our sexual lives.' (BB)*

Double victimisation. Hiding the hurt and shame. *'The pain and the damage has been so great that for more than thirty years we could not tell anyone – not our families, not our partners, and not our psychologists. The traumatic effects last over time and only now, in the group, have we been able to put them into words (perhaps because of the bonds of affection and caring that now exist between us, that bind us strongly despite the differences in our lives and our political and generational differences); we remember and relive the horror with trembling voices and tears in our eyes. In this long and painful process of denouncing and redress, which has lasted more than two years now, we hear stories of the most cruel, unimaginable, and horrifying acts of sexual violence against women prisoners. (. . .). If we don't talk about it, it doesn't heal. After [the preliminary hearing] before to the judge, many of us feel the immense relief of "mission accomplished," of "finally sleeping in peace" (. . .).' (BB)*

The value of justice. *'We also believe in the potential restorative capacity of the judicial sentence, and fervently hope that they are punished and sentenced for sexual violence, crimes against sexual integrity, and crimes against humanity.' (BB)*

Elements for a definition of psychological torture based on the testimonies of Gurruchaga and Brenzano

1.   The purpose of sexual torture is to demonstrate **omnipotence** and **absolute control** even in the most intimate spheres. This includes access to the most inviolable parts of a human being.
2.   Torture is finding where each detainee has his or her own **limits**, so as to break these limits.
3.   Torture becomes an **indelible memory in the body**. The damage is for life, and is sometimes expressible in words, but in most cases expressed through the body.
4.   Sexual torture involves feelings of **humiliation and shame**. Rape often brings social shame on victims and their relatives or other members of their community. Victims may

also feel political shame because they survived and other activists did not. Both social and political shame may cause the person to remain silent and internalise the damage suffered, often for life. This shame is filed away inside the person under 'do not remember', amplifying its impact. Because sexual torture cannot be fixed or changed, the victim may not discuss it in order to avoid offending or embarrassing others. But in the end, bearing witness to survivors' experiences creates a space in which the damage can begin to be repaired, and the search for justice becomes one of the few ways for victims to regain balance in their lives.

Mario Villani – *Disappeared: Memories of Captivity*

Mario Villani, a physicist and activist in the Argentine left, was kidnapped by the Federal Police in 1977 when he was 38 years old. He remained disappeared until 1981; during that time he was tortured for months and was forced to work as a slave in five clandestine detention and torture centres: Athletic Club, Banco, El Olimpo, Pozo Quilmes and the Escuela de Mecánica de la Armada (ESMA). His testimonies, mostly collected in his book *Memories of Captivity*, offer unique portraits of each torture centre and the dynamics therein, and he worked extensively to cross-check his memories with the facts. His testimonies have been a keystone in the trials of many former torturers in Argentina (Villani, 2011).

Softening. '*I was thrown into the "lion's den,"[2] chained together with other people, not yet aware that that place temporarily housed the newly kidnapped during the "softening" time. In addition to torture sessions, this period also brought the terror of being in a strange place. Lying on the mat dread started to churn around in my mind. I was thinking of everything a mile a minute. It was difficult to estimate the time since the kidnapping: there were moments that seemed eternal and others were like snapshots. In the "lion's den" I heard the first screams of people being tortured and the clamor of the guards going in and out to control the prisoners, punching and kicking them when they moved or raised a hand to touch the blindfold. It was an eerie and frightening environment (. . .). During my stay in the "lion's den" they did not feed me. (. . .) In this and other fields where time does not exist, measuring it became an obsession for me. While blindfolded and isolated, I tried to keep track of the days to know the exact date. (. . .) As I received no food in the "lion's den," I could not go to the bathroom*' (p. 43).
'*Inside, the light was always on and I could not distinguish day from night (. . .). I guess that was also part of the process of destruction of our personality; it is very difficult to maintain one's internal clock*' (p. 65).

Uncertainty. '*Uncertainty itself was a torture method and an important part of this stage. Sometimes it is worse to imagine torture than to suffer it. You try to imagine the pain, but it is never the same as real pain*' (p. 44).

Cognitive and emotional exhaustion. '*At first I killed time thinking about my life, why I had been kidnapped, if I had taken unnecessary risks or if being an activist had been a mistake. But soon I realized that it was not worth it. (. . .) The only plans I could afford were those that had to do with trying to live until tomorrow. (. . .). This constant struggle to live to see the next day was exhausting, and yet it also formed a sort of callus on the spirit*' (p. 65).
'. . . *In the fields, there wasn't something that could be called a "normal day." Every day could be repetitive and identical to many others, but it could also be the last. That's what made the system cruel: repeating a routine hundreds of times in which each "normal" day is the same, but at the same time may be the final day, is a sophisticated system of torture. Such a system did not even need to lay a finger on the victim to cause him to despair*' (p. 67).

Intellectual and emotional struggle to maintain spaces of control. *'I never liked to feel that things happen regardless of my will; it's not that I consider myself omnipotent, but I hate to give up on my personal integrity. I wanted to feel that I was myself, but everything in the detention center – in particular the ambiguity of roles and the uncertainty about where everyone stood – was aimed at destroying the identity of the detainee. Am I myself? Am I the torturer? And if I'm neither the torturer nor myself, who am I?'* (p. 78).

Dissociation and apparent acclimation to atrocity. *'Listening to the screams of the tortured (. . .). Oddly enough, this is also part of that kind of non-routine routine, the repeated uncertainty that ends up becoming routine. (. . .). In such a place, it is impossible to ignore the heart-wrenching screams of people being tortured every day, at any time, but you end up "getting used to it"; you can't get earplugs so you end up bitching silently and continuing to work'* (p. 81).

Living with sudden bursts of brutality and sadism. *'From my working place, I heard the screams of pain of the tortured and the excitement of the guards who had stopped considering it a "softening" routine and lashed out to the point of becoming sadistic. I could see some terribly beaten detainees, especially those who were beaten in the face with iron chains. (. . .). When the beating began they had clothes on, but after a while the clothes looked torn and bloody; later, they were naked bodies with marks everywhere. They began to take them one or two at a time to the "quirófanos"[3] for interrogation, while still beating those waiting their turn with chains while they lay still on the floor. By the end they were just a mass of motionless bodies (. . .). A few of them had to be taken directly to the infirmary because of the terrible state they were in. I do not know how many hours all of that lasted'* (p. 82).

Guilt. Awakening the internal enemy. Forced choices. *'Another persistent memory I have of incidents that interrupted the camp routine is a dilemma that I faced in* El Banco *when I had to repair a cattle prod ["picana"] (. . .). When [the torturer] told me to fix it I dared to answer: "I cannot." "How can that be if you've repaired a lot more complicated things?" he asked me. I replied, "It is not that I cannot technically; it's that is that I cannot fix an instrument of torture." I had not finished speaking, when I got scared and thought: "Right, it's all over now (. . .)." "You can't? Okay, from now on I'm going to torture with the* Variac *[electrical transformer] (. . .)." As the days passed, I saw people coming out of the "quirófano" in terrible conditions, including comas. (. . .). I endured this spectacle for about a week until I could not take any more and said, (. . .) "bring me the* picana *so I can fix it"'* (p. 84).

Absurdity and loneliness. *'When the World Cup was held in Argentina in June 1978 [we were obliged to see Argentine matches on TV] (. . .). I could not help thinking that those thousands of Argentines knew nothing of my existence as a disappeared person. The prisoners did not exist for them; and at the same time they and the outside world had disappeared from our lives. (. . .). This made me feel powerless and I found it maddening (. . .). It was part of the basic principles for de-structuring the personality'* (p. 86).

Manipulation of affection. Emotional breakdown. *'Suddenly the door opened and Cobani entered to tell me insidiously: "Flaco, Juanita [a prisoner with whom I felt a deep emotional connection] leaves in this 'transfer'"[4] (. . .). In a flash, I saw how I had to react (. . .). I tried to appear strong and swallowed, despite the terrible lump in my throat. I looked into his eyes and I said with simulated indifference, "Cobani, there are many women [in the world] . . ." (. . .) Part of the process of destroying one's personality includes removing any feeling of affection and compassion for others. (. . .) The lump in my throat that I felt for Juanita was added to the fear for my own life. I felt like I was walking a tightrope. But the scariest thing was yet to come. Cobani suddenly asked, "Do you want to say goodbye to her?" I said yes. (. . .). I hugged Juanita, crying. While I hugged her, I felt Cobani's mocking face* *being etched into me. (. . .). To this day, I think about what happened that day (. . .) it was one of the worst things – worse than physical torture – that I experienced in the camps. One of the worst and one of the deepest (. . .). The memory of Cobani haunted me for a long time. I even fantasized about my release and about looking for Cobani in order to torture and kill him'* (pp. 89–93).

Torture as a social fact. *'Do not forget that torture was not an individual act: they sought to torture the entire society by torturing the victims. Rape, or turning an activist into a torturer, extend the suffering to their children and to the society around them'* (p. 95).

Internal police. *'Why didn't I try to escape in that restaurant with, for example, the excuse of going to the bathroom? It wasn't just because of the fear that they would shoot me. I repeat now what I said then: the limits of the prison were not those of El Olimpo; the whole country was a prison. So where could I run? And if I escaped, how could I find a way to take my family to another country? (. . .) I had no answer to the question of how to avoid the consequences of my escape. Maybe I would not have escaped even if the guards had gone for a walk and left me alone for a while (. . .). Beyond these rationalizations, there is the question of the internal police that everyone carries inside: at that point, terror paralyzes. An example of the terror that infiltrates a person is what happened to me in 1985 when (. . .) I was asked if I wanted to be interviewed by a journalist. My first reaction was panic because I was going to be on TV – everyone would see me, including the repressors, who were free. They would know that I was denouncing. Just before saying no, I looked around and realized that this time there was no one at my side with raising their finger and saying, "Look, if you talk, I'll bust you." Suddenly I realized that the person who raised his finger and threatened me was inside me. (. . .). At that moment I felt I was starting to get rid of the internal police; this was four years after having been released! This is why even today, many people do not dare testify against the perpetrators. (. . .) Such is the power of the internal police that still terrify us'* (pp. 109–110).

Breakdowns and detainee collaboration. *'Of the members of the Council[5] who were detained in Pozo de Quilmes, I especially remember Tano and Cristoni for their collaboration in intelligence work (. . .). They were dangerous and [other prisoners] should have been wary of them, but at the same time they were human beings and were still prisoners like the rest. (. . .) Tano and Cristoni started doing tasks in the Club Atlético such as distributing food or bringing people to the showers, until at some point they began to participate in interrogations. (. . .). They went to work on the immense papers spread out on the wall of an office where the charts with contacts from organizations were drawn, with a huge number of noms de guerre, addresses and arrows. (. . .) Perhaps at some point they offered to be present during the interrogation of someone they knew to check that the information they extracted from him was correct; from there it was easy to convince themselves that the best thing for each person being tortured was to talk, so that the war would end soon. Indeed, they argued – I heard it from their own mouths – that we were defeated, but could help end the war and help stop the deaths. Did they really believe that they cooperated to save lives? I can only guess; it would be important to understand how they rationalized their actions (. . .). They contributed to sending many ex-comrades to their deaths. (. . .). But for me, they are not the real culprits, but rather another kind of victim (. . .). Today I can say without any doubt that I would have never collaborated with torture. But I really do not know what circumstances pushed them to do so (. . .)'* (p. 132).

'After being freed, "Ratón" continued to work with people from the Intelligence Service. When democracy was established [in Argentina] he began working with a former torturer from ESMA (. . .) with whom he collaborated at an agency that offered private investigation and protection to individuals (. . .). Even though I don't think "Laura" helped torture, everyone from the South Column of Montoneros fell because of the dates [she went on with interrogators] and the contacts that she turned in.

In the intelligence office, she helped to choose the targets, and they often took her out to identify people on the street (. . .). When Laura was released, she started dating a civilian member of one the ESMA taskforces' (pp. 133–137).

Totalising environment. *'ESMA was the kingdom of helplessness, of evil, of "damned if you do and damned if you don't." In that situation, a prisoner comes to think that the camp is the world'* (p. 154).

Hope as a painful feeling. *'My perception of time began to lengthen, paradoxically, from the moment I sensed that I could get out alive. Since I began considering that possibility, the long-awaited moment never came, and sometimes I got desperate. I was wrapped in a routine where every day was the same as the previous one. And strangely enough, at that point, that exhausted me more than the struggle to live to see the next day'* (pp. 154–155).

Upon release.

Distrust. *'At first I found it difficult to approach the relatives of the disappeared to give them information or ask about details that confirmed something I already knew, because there was always suspicion and distrust. "My son (or my brother, my cousin) disappeared," they said. "Why are you alive?"'* (p. 168).

Sequelae of torture.

Exhaustion. *'Since I was released, I faced the difficulties of the survivor traumatized by his experiences. (. . .). [I had] the face of a weathered old man, [but] I was just over 40 years old. (. . .). Add to this the feeling that people I knew crossed the street to avoid me, either because of the fear that endured, or because they didn't know what to say. When one comes out of the detention center, it is impossible not to feel relief, but one also feels an immense exhaustion. (. . .). The psychological torture of the possibility of being tormented again – in which there were no exceptions or pardons for "good behavior" – was worse than physical torture'* (p. 177).

Distrust. *'Living day to day, with the stress of always being alert in order to distinguish between the torturer, the collaborator, and the fellow comrade, leaves you exhausted. (. . .). This produces a constant tension between the immense need for affection felt in there and distrust as an instinctual precaution. It's exhausting, but you can't give up because that would be tantamount to throwing up one's hands, to committing suicide (. . .). I'm alive, but only because of years of that crushing exercise: trying to survive'* (p. 177).

Being ill. *'I don't know whether to attribute it to the living conditions in the prison, but after my release I suffered from ongoing illnesses and serious physical problems'* (p. 178).

Trauma. *'But the psychological traces [of torture] are deeper than the physical ones. (. . .) Three and half decades after my abduction, I still have dreams related to the Camp, and if someone wakes me I lift my arms and cover my face defensively. They are not exactly nightmares, but dreams about everyday situations in the clandestine centers, "normal" times, not always the most horrific. (. . .). That's why the word that best defines my memory of the centers is anguish. (. . .). Today, after many vicissitudes, I have symptoms that led me to turn to professional help, resulting in a diagnosis of PTSD'* (p. 178).

Remembering and forgetting. *'Some memories, such as the impact of torture sessions, are impossible to banish, but others fade. (. . .). I would like to have a perfect memory, to be able to hold on to all the details. It distresses me that this is not possible. Maybe it is a defense mechanism that appears in anyone who has experienced extreme situations. The mind cannot hold on to every little detail. (. . .). With the passage of time, forgetfulness does its work and that's also a torment. Is forgetting a sin or is it salvation? I would like to forget, but the imperative to remember is stronger'* (p. 179).

Dissociation, emotional detachment, and resistance. '*[My wife] Rosita has trouble under-standing that survivors find humor in certain memories from the past. We have learned to de-dramatize our story, to use dissociation as a coping mechanism, and this can cause great distress in those who hear us. (...) We are aware that burying emotions is negative and that dissociation is a sign of ill health, but in the Camp we were used to it to avoid suffering, until it ended up becoming a way of life that may harm us now. Whenever I feel that I must suppress my feelings, it is then that I begin to feel the beginning of something pushing its way to the surface: perhaps there lies the possibility of overcoming the petrification of emotions*' (p. 181).

Dilemmas and guilt. Absurdity. Questioning identity. '*Life in the camps was fraught with dilemmas: what was right or wrong, where the boundaries between normal and aberrant were, what distin-guishes a torturer from a person forced to denounce his or her fellow prisoners. For me, the quintessential con-troversial situations were repairing the "picana" so that the torturer did not continue torturing with a bare wire, giving artificial respiration to a dying companion knowing that if he did not die he would soon return to being tortured, and preparing "mate" [tea] for the interrogators while they were torturing*' (p. 181).

Life and death. '*Why am I alive today? I don't know, it wasn't me who decided. I can assume that I am alive for two reasons: I offered useful electrical repairs and maintenance, a collaboration which I believe did not go against my ethical principles; and they wanted to leave some of us free – based on a mostly random selection – so that when we got out, our stories disseminated terror in society as part of a methodology of social control*' (p. 182).

Nothing has changed. '*When I see what happened in Iraq, the torture of prisoners in Abu Ghraib prison, I infer that history repeats itself (...). In the photos of Abu Ghraib in the press, I see the same dingy corridors, the same cells with barred doors, the same expressions of horror on the faces of the prisoners I met; in those pictures I see my own face and the faces of my old compañeros from captivity. Those naked, hooded prisoners remind me of my hood and my humiliation. I smell the unmistakable scent of fear once more. I see the pictures of prisoners stacked up, some covered in blood. And I remember myself in a similar pile, hooded and beaten by guards who mocked us as they stood and walked on this human mountain with their army boots. (...). The executioners seek the pain, suffering, and death of their victims even more than the information that comes from them – the corpses do not confess. Combating terrorism with terror is like fighting cannibals by eating them. If torture is not only useful to obtain reliable informa-tion: what else is it good for? Perhaps it terrorizes victims and, above all, the population of which they are part, leaving the existence of torture to transcend while officially denying it. Terror as a tool of social control makes the indifference and individualism of "every man for himself" spread through society. The impunity of perpetrators sows suspicion among everyone, we don't know if the person sitting next to us in a cinema is in fact a torturer. These regimes will generate torturers again whenever they need them*' (p. 182).

Elements for a definition of psychological torture based on Villani's testimony

1. **The process.** There is a carefully studied *torturing process* that includes several constant elements. It begins with a *softening period* of isolation and uncertainty that produces anguish, ruminated dreading. This is alternated with physical maltreatment. When the interrogation officially begins, the torturer has *already established the conditions* for rapidly breaking down the individual with minimal effort.

2. **Attacking identity. The unconscious search for closeness and affect.** Isolation fosters the need for closeness, for someone who talks to the prisoner, who explains, provides logic, and perhaps even cares about him or her. The relationship with the torturer constantly oscillates between ruthless cruelty and the emotional closeness and

intimacy of the confessional. Human beings seek love to preserve their identity; the duality between closeness and violence can destroy a person seeking protection and affection. The dilemma has no solution, and results in psychological exhaustion: if detainees close themselves off to affection, they may feel that they have lost the opportunity to stop or ease their suffering. But if they open themselves up to affective closeness they become vulnerable, and any sudden switch to cruelty is devastating. These oscillations, like everything else in the torture system, are usually unpredictable and illogical.

3. **Isolation. Nobody knows, nobody cares.** Part of the process is instilling the feeling of abandonment, of nobody knowing where the person is, and of society ignoring what is happening or even justifying it. Feelings of social detachment deepen hopelessness and promote bonding and vulnerability at the smallest sign of affection from the torturer.

4. **Psychological struggle.** In the struggle to maintain one's integrity, different strategies arise, including dissociation, 'habituation' to horror, and emotional detachment to the suffering of others. Hope is demoralising, and living from one day to the next without expectations or hope often appears to be the best approach. Small and subtle acts of resistance and dignity serve as affirmations of the self.

5. **Cooperation.** Resilience sometimes implies partial compliance with the demands of the torturers, which causes anguish over whether to consider compliance to be 'survival' or 'cooperation'. Guilt is unavoidable.

6. **Consequences.**
   - In the long term, torture leads to the interiorisation of fear and the development of internalised policing in the detainee.
   - Survivors may also feel permanent distrust towards others, or minimise the suffering of others.
   - Trauma ensues and is mostly experienced through nightmares and flashbacks.
   - Psychosomatic disorders are frequent bodily expressions of suffering.
   - Survivors of torture may feel many kinds of guilt, mostly related to surviving or to minute decisions made during captivity.

7. **Memory** is outside the realm of one's control. Forgetting may produce guilt, while remembering may cause trauma to be revived. Lack of control over the ability to remember or to forget causes further anguish.

Henry Engler – *The Circle*

Henry Engler was arrested and held in isolation for thirteen years during the Uruguayan dictatorship. During those years of solitary confinement, he developed a hallucinatory psychosis, and was diagnosed with schizophrenia and delusional disorder. Upon release, his psychotic symptoms slowly disappeared. He describes psychosis as a psychological fight against himself as a product of torture (Engler, Charlo and Caray, 2012).

'The treatment in Colonia was brutal. I could never see anything because the cell was completely walled, with the light permanently on. They took me, hooded, to the courtyard, I could never see the sky and I have no idea what the place was like, not even the prison cell. Nothing' (p. 59).

'I lost track of time (. . .) I couldn't tell day from night, except for the sounds of trumpets (. . .) I didn't leave, not even to go to the bathroom. I had a bucket to defecate in (. . .)' (p. 69).

'Shortly after, (. . .) I started to hear voices. Before, in the interrogation period, I had problems and confused reality with what was happening in my head. But in Paso de los Toros the issue becomes more acute. I hear them torturing Rosencof and Antonio Mas, dragging them across a concrete floor, interrogating *them. This is happening night and day, it's a torture that has no end. It is repeated again and again; I'm sure it is real, it is happening. It is a very fucked-up situation, so I tell them to torture me and to leave Rosencof and Mas alone. Some officers come and ask me, "Where are we torturing?" and I reply, "back there." "But look, what's back there is an ironworks," says an official. I was sure he was lying but he left me with doubts. These voices became more and more aggressive until finally they began to attack me. From that moment on, I entered a hallucinatory period that lasted practically the entire time I was imprisoned. It started in '72 and lasted almost until the end; just imagine how many years that was"* (p. 53).

'At first I was convinced that when they removed the bullet, they placed an implant somewhere in my brain and that the CIA could read my thoughts. So I'm desperate not to think because I figure that if I think about this thing or that, they will go look for this person or that person. This fills me with a terrible fear, a fear that produces an almost unbearable pain. Being unable to hide my thoughts terrified me. Later, it's not the CIA that dominates my thoughts, but extra-terrestrial beings who send me messages and control my brain. They are very aggressive voices that first project from the walls and then I start feeling that they come from inside my brain. (. . .). The voices start electrocuting me. If I eat, for example, it triggers an electric current to my brain and gives me some kind of seizure – I have seizures. It is an impressive pain. So I start to eat less and less. They also manipulate my heart, it seems they can grab it and make it stop. The fear and panic that I felt when the voices invaded my brain is indescribable. I'd never had a feeling like that before. It was the worst terror' (pp. 56–58).

'My brain hurts, so I try to turn off the voices. My struggle is to stop the thoughts and turn the voices off. I begin to spend all my time standing motionless, staring at a spot on the wall ["the circle"]. At first I tried to do it sitting, but I fell asleep. So I stand. I learned not to blink to not lose sight of that spot . . .' (p. 69).

Elements for a definition of psychological torture based on Engler's testimony

*   **Isolation** per se can destroy a person. In Engler, it induced a full psychotic syndrome that lasted over four years. Voices appear as an extreme form of threat. This threat becomes part of the person's psychic system, causing extreme terror. The enemy is inside one's mind, and is none other than oneself.
*   Engler was able to stay mentally grounded by focusing attention on 'the circle', or a specific spot on the wall. This represents the obsessive fight against invasive voices, against psychological torture, and to regain control over the integrity of the self.

Marcelo Viñar – *Fractures of Memory*

Marcelo Viñar, psychiatrist and psychoanalyst, was arrested and tortured daily for more than three months as a suspected collaborator of the Tupamaros. Years later, in exile, he wrote a book (Viñar and Ulriksen, 1990) with his thoughts regarding the elements that define torture, and it is one of the best books on the subject in Spanish. It also includes the story of his own torture, described in the third person. The following are not parts of the book, but transcribed excerpts from a personal conversation with him.[6]

Waiting breaks the person. *'Upon arrival they applied the submarine[7] for weeks. Without asking anything. Nothing at all. They left me, they took me back to the water tank, they returned me to the cell . . . they hardly talked to me . . . just the torture and the waiting. So for days, no matter how much you thought about it, you didn't know the reasons for the detention, or what awaited you (. . .). The waiting was terrible. In my case, I was arrested and no one said anything to me for at least three weeks . . . I had to stand for three weeks, blindfolded, while they hit me from time to time . . . without saying so much as a word to me. The fact that it took over three weeks to tell me why I was arrested made my anxiety reach extreme [levels], [it was] overflowing . . . .'*

Uncertainty. '*Not knowing is terrible. You feel that you're in their hands, because the reason for your detention could be anything and you turn it around and around in your mind because you're never sure of what they know . . . or what they imagine they know . . . In my case, they suggested that I had been arrested on charges of being a "Tupa" leader. In reality, I had simply met a boy who was "Tupa" who was underground and he had a psychotic breakdown. I went to see him and I prescribed, as a psychiatrist, a neuroleptic. That was all. Well, something else, but they didn't know that. The important thing is that those three weeks waiting, waiting without knowing anything, destroy the person. Nothing other than waiting is needed. (. . .). To me what defines torture is waiting.*'

Bodily functions. The body as an enemy. '*If I had to elaborate, I'd say that beyond waiting, what defines torture is everything that the arbitrary interruption of bodily functions provokes – sensory deprivation, sleep disruption, and the impossibility of controlling the sphincters. In other words, those two things go hand in hand, and the arbitrary disruption of physiological functions turns time into a constant waiting period. Something as seemingly banal as defecating. (. . .). It is difficult to imagine what the struggle to not defecate or urinate on oneself can mean. When you stand for hours . . . trying to resist without knowing whether they will allow you to go to the bathroom in an hour or a day . . . combined with the hunger, sleep, thirst.*'

The unpredictable, the illogical and the uncertain: terror. '*Unpredictability also has to do with what will happen in the next hour. When they take you to the bathroom you do not know if they're taking you to the bathroom, or to your death (. . .). It is hard to imagine that such terror is generated by seemingly minor elements. For example, going to bathroom while hooded. You know that there are several stairs along the way to the bathroom. Every step you take is a step into the abyss, [causing] anguish, because you never know if the guy who takes you by the arm takes you right to the bathroom or to death, or if the guy is behind you, or if he will push down the stairs or hit you with a door. So you were forced to go to the bathroom. If you went, you had to achieve defecation even if you didn't want to (. . .). To get from one place to another hooded, and feel you'd come back alive was something like being a national hero . . . That is terror's permanent mark. No punching is needed (. . .).*'

To torture does not mean to produce pain: it is the manipulation of expectations and the production of terror. '*A torturer told me, "I've tortured someone with this" (and he showed me a ballpoint pen). "He is hooded, and you bring this up to one arm and softly touch the skin; he will tell you everything he knows." This is possible because it's added to the bureaucracy of horror, to the pseudo-medical examinations, to the pictures on the wall when you enter a room . . . to the fact that you knew that they killed someone by pushing him down the stairs that you had to go down when going to the bathroom or to an interrogation. And when you walked while hooded, you felt the terror of taking 200 steps without knowing if the next step would be into an abyss . . . It's terrible (. . .). That's how you can break someone by simply gently touching his knee with a pen.*'

We have all the time in the world. '*The next step is that one day the "good" interrogator, the persuasive one who speaks as if he were not part of the system, finally comes for a visit. You're waiting and looking forward to his visit. And he says this, literally: "They have to rip information out of you. They're going to do it anyway." And then he begins to threaten in a subtle way and says, "Everybody talks. Some may need a day, others need three, [or] a month, or six months. Here, none have made it past nine. But no one has not talked. If you collaborate now, you can save yourself from all that suffering, because in the end there has never been anyone who has not talked. We have all the time in the world to make you talk."*'

'*And that's the phrase. The worst phrase they can say is, "We have all the time in the world." That draws an infinite, endless scenario, in which time is inexhaustible. They say it as fatherly advice. But what they are saying is that time is infinite. And this idea that time is infinite – when overcoming every day is so difficult in this context of helplessness – is unbearable.*'

Constant doubt: the enemy within. *'One day they burst in on me at night. Everything was icy, it was extremely cold. They took me, hooded, to a room. There, they gave me a piece of paper and a pen and said, "Write your story." I sat a long time thinking that if I wrote something, they'd be satisfied. But at the same time, I also thought that it would be worse because then they would actually believe that I knew something . . . ultimately, I left the paper blank. (. . .) When they came back and saw it blank, they shouted and insulted me. [They said] "Now you will know how things can go wrong," and took me to my cell. From that time on, the "waiting" began, waiting for the next torment, the consequences of my decision to leave the sheet blank, which, as announced, would be terrible. And you question if you were wrong to leave that sheet blank, if you missed the opportunity to do something.'*

Progressive physical wearing-down, which is also psychological. *'There is a cumulative factor. The horror is cumulative. The second month is worse than the first, and the third worse than the second. There is a progressive wearing-down that becomes faster as time passes. And you have less ability to resist, to restart physically because you are malnourished, exhausted . . . And this takes a psychological toll. They go together – often death is desired. It is a thought that appears on a recurring basis. If I had to define it, I would say that the fear of agony is worse than death, and causes death to become desirable.'*

Fear as an indelible mark. *'Fear will accompany you forever . . . the proof of fear's damage is that it no longer disappears. The fear that they detain you again, for example, is terrible. My torture ended in 1972. During [the next] three years, I had various psychiatric diagnoses: dyspepsia, sleep disorders, anxiety . . . One day, while attending a patient, several people in uniform showed up. In fact, they were not coming to detain me but were there for some other banal reason, but when they left I had to ask the patient who was with me to leave. I could not listen to him because of the enormous stress I felt. (. . .) That day was when I decided I had to go into exile. Because I could no longer listen to my patients. It was 1975 and it had been three years since my torture. That is the effect of fear. Waiting for renewed detention and horror . . . the waiting gets inside you. When I came to Paris, after a few months all my diagnoses disappeared. I never had problems again. It was anxiety and the tension of waiting.'*

'This adds to other psychological elements that break the person. You know that your mother punishes you. It makes sense. There's something you've done, and this entails a punishment. You understand and accept it. Here there is no "punishment". Here the core is the "illogical". Or in your social life . . . in your social life you expect a "logic", a "meaning" to your interaction with others. Here, instead, the "illogical" and the arbitrary dominate. And this breaks you. This is the case, for example, of the relationship with the torturer: there is a constant oscillation between seduction and torment.'

Elements for a definition of psychological torture based on Viñar's testimony

1. **Torture is always psychological.** Torture is physical, of course, but above all, it is psychological. Torture does not equal pain, though pain is often present. Torture is a process of breaking a person. And the best way to understand this, for Viñar, is to understand the concept of 'waiting'. It is a key concept in that it shows that the 'wait' is more devastating than the torture itself, to the extent that physical beating may even come as a relief.
2. **Waiting time and uncertainty.** The wait is devastating because it is associated with uncertainty, doubt, inability to control, constant questioning and confronting one's fears. It is associated with constantly thinking about what has happened – magnifying every detail and reaction, every piece of information – in an attempt to find spaces of control that allow survival.
3. **Terror as the keystone of torture.** All torture systems create a situation in which each element is designed to create terror. That terror does not necessarily involve physical

pain. The indelible mark is not the beating; memories of terror are deeper than memories of physical pain.

4. **Every banal aspect can destroy you.** The importance of the arbitrary disruption of bodily functions (sight, sleep, food or liquid intake) is an example of how the most seemingly banal aspects of detention (even those which might be not considered to be torture on their own) can destroy the detainee. Torture entails the combination of attacks on dignity and on identity, feelings of helplessness and lack of control, the stress of waiting and the weakening process.

5. **Torturers control time.** The message is 'there is no reason to hope'. Nobody knows what is happening, and nobody can do anything to avoid what will happen if the person does not speak. When the time between torturing sessions finally arrives, it is a time of wearing down the detainee, of psychological exhaustion from the effort to maintain control, and of constant self-questioning and obsessive rethinking of one's actions.

6. The processes of weakening the detainee physically, emotionally and mentally go hand in hand.

Jean Améry – *At the Mind's Limits*[8]

The classic text of philosopher Jean Améry (2009), who was tortured by the Gestapo and was a survivor of the Auschwitz and Buchenwald camps, is probably the most frequently quoted when presenting a subjective definition of torture. He recounts that his torture lasted for only a few days because he was quickly transferred to a concentration camp, but that those days will forever mark him.

Torture is not equivalent to pain. *'If one speaks about torture, one must take care not to exaggerate. What was inflicted on me in the unspeakable vault in Breeridonk was by far not the worst form of torture. No red-hot needles were shoved under my fingernails, nor were any lit cigars extinguished on my bare chest. What did happen to me there I will have to tell about later; it was relatively harmless and it left no conspicuous scars on my body. And yet, twenty-two years after it occurred, on the basis of an experience that in no way probed the entire range of possibilities, I dare to assert that torture is the most horrible event a human being can retain within himself'* (p. 22).

Rumination and the search for logic leads to self-destruction. Torture breaks all logic and basic beliefs about human beings, leading to acceptance and surrender. *'Who was governed by the spirit was unable to understand that the logic had changed. Not only was rational-analytic thinking in the camp, and particularly in Auschwitz, of no help, but it led straight into a tragic dialectic of self-destruction. (. . .). In regard to him, the prisoner, the SS was employing a logic of destruction that in itself operated just as consistently as the logic of life preservation did in the outside world. You always had to be clean-shaven, but it was strictly forbidden to possess razors or scissors'* (p. 10).

'The intellectual, however, revolted against them in the impotency of abstract thought. In the beginning the defiant wisdom of folly held true for him: "What surely may not be, cannot be." But only in the beginning. (. . .). The rejection of the SS logic, the revolt that turned inward, the muted murmuring of such incantations as: "But that is not possible," did not last long. After a certain time there inevitably appeared something that was more than mere resignation and that we may designate as an acceptance not only of the SS logic but also of the SS system of values' (pp. 10–11).

'Not much is said when someone who has never been beaten makes the ethical and pathetic statement that upon the first blow the prisoner loses his human dignity. I must confess that I don't know exactly what that is: human dignity. (. . .). Yet I am certain that with the very first blow that descends on him he loses something

we will perhaps temporarily call "trust in world." Trust in the world includes all sorts of things: the irrational and logically unjustifiable belief in absolute causality perhaps, or the likewise blind belief in the validity of the inductive inference. But more important as an element of trust in the world, and in our context what is solely relevant, is the certainty that by reason of written or unwritten social tracts the other person will spare me – more precisely stated, that he will respect my physical, and with it also my metaphysical, being. (. . .). It is like a rape, a sexual act without the consent of one of the two partners. Certainly, if there is even a minimal prospect of successful resistance, a mechanism is set in motion (. . .). If no help can be expected, this physical overwhelming by the other then becomes an existential consummation of destruction altogether. The expectation of help, the certainty of help, is indeed one of the fundamental experiences of human beings' (p. 28).

'All your life is gathered in a single, limited area of the body, the shoulder joints, and it does not react; for it exhausts itself completely in the expenditure of energy. But this cannot last long, even with people who have a strong physical constitution. As for me, I had to give up rather quickly. And now there was a crackling and splintering in my shoulders that my body has not forgotten until this hour' (p. 32).

'Whoever has succumbed to torture can no longer feel at home in the world. The shame of destruction cannot be erased. Trust in the world, which already collapsed in part at the first blow, but in the end, under torture, fully, will not be regained. That one's fellow man was experienced as the anti-man remains in the tortured person as accumulated horror. It blocks the view into a world in which the principle of hope rules. One who was martyred is a defenseless prisoner of fear. It is fear that henceforth reigns over him. Fear – and also what is called resentments. They remain, and have scarcely a chance to concentrate into a seething, purifying thirst for revenge' (p. 40).

The torturer as a god. *'With heart and soul they went about their business, and the name of it was power, dominion over spirit and flesh, orgy of unchecked self-expansion. I also have not forgotten that there were moments when I felt a kind of wretched admiration for the agonizing sovereignty they exercised over me. For is not the one who can reduce a person so entirely to a body and a whimpering prey of death a god or, at least, a demigod?'* (p. 36).

Psychological torture. Sequelae. *'[Torture] has an indelible character. Whoever was tortured, stays tortured. Torture is ineradicably burned into him, even when no clinically objective traces can be detected'* (p. 34).

'A slight pressure by the tool-wielding hand is enough to turn the other – along with his head, in which are perhaps stored Kant and Hegel, and all nine symphonies, and The World as Will and Representation *– into a shrilly squealing piglet at slaughter. When it has happened and the torturer has expanded into the body of his fellow man and extinguished what was his spirit, he himself can then smoke a cigarette or sit down to breakfast or, if he has the desire, have a look in at* The World as Will and Representation' (p. 35).

Torture seeks a person's limits. *'One can shake off torture as little as the question of the possibilities and limits of the power to resist it. I have spoken with many comrades about this and have attempted to relive all kinds of experiences. Does the brave man resist? I am not sure (. . .). Where does the strength, where does the weakness come from? I don't know. One does not know'* (pp. 36–37).

Elements for a definition of psychological torture based on Améry's testimony

1. **No pain**, much less extreme pain, is required for torture to have taken place. After hearing the sound of one's bones 'crackling and splintering' for the first time, from then on even slight pressure from a torturer's hand is enough to make the victim subhuman.
2. Terror is left as an **indelible mark** which will turn into deep, permanent anguish with time.
3. The **victim's view of the world** as they know it will change: he or she may lose trust and faith in the world and assume that there is no limit to the damage others

can exert. This can be defined as the deterioration of one's belief in logic and kindness, the termination of the social contract and absolute helplessness. Améry writes that the damage to the victim is intangible and irreversible and offers no hope for recovery.

Aleksandr Solzhenitsyn – *The Gulag Archipelago*[9]

Written over the course of more than a decade and published in three volumes (Solzhenitsyn, 1975), *The Gulag Archipelago* is one of the deepest and most complex descriptions of torture ever written. It is based on Solzhenitsyn's personal experience and interviews with 227 survivors of Soviet labour camps, or gulags. The book provides a unique view on a system of integral torture, with an emphasis on psychological methods.

'Let us begin with psychological methods.' (. . .)

Confusion, exhaustion and vulnerability. *'First of all, night. Why is it that all the main work of breaking down human souls went on at night? (. . .) Because at night the prisoner torn from sleep, even though he has not yet been tortured by sleeplessness, lacks his normal daytime equanimity and common sense. He is more vulnerable.'*

Humiliation. *'Preliminary humiliation was another approach. (. . .) At the Lübvanka, Aleksandra Ova refused to give the testimony demanded of her. She was transferred to Lefortovo. In the admitting office, a woman jailer ordered her to undress, allegedly for a medical examination, took away her clothes, and locked her in a "box" naked. At that point, the men jailers began to peer through the peephole and to appraise her female attributes with loud laughs. If one were systematically to question former prisoners, many more such examples would certainly emerge. They all had but a single purpose: to dishearten and humiliate.'*

Deception. *'The lie. We lambs were forbidden to lie, but the interrogator could tell all the lies he felt like. (. . .) Intimidation through enticement and lies was the fundamental method for bringing pressure on the relatives of the arrested person, when they were called in to give testimony. "If you don't tell us such and such" (whatever was being asked), "it's going to be the worst for him. You'll be destroying him completely." (How hard for a mother to hear that!) "Signing this paper" (pushed in front of the relatives) "is the only way you can save him" (destroy him).'*

Threats to family and loved ones, and intimidation. *'Playing on one's affection for those loved was a game that worked beautifully on the accused as well. It was the most effective of all methods of intimidation. One could break even a totally fearless person through his concern for those he loved. (Oh, how foresighted was the saying: "A man's family are his enemies.") Remember the Tatar who bore his sufferings – his own and those of his wife – but could not endure his daughter's! In 1930 Rimalis, a woman interrogator, used to threaten: "We'll arrest your daughter and lock her in a cell with syphilitics!"'*

Fake situations and trickery. *'They would threaten to arrest everyone you loved. Sometimes this would be done with sound effects: Your wife has already been arrested, but her further fate depends on you. They are questioning her in the next room – just listen! And through the wall you can actually hear a woman weeping and screaming. (After all, they all sound alike; you are hearing it through a wall; and you are under terrific strain and not in a state to play the expert on voice identification. Sometimes they simply play a recording of the voice of a 'typical wife' – soprano or contralto – a labor-saving device suggested by some inventive genius.) Then, without fakery, they actually show her to you through a glass door, as she walks along in silence, her head bent in grief. Yes! Your own wife in the corridors of State Security! You have destroyed her by your stubbornness! She has already been arrested! (In fact, she has simply been summoned in connection with some insignificant procedural question and sent into the corridor at just the right moment, after being [told]: "Don't raise your head, or you'll be kept here!"). Or they* *give you a letter to read, and the handwriting is exactly like hers: "I renounce you! After the filth they have told me about you, I don't need you anymore!" (And since such wives do exist in our country, and such letters as well, you are left to ponder in your heart: Is that the kind of wife she really is?)'*

'The interrogator Goldman (in 1944) was trying to extort testimony against other people from V.A. Korneyeva with the threat: "We'll confiscate your house and toss your old women into the street." A woman of deep convictions, and firm in her faith, Korneyeva had no fear whatever for herself. She was prepared to suffer. But given our laws, Goldman's threats were all too real, and she was in torment over the fate of her loved ones. When, by morning, after a night of tearing up rejected depositions, Goldman began to write a fourth version accusing Korneyeva alone, she signed it happily and with a feeling of spiritual victory. We fail to hang on to the basic human instinct to prove our innocence when falsely accused. How can we be there? We were even glad when we succeeded in taking all the guilt on our own shoulders.'

Sensory, emotional and cognitive exhaustion. *'Just as there is no classification in nature with rigid boundaries, it is impossible to rigidly separate psychological methods from physical ones. Where, for example, should we classify the following amusement?'*

> **Sound effects.** *'The accused is made to stand twenty to twenty-five feet away and is then forced to speak more and more loudly and to repeat everything. This is not easy for someone already weakened to the point of exhaustion. Or two megaphones are constructed of rolled-up cardboard, and two interrogators, coming close to the prisoner, bellow in both ears: "Confess, you rat!" The prisoner is deafened; sometimes he actually loses his sense of hearing. But this method is uneconomical. The fact is that the interrogators like some diversion in their monotonous work, and so they vie in thinking up new ideas.'*
>
> **Tickling:** *'This is also a diversion. The prisoner's arms and legs are bound or held down, and then the inside of his nose is tickled with a feather. The prisoner writhes; it feels as though someone were drilling into his brain (. . .).'*
>
> *'**The effects of lighting** involve the use of an extremely bright electric light in the small, white-walled cell or "box" in which the accused is being held – a light which is never extinguished. (The electricity saved by the economies of schoolchildren and housewives!) Your eyelids become inflamed, which is very painful. And then in the interrogation room searchlights are again directed into your eyes.'*
>
> *'Here is another imaginative trick: On the eve of May 1, 1933, in the Khabarovsk GPU, for twelve hours – all night – Chebotaryev was not interrogated, no, but was simply kept in a continual state of being led to interrogation. "Hey, you – hands behind your back!" They led him out of the cell, up the stairs quickly, into the interrogator's office. The guard left. But the interrogator, without asking one single question, and sometimes without even allowing Chebotaryev to sit down, would pick up the telephone: "Take away the prisoner from 107!" And so they came to get him and took him back to his cell. No sooner had he laid down on his board bunk than the lock rattled: "Chebotaryev! To interrogation. Hands behind your back!" And when he got there: "Take away the prisoner from 107!"'*

Elements for a definition of psychological torture based on Solzhenitsyn's testimony

1. **The possibilities for torture are endless.** The only limit is boredom of the torturers or their desire to be distracted by the prisoners.
2. **Systematic sensory confusion** is created through:
   - The psychological exhaustion associated with physical and sensory fatigue. Using sensory overload or environments that produce symptoms similar to psychosis.
   - Using deception and lies; manipulating information and the environment.

3. **Threats**, especially to family members, are very effective torture strategies, even more so than physical torture.
4. Torture is based on constant attacks on **identity**, including nudity, mockery, humiliation and sexual abuse.

Javier Larreta Aldazíbar – *Incommunicado detention and torture in Spain*

In the Basque Country there are an estimated 10,000 people who have been subjected to incommunicado detention, many whom have been interrogated using coercive methods under the Anti-Terrorism Law (Arzuaga, 2012; Carmena, Landa, Múgica and Uriarte, 2013). This law allows detainees to be held in an unknown place for five days (extendable to thirteen) without contact with lawyers, friends or relatives, and permits interrogation by the national police, the civil guard or the Ertzantza (Basque regional police) with no right to habeas corpus. Many of these people later reported abuse and torture.

This is the public testimony of a priest, Javier Larreta Aldazíbar (Larreta, 1998).

'I am a priest, and the pastor of Arellano, a small village located (. . .) near Estella, and director of Mondragon High School (. . .). I was having lunch, [and was returning] to Mondragón to continue classes when the doorbell rang. My brother came down and met with the police again (. . .). Then I went down, and said that I was the man who they had come to detain [the previous day] and I asked what was happening. Then they told me that there was barely anything to do, that they just had to ask me a few questions and I had to go to Pamplona, and that it was a simple procedure that would be finished within a couple of hours. I tried to drive my car to get back to class, but they did not let me. I went up to say goodbye to my elderly parents and told them not to worry, that I would soon return, and [with just] a sweater, blue jeans, and a few coins in my pocket, they took me to Pamplona. There, they applied the Anti-terrorist Law and interrogated me exactly three times.'

Physical torture: beatings. *'In these [interrogations] I would like to highlight three aspects: first, abuse, beatings to the head, neck, stomach etc. Strong and almost constant beatings. (. . .) Second, the "torture" as such – and I understand by that the calculated pain and torment, studied, applied with cold blood and even I would say, cynically; like for example when they first applied the "quirófano." They said to me: "Come on, get on the table, sit there [on top]. We call what we are going to do to you 'the table,' but your buddies call it the 'operating room.'"'*[10]

Psychological torture: fear. *'Third, the psychological torture is very difficult to explain because it includes many factors. For me specifically, I think that this was what made me suffer the most; that internal suffering that is corroding you, that can go on destroying. That can make you lose everything inside yourself that has genuine worth. (. . .) Many things are involved; for example, fear. Fear is something so big and so subtle that it invades your whole being, and it is primarily caused by physical fear; you are receiving beatings, torture, you do not know when all of this will end. It is the fear of death. I realized that they could kill me with absolute impunity. You have no one to witness that you are there or what is happening to you, and they can offer any justification for your death. They are also the ones who will be believed: the "Law." You are the "terrorist" to be removed from the face of the earth. There is also the fear of losing the most valuable things you have, and that somehow you become so broken inside that you could confirm or say things that are completely false, involving third parties – persons you might not even know who are innocent.'*

Psychological torture: uncertainty. *'Another element involved in psychological torture is uncertainty. The uncertainty of not knowing what will happen the next minute. They could offer you a cigar or torture you again, cynically and in cold blood. The uncertainty of not knowing what time of* *day or night it is. At the police station all time is the same: day, night, morning, evening. They take your watch, the light is artificial, the places where you are, if there are windows, they are fully enclosed. Your time in the police station is not a chronological time but an intensive time. There is also the uncertainty of not knowing how your parents are, or your friends; if they are doing something to get you out, if they know where you are.'*

Psychological torture: attacks on dignity and identity. *'Another element involved in psychological torture is their contempt for and derision of the values that are important to you. In my case, specifically, they constantly messed with my priesthood. I could quote many more things involved in the psychological torture. For example, they force you to do many things that make you feel completely ridiculous; you are a clown who makes them laugh and provokes their contempt. You're some kind of worm, an object which they are constantly crushing and humiliating.'*

Psychological torture: perplexity, helplessness, and no rule of law. *'Finally, I want to highlight another element greatly involved in creating this mental torture: the application of the Anti-Terrorism Law. Suddenly you find yourself helpless and totally unprotected by the law, all alone, alone with your interrogators who are representing the law. Their will is the only valid will at the time, but it is also a capricious will.'*

Psychological torture: attitude of the interrogators. *'You discover in them a hostile attitude, a strong aggressiveness against you, and a load of intense hatred – all at the same time. And you realize that the only way to get away from that situation is to maintain and develop your own alertness. Alertness to avoid falling into the fallacies and traps that they constantly lay for you. There are many more things that I could recount, such as the system used at the police station when they put you in solitary confinement; the heavy sound of the keys and locks, [or the fact that they are] constantly asking you for your ID. It is a system that tends to maintain a level of anxiety, permanent anguish, and the uncertainty. Its ultimate purpose is to prevent the detainee from resting, to exhaust him (. . .). From Pamplona they took me to Madrid. I arrived there at night (. . .). Then they moved me to the court (. . .). I was again put in solitary confinement (. . .). By noon or thereabouts I stood before the judge, who ordered my unconditional release without any kind of charge (. . .). The sequelae after the detention can be roughly summarized in two types: one type physical, a pretty severe pain in the spine that has not left me since then (. . .). Another psychic: every day, around two or two-thirty in the morning I suddenly wake up and I am rigid in bed, flooded by a kind of fear, terror, and I carefully listen to all the noises around me, footprints, cars; I stay in that state for a while until I manage to go back to sleep.'*

Elements for a definition of psychological torture based on Larreta's testimony

- Endless torture is devastating, but intensive and focused short-term incommunicado detention by a team of interrogators can also have devastating effects. A **time-limited**, short incommunicado detention (three to five days long) **can have long-lasting effects on the person**.
- **Fear and terror** are keystones of torture, more than pain itself.
- Fear and terror result from **threats**, uncertainty and isolation combined with humiliation, debasement and attacks on dignity and the self.
- Detainees also feel disbelief at their own helplessness and at the lack of rule of law. 'They are the law, the ones who are supposed to be trusted and believed, the honest and good ones.' Impunity and lack of redress increase the impact of torture.

Summary and conclusions: defining psychological torture in the experiences of torture survivors

The above elements for a definition of psychological torture, taken from each survivor's testimony, are summarised in Tables 2.1 and 2.2. They offer a bird's eye view of the complexities of each of the testimonies and their common elements. We find striking commonalities across different experiences, historical and cultural contexts, and conditions and purposes for detention.

To simplify the analysis we then combine these elements into three mindsets (Figures 2.1, 2.2 and 2.3) affording an integrative view. The result is a complex, interrelated map of multiple factors that can be combined in almost infinite ways to constitute torture.

The survivors make no distinction between *torture* and *psychological torture*. Most say that torture *is* psychological and that pain is one of the ways to produce terror and compliance, which are the core aspects of torture.

The three mindsets represent three different degrees of depth into the strategy and impact of the torture inflicted.

The first mindset represents conventional physical torture based on pain (Figure 2.1). It has no other aim than to intimidate, punish or set an example. The perpetrator abuses the body, hits it, disfigures it or mutilates it with the sole purpose of taking the person beyond his or her tolerance threshold, reducing him or her to the state of an animal, as Jean Améry said, or depriving the person of everything that makes someone human, to use Van Nath's expression. The person is confronted with his or her own survival instincts, beyond reasoning. Only pain. Brutality, defencelessness, incredulity and inescapability amplify the body's experience in confronting pain. Torture here may be intended as a punishment or annihilation or as preparation for a subsequent stage.

Figure 2.2 represents this more advanced stage based on the victims' testimonies. The crux of this stage is no longer pain itself but rather a combination of pain and anticipation of pain. It is about handling time and waiting. The prospect of pain and unending waiting time becomes more devastating than pain itself, we are told. It involves the likelihood, which in the mind of the victim is always real, of irreversible damage, unbearable pain, rape or death. This is stoked by thoughts during the waiting time that the perpetrator leaves knowing that, as Villani said, the person will fall apart immersed in his or her thoughts (see Figure 2.2): endless time; another person owns and controls the situation; uncertainty; disorientation; perception of loneliness, that no one knows what is happening; the lack of rules and arbitrariness of the situation; the feeling of the unreal, incredulity; the need for hope and the destructiveness of each thwarted hope. Plus – according to the voices of survivors – these dichotomies have no ostensible solution. One's own body is both one's own enemy but at the same time one's only support. The mind is both a source of anguish and rumination and of one's identity. The torturer is both the cause of pain and the key to relief. All of this often plays out in a sensorially altered environment where the victims are disoriented and confused, physically and psychologically exhausted.

The pain, expectations and fear generated are combined with attacks against one's dignity and identity (Figure 2.3). Destructive messages, being under someone else's control in every way (including one's sexual integrity), being treated as odious, dirty, unworthy, stupid and wrong, stinking, babbling and sub-human, undermine one's identity and awareness of the self. Shame and guilt, which may arise as sequelae, take hold and the person is led to question his or her world values and life project. The person is confronted with him or herself.

TABLE 2.1 Torture/psychological torture: key elements for a definition according to the experiences and testimonies of torture survivors

Survivor	Key elements for a definition of torture/psychological torture
Vann Nath (Cambodia)	• Torture is not an isolated event. It is always part of a *torturing system*. The person knows this and what this implies. • *Hunger.* The use of the painful, slow death of the body as a way to break the psyche and obtain absolute submission. Self-incrimination or false accusation of 'comrades' is the ultimate goal. • *Hopelessness.* Infinite time for torturing. Believing that in the end, everybody dies.

Carlos Liscano (Uruguay)	• *Relationship with the torturer:* torture as a psychological struggle against the torturer. Physical pain as the space in which that struggle is settled. Mutual dependence between the torturer and his or her victim. The interrogator *needs* information.
	• The prisoner's *relationship with his or her body*:
	  – Torture is a painful process of self-awareness. Pain as an extreme form of knowledge that pushes the victim's mind to its limit.
	  – Ambivalent relationship with the body: it is both abject and the only thing one has.
	• Banal things (like defecating) can become the absolute center of one's thought. The torturer designs seemingly minor situations that foster (a) absolute dependence on the torturer and (b) an internal and exhausting battle for dignity and against humiliation. Victims feel shame and question their identity.
	• The torturing system creates an illusion: victims feel that they are in a *battle with themselves.* This causes (a) devastating physical and psychological exhaustion, and (b) nearly unavoidable guilt.
	• No part of torture happens by chance. As a process, *its mechanics are perfectly defined.* It is 'professional work' and interrogators are 'professionally trained' to execute it.

Jacqueline Gurruchaga and Beatriz Brenzano (Uruguay)	• Torture is locating the *limits* of each detainee, so as to break these limits. • The purpose of sexual torture is to demonstrate *omnipotence and absolute control*, even in the most intimate and seemingly untouchable spheres. • Sexual torture involves elements that have to do with *humiliation and shame* (social shame, familial shame and political shame). Multiple types of shame may lead to lifelong silence and the treatment of damage as an individual, private problem.
Mario Villani (Argentina)	• *The process.* There is a carefully planned *torturing process.* It begins with a *softening period* that creates conditions for the rapid breakdown of the individual. • *The unconscious search for closeness and affection.* Human beings seek love to preserve their identity; the duality between closeness and violence destroys the victim. This dilemma has no solution. • *Isolation.* Part of the process is instilling feelings of being abandoned, of nobody knowing what is happening, of society pretending to ignore what is happening – or even justifying it. • *Psychological struggle.* Dissociation, adaptation to horror, emotional detachment from the suffering of others. Hope is demoralising. Living one day at a time. • *Cooperation.* Resilience may require partial compliance with the demands of the torturers, causing anguish about whether such compliance is part of 'survival' or if it is 'cooperation'. *Guilt* is unavoidable.

Survivor	Key elements for a definition of torture/psychological torture
Henry Engler (Uruguay)	• *Isolation* destroys the person. It induces a full psychotic syndrome that lasts more than four years. 'The enemy is in your mind, it is you.' • 'Fighting against the circle': focusing attention on a spot on the wall as a kind of mental anchor. This represents the obsessive fight against psychosis, against psychological torture, and to regain control by maintaining the integrity of the self.
Marcelo Viñar (Uruguay)	• *Torture is always psychological.* Torture does not equal pain, though pain is an element. Torture is fracturing, 'demolishing' the person. • *Waiting time and uncertainty* are devastating. They are associated with doubt, loss of control, constant questioning, amplifying every detail and reaction, and being forced to confront one's fears. • *Terror as the keystone of torture.* All torture systems create a situation in which each element is configured to create terror. That terror does not necessarily involve physical pain. Memories of terror are stronger than memories of physical pain. • *Every banal aspect destroy a person.* It is an error to limit one's understanding of torture to beating and ill-treatment. For example, the arbitrary disruption of bodily functions (vision, sleep, food or liquid intake, or defecation), is of central importance and reveals how even the most apparently banal aspect of detention can demolish a person – even aspects not normally considered 'torture'. Torture includes the combination of: attacks on dignity and identity, feelings of helplessness and lack of control, the stress of waiting, and the weakening process. • The torturer controls time. There is infinite time for torturing. Lack of hope. • Physical, emotional and mental weakening go hand in hand.
Jean Améry (Austria)	• *Torture is not equivalent to pain.* After the 'crackling and splintering' of one's bones, slight pressure from a torturer's hand is enough to make the victim subhuman. • *Torture is equivalent to terror.* Terror leaves an indelible mark on the victim, and will turn into deep, permanent anguish with time.
Aleksandr Solzhenitsyn (Russia)	• *The possibilities for torture are endless. It is useless to classify torture according to types or techniques.* The only limit to torture is the boredom of the torturers and their desire to be distracted by the prisoners. • Systematic creation of *sensory confusion* through: – Psychological exhaustion associated with physical and sensory fatigue. Environments that produce a distorted perception of reality leading to psychotic symptoms. – Deception, lies and manipulation of information. – Threats (especially to family members) are an even more effective torturing strategy than physical torture. • Torture is based on constant attacks on the dignity of the person, including nudity, mockery, humiliation and sexual abuse.
Javier Larreta (Spain)	• Endless torture is devastating, but intensive and focused short-time incommunicado detention by a team of interrogators can also have devastating effects. • Although pain is involved, *fear and terror are the keystones of torture*; over time, fear and terror endure more than pain. • Torture is based on *threats*, uncertainty and isolation, combined with humiliation, debasing attitudes and attacks on dignity and the self.

TABLE 2.2 Torture/psychological torture: impact and consequences according to the experiences and testimonies of torture survivors

Survivor	Impact and consequences
Vann Nath (Cambodia)	• Permanent changes in worldviews. 'They have taken everything that is human from me.' • Introjection of fear for the rest of one's life. Lack of logic, permanent fear. • Forgetting is impossible. *'Everything comes back to me.'*
Jacqueline Gurruchaga and Beatriz Brenzano (Uruguay)	• Torture leaves an indelible memory in the body. The damage is for life. • Silence amplifies the impact. The search for justice becomes one of the few ways to heal.
Mario Villani (Argentina)	• Interiorisation of fear, internal policing. • Permanent distrust of others. • Trauma (mostly expressed through nightmares and flashbacks). • Bodily expressions of suffering. • Many kinds of guilty feelings, mostly related to surviving or to minute decisions made during captivity. • Forgetting is impossible.
Marcelo Viñar (Uruguay)	• Fear is introjected. It takes years to escape fear.
Jean Améry (Austria)	• One's very understanding of the world changes: one assumes that there is no limit to the damage others can exert. This can be defined as the deterioration of one's belief in logic and kindness, the termination of the social contract, and absolute helplessness. The damage is intangible and irreversible, with no hope for recovery.
Javier Larreta (Spain)	• Disbelief of the lack of rule of law and of one's own helplessness. Impunity and lack of redress increase the impact of torture.

FIGURE 2.1 Pain-based torture.

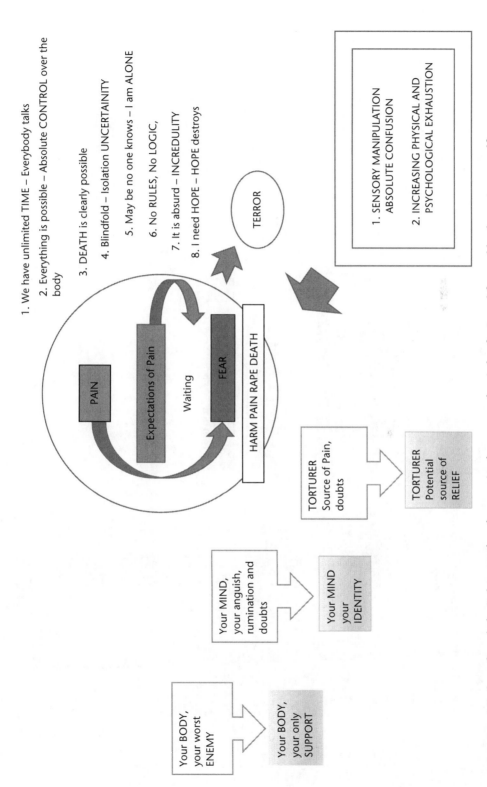

FIGURE 2.2 Mindset of psychological torture based on survivor's accounts: the circle of pain and fear, and battles against oneself.

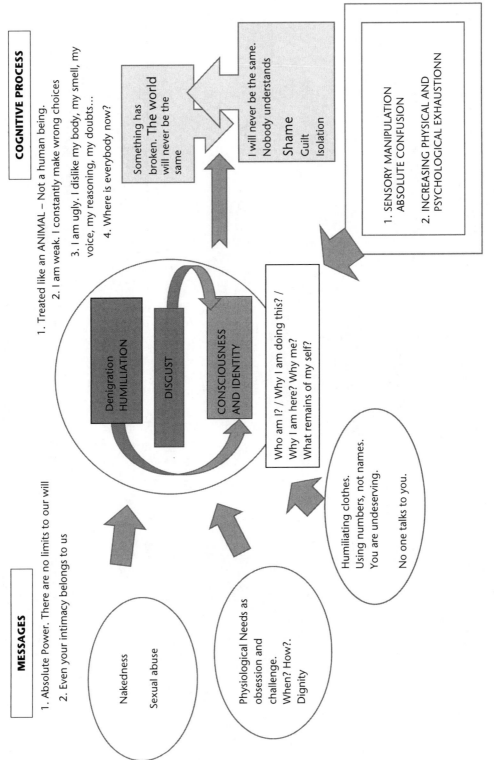

COGNITIVE PROCESS

1. Treated like an ANIMAL – Not a human being.

2. I am weak. I constantly make wrong choices

3. I am ugly. I dislike my body, my smell, my voice, my reasoning, my doubts…

4. Where is everybody now?

Something has broken. The world will never be the same

I will never be the same. Nobody understands

Shame
Guilt
Isolation

1. SENSORY MANIPULATION ABSOLUTE CONFUSION

2. INCREASING PHYSICAL AND PSYCHOLOGICAL EXHAUSTIONN

Denigration HUMILLIATION

DISGUST

CONSCIOUSNESS AND IDENTITY

Who am I? / Why I am doing this? / Why I am here? Why me? / What remains of my self?

Humiliating clothes.
Using numbers, not names.
You are undeserving.

No one talks to you.

MESSAGES

1. Absolute Power. There are no limits to our will

2. Even your intimacy belongs to us

Nakedness

Sexual abuse

Physiological Needs as obsession and challenge.
When? How?.
Dignity

FIGURE 2.3 Mindset of psychological torture based on survivor's accounts: the circle of consciousness and identity.

Depending on the context and the situation, this breaking of a person's identity is generated by varying combinations of the three circles (pain, fear and dignity – identity). Prolonged
over time, they can actually go beyond breaking a person's identity and cast a new identity
according to the torturer's designs. Here, what comes into play is a human being's capacity
to adapt and when placed before his or her utter limits, either consciously or subconsciously
seek survival if not also identification with the perpetrator and, when doing so, generation of
a new, more adapted identity to survive under those conditions.

We now put forward a definition of torture, which for some survivors is also a definition
of psychological torture (because, as we found from their integrative perspectives, all torture
as psychological):

Torture is the manipulation of a human being through terror produced by the infliction of
pain and harm, the disruption and control of bodily functions, and the manipulation of time,
the environment and the senses in order to break the individual, to instill fear, to physically
or psychologically punish, to produce information, to attain self-incrimination, or to change
the detainee's identity or worldviews to accommodate the will of the perpetrator. Although
it is the torturer who makes the rules, torture is experienced as a physical, intellectual and
emotional battle against oneself that leaves permanent marks on the individual (usually in the
form of guilt, shame, recurrent memories and the inscription of pain in the body).

Implications for the legal definition of torture

The above definition contrasts sharply with the current legal definition of torture in the
UNCAT:

1. **Torture is not equivalent to pain.** It is true that pain has been the most widely used
   method to induce fear and terror, and it is still used in many countries: torture almost
   always involves at least some physical pain. However, pain is only one of many elements
   employed to induce fear. This is echoed in the testimonies of Améry (the torturer establishes control through fear after the first 'crackling and splintering' of one's bones), Viñar
   ('Torture is not pain. Torture is about demolishing, fracturing the person.') and Larreta
   ('Although there is pain, the point is fear . . .').
2. **Torture is equivalent to terror.** Terror leaves an indelible mark on the victim, and
   will turn into deep, permanent anguish with time. We find this in the experiences of Van
   Nath ('You are afraid for your whole life. There is permanent fear, and no logic.'), Villani
   ('Fear is forever. You realize that in the end the police are inside of you . . .') and Viñar
   ('Fear is introjected. It takes years to escape from it.').
3. Emphasising the **severity of suffering** in an attempt to distinguish low-level
   (ill-treatment) and high level (torture) abuse does not make sense, because the torture
   process does not impact all victims equally. It is impossible to define a limit for 'extreme
   suffering' or 'extreme psychological suffering', because that limit depends on each individual. Torture is based on the battle that takes place within the victim. The impact of torture
   also depends on the physical characteristics of the detainee and his or her physical endurance. In defining torture, the emphasis should be placed on the *purpose*, not the method.
4. **Torture as an 'art'.** The torturer seeks the 'limits' of the detainee. But what are the
   'limits' – and is it even possible to find them? The only true limit is death. What the interrogator purports to monitor (with or without professional help) is that the detainee does
   not suffer permanent damage or die before he or she has offered information. In this 'art',

psychological damage is not taken into consideration. It is irrelevant. It can't be seen, it might appear a long time after detention, it can be written off as 'exaggerated', 'subjective', and debatable; rarely will it have any legal implications for the torturer.

5.   **The method does not matter.** While tortured, Liscano was subjected to the tank ('tacho'), the stand ('caballete'), to blows and beatings. The catalogue of torture methods, he wrote, is inexhaustible. Solzhenitsyn's testimony shows that the possibilities for torture are endless. The only limit is the boredom of the torturers and their desire to be distracted by the prisoners. As Liscano reminds us, each center will 'specialise' in a specific method. In his detention center, it was wet suffocation and waterboarding (the 'tacho'). In others, it was the prod (the 'picana'). Torture methods cannot be conceptualised as more or less humane; each causes a different type of pain and awakens different personal fears. Different methods challenge different psychological and physical limits, but in the end, all methods are simply specific strategies within the broader game of domination and subjugation that lies at the heart of torture. When judicial procedures evaluate the severity of torture based on the method used (e.g. breaking one's legs is deemed worse than stress-positions or hunger), they ignore – as Viñar and Liscano remind us – that the most banal technique can destroy a victim if properly applied. It makes more sense to evaluate the aims and targets of torture, and the different pathways involved in the breaking the individual. In other words, to understand torture one should focus on the psychological mechanisms it puts into motion.

6.   **Time and reiteration** are not the most relevant criteria. Although detention without time constraints is more damaging, even very short detention periods can have long-lasting effects. It is misleading to distinguish ill-treatment from torture using length of detention or reiteration of abuses as the primary criteria.

Notes

1   Mr. Nath survived because somehow the guards knew that he was a painter, and he was assigned the task of making large oil paintings of Pol Pot.
2   A small cell where new detainees were piled up upon arrival.
3   'Quirófano' (literally, operating room) is a euphemistic expression for the torture room were detainees are interrogated.
4   'Transfers' were what are known as death flights. As Alfredo Scilingo and other torturers have declared in trials, prisoners were disappeared by being boarded in groups onto military flights, and then handcuffed, tied up, drugged and thrown alive into the ocean.
5   Group of detainees appointed to serve as aids in organising the camp.
6   Montevideo, October 2012.
7   Waterboarding.
8   *At the Mind's Limits: Contemplations by a Survivor on Auschwitz and Its Realities*, Améry, Jean. Sidney Rosenfeld and Stella P. Rosenfeld, translators. © 2009, Indiana University Press. Reprinted with permission of Indiana University Press.
9   The selection of paragraphs was made by William F. Schulz, editor of the collection *The Phenomenon of Torture: Readings and Commentary*. University of Pennsylvania Press. 2007 (pp. 63–7). Text from *The Gulag Archipelago* by Aleksander Solhenitsyn. Published by Harvill Press. Reprinted by permission of The Random House Group Limited.
10 Larreta uses the word 'quirófano' in this case to describe a technique of torture in which the person is put on a table with half of his or her body hanging in the air. While some interrogators hold the person down, others bend his or her body using the edge of the table.

3

THE DEFINITION OF PSYCHOLOGICAL TORTURE IN THE TESTIMONIES OF HARSH INTERROGATORS AND TORTURERS

There are few testimonies of perpetrators. Most are self-exculpatory texts in the context of judicial procedures, making it difficult to gauge the extent to which they reflect the actual thoughts of the interrogator. Different studies have shown that these texts mostly offer rational-isations of actions, or false requests for forgiveness (Payne, 2009). The purpose of this chapter is not to reflect on how an ordinary person becomes a torturer, or the psychological mechanisms that allow him or her to practice torture, but to examine *how torturers conceptualise psychological torture*. This will complement our analysis of interrogation techniques in later chapters.

Our reflection is based on the texts of three Uruguayan torturers (Jorge Néstor Troccoli, Gilberto Rivas and Hugo García); Bruce Moore-King, a member of a Rhodesian paramilitary group; and Damien Corsetti, an American interrogator at Bagram Airbase and Abu Ghraib prison. All of them admit to torturing detainees. Given that the psychological component of torture lies at the heart of so-called harsh interrogation techniques (recognised as torture in a 2014 report by the US Senate and by President Obama himself), Damien Corsetti's testimony helps us understand the views of the Behavioral Science Consultation Team, the group of professionals responsible for the design and implementation of these techniques.

Jorge Néstor Tróccoli – *The Wrath of Leviathan*

Jorge Néstor Tróccoli, Uruguayan Chief of Intelligence of Naval Fusiliers (FUSNA) and coordinating officer for the Uruguayan Army during Operation Condor, wrote a book called *The Wrath of Leviathan* (Troccoli, 1996). In it he publicly recognised having tortured detainees, but claimed that he considered torture necessary in the context of war because it was imper-ative to obtain life-saving information from the enemy. Some considered him a hero because he was the only officer who admitted having been a torturer. He escaped the warrant issued for his arrest, and was later located in Rome in December 2007. In what was seen as the result of a secret agreement between the military and political establishment to avoid his prosecu-tion, Uruguay failed to extradite him because of a bureaucratic error. His book ostensibly attempted to explain the events of the past, but was ultimately revealed to be a media stunt for his social and legal exculpation. What follows are extracts from his book organised by subject.

In some instances Tróccoli himself is writing [T], in others he interviews fellow ex-torturers (who were probably his subordinates) who used the aliases Joaquin [J] and Pedro [P].

[T] Obedience. *'Honor is the military virtue par excellence, it is a religion, the religion of duty indicating imperatively how to face every situation (. . .). Daily behavior . . . comes from the religious-military mystique. (. . .). It is important to remember that the military profession is called "castrense" [in Spanish] due to its own nature of castrating the free exercise of ordinary behavior'* (p. 15). *'All this to fulfill the mission – one could call it sacred – to guard the spiritual and material wealth of the nation'* (pp. 16–19). *'The guerrillas wanted to change society . . . even though society did not want to be changed. Through armed struggle, the Movimiento de Liberación Nacional (MLN) sought to create the conditions in which society would ask for change and revolution. We, the institutional military, wanted to defend the country, and we did'* (p. 20).

Peer pressure: the enemy

[T] *'Was it better to be killed, or to kill or torture someone to avoid being considered a wimp?'*

[J] *'Before I came to the security force I was a fearful man, and there I learned to act even when I was afraid. The worst thing that can happen to you is to not overcome your fear, anything is better than that. (. . .) Then I began to think of how to get rid of my fear. I thought, fear disappears when you know your enemy. I went to where the prisoners were, women and men, and I stood next to a Tupa.[1] I saw that he and I were the same (. . .). The next day, I was interrogating someone without knowing what to ask; they were talking about "the irons" [torture implements] and I had to stop and ask another interrogator what "the irons" meant. That's how I learned. We put all of the statements together, and they sold each other out. (. . .) The group provided other initiations: individual merit was manifested by ascending the hierarchy. Good performance made the hierarchy of the group grow. The group is always the priority. (. . .) The urge to demonstrate unity and the reason for being in the group structure is high. You feel constant observation and judgment from your group'* (pp. 24–28).

[T] *"Every group needs an enemy, even just a hypothetical one (. . .). The materialization of the enemy provides the necessary opposition so that the conflict can be solved through arms. (. . .) The enemy is no longer granted humanity, they are merely your reason for being, the obstacle that must be overcome as the greatest rite of initiation; then true membership is acquired, even if such dominance must be demonstrated at all times (. . .). An enemy is someone capable of killing me'* (pp. 27–28).

[T] The lesser of two evils. *'They were acts of war . . . that you cannot qualify with value judgments. Just as one cannot label the bombing of civilian populations during conventional war, or the use of napalm, or any of acts of war'* (p. 55). *'In the context of a war, [torture] is necessary and therefore legitimate. (. . .) There was torture in every war in the history of the world'* (pp. 60–62). *'Nobody stops a war to analyze how you are fighting, especially if you are winning'* (pp. 69–70).

[T] Isolation and alienation from society. *'The situation was unreal for me, violent (. . .). The rift between society and me was deepening, the same thing was happening to all of us. Days later, when we returned to our homes, the separation continued as our friends and family rebuked or challenged us about "what we did." At the age of 22, [the difference between] "us" and "them" was increasingly common'* (p. 32).

[T] Doublespeak: hypocrisy. *'Social institutions shifted (. . .). The whole system of social interaction was unstable (. . .). The executive branch shook with every minister's resignation. (. . .). Of all the branches of state power, only the military remained. (. . .). None of the institutions of the state complained when the military began to be used to control the population'* (pp. 34–35).

[T] Torturous system: impunity. *'Several times my superiors were present during interrogations; they were just another official entity. (. . .) Whoever claimed to be ignorant of what their subordinates were doing during an interrogation would be in a very sad position'* (p. 66).

[T] *'[For some] the struggle offered an escape from mediocrity . . . and they refused to go back to the way things were. Every day they appeared with a new revelation or piece of information, and they magnified its importance. So it was that bulky charts were drawn to report on the "functioning" of "organizations" that were sometimes no more than seven or eight individuals. In the struggle, success had become a sign of prestige, control, efficiency, and personal fame'* (p. 96).

[J] *'One had to ask the judge for a search warrant, and you could not hold detainees for over 24 or 48 hours without notifying the judge. Then we had him for 7 or 8 days until he talked, and we wrote down whatever day we had to in order to keep it under 48 hours (. . .). It was well known that the judges were threatened. The slightest abnormality would make the judge release [the detainee]. (. . .) Then Military Justice took over and provided another level of security'* (p. 53).

[T] *'At times, the justice [system] left no room for nuance, or for analyzing personal circumstances (. . .). On occasion when we went before a judge . . . he replied that he acted based on what we wrote. The solution was simple: we had to write up the reports according to the punishment we thought was adequate, and that's how it was done on innumerable occasions. Justice was largely in our hands'* (p. 97).

[P] Torture. *'Obtaining information was a premise, which is to say that the point was to obtain information in order to know precisely on which battlefront we could go and capture the enemy. (. . .). Once the enemy was captured, the idea was to obtain information'* (p. 52).

[P] *'We learned a great deal from the enemy, not only from their actions, but mainly through interrogations. It is difficult to analyze the issue of interrogations because it carries such strong connotations (. . .). We must, with great effort, break free from these connotations and see, objectively if at all possible, human beings acting under extreme conditions. (. . .). It is with these precautions that we have to address the issue of interrogations, which are very strongly conflated with torture. Torture is, in a purely literal sense, suffering or anguish. However, the meaning attributed to the term is different. Torture has come to mean gratuitous suffering, disguised as sadism, usually committed against an innocent victim by a completely twisted person'* (pp. 59–60).

What is torture?

[T] *'Where is the limit of what is and is not torture? Why do we torture each other?'* (p. 63).

[P] *'This was largely a war of information, a war of intelligence. That is, the point was to obtain information (. . .). Information was obtained through interrogation. A typical interview involves stripping people (. . .), verifying their documents, trying to verify their data, and asking them things. At first it was – let's just call it a one-on-one, face-to-face interaction. Later, we had to respond to the possibility that we might be identified, and face-to-face interactions were no longer used'* (p. 63).

[T] *'Did you use pressure? Torture, as they call it, was it used or not?'*

[P] *'Well . . . the people who came in, came in hooded. They stayed naked for a long time, and were kept standing, they would get hungry or thirsty and were not fed well [for days]. Yeah, that was a kind of pressure'* (p. 63). *'I always wondered where the boundary is between what's considered torture and what isn't. Because I've seen people after three, four days of constant standing, of being on "plantón." Their feet were extremely swollen, and they could not go more than five days without water because they could get dangerously dehydrated'* (p. 63).

[J] *'At that time, even though it was said that torture didn't occur, the person was kept standing for five days, with water and one biscuit a day, blindfolded. That's not torture? Or threatening their daughter, sister, mother, or father? And that was not considered torture. What's the limit then? (. . .) In other places I also saw torture methods applied for days. Over the years we learned that a cup of coffee at a specific moment after having suffered could make them start talking (. . .). Torture is everything, it's everything that the prisoner goes through, it is a means to reach the objective (. . .). If you are in a war, your main concern is the objective (. . .). But when he started talking, he was no longer an enemy, he was a collaborator'* (pp. 64–65).

[T] Types of torture. *'There is no other way to get information. There is no other way'* (p. 63). *'I didn't undress a person for the sake of seeing how beautiful she is, I did it to search her completely; (. . .) I didn't take pleasure in observing a person's physique, or enjoyment in seeing him get screwed over. I wanted to obtain information, one way or another. And the idea was to get information as quickly as possible. (. . .) And I think that the information within the navy was, well, it was much more . . . let's just say that physical pressure was applied to a person only to obtain information, nothing more. I believe that in other sectors of the armed forces, that wasn't the case. (. . .) Actions were taken just to . . . not to obtain information, but to punish the person. I was never interested in punishing anyone'* (p. 64).

[T] *'There were people trying to punish them. Punish them for what they had done, that's the difference between taking it personally and to keeping things within institutional norms'* (p. 64).

[P] *'I was doing my job, obtaining information. I didn't doubt that I was doing things in the best possible way. I had no doubt'* (pp. 63–64).

[T] *'I saw everything . . . I saw the interrogator trying to get information . . . and I saw others who took the fight personally and tried to punish the detainee'* (p. 64). *'They were easily recognizable because they said to the prisoner, "You did such and such to us, you killed so and so" and then they hit him. (. . .). I also saw the others, the sadists. But of the hundreds of people who interrogated detainees, they were a tiny minority. They can be found in any other activity or role'* (p. 64).

[T] Psychological elements of torture. *'During an interrogation a detainee spoke many times, as he had never spoken to anyone before. In the privacy of the room, without physical violence, the worst thing was contact with the greatest levels of human misery (. . .). Secret longings, unconfessed desires, the most vile acts of betrayal, and acts of loyalty and incredible bravery (. . .). Those situations were so violent that they even surpassed physical violence'* (p. 65).

[T] Victims and family. *'Allegations of torture of detainees increased, and the Committee of Relatives of Political Prisoners was formed, a name that astonished us. (. . .). Disappearances and torture are a long-standing part of our history and each side violated the other's human rights almost daily'* (p. 55). *'No one is indifferent to the death of friends, to prison or torture, but any fighter who is worthy of the name knows that this could happen to him. That's why I don't understand some people's self-pitying expressions when they complain about "what they did to us"'* (p. 95).

[T] Torture is what *we* are experiencing now. *'If torture is suffering, anguish – which can be both physical and mental, or moral – then who endured that suffering in the years we're talking about? Maybe we should ask who did not suffer'* (p. 60). *'What all of us tend to forget is that labeling people makes them suffer – one could even say that they are tortured – without giving them the opportunity for personal change. Because what isn't recognized is that any person in the same circumstances is capable of reacting in the same way'* (p. 61).

Elements of analysis for a definition of psychological torture based on Tróccoli's The Wrath of Leviathan

From the point of view of the interrogators:

1. **Context is important.** Torture is as an exaggerated, biased term that should not be used, which should be understood in the context of: (1) unquestionable obedience ('castrense'[2]) and honour as core values; (2) times of war that should be declared and understood as such; (3) conflict in which the enemy operates with the same or even more lethal weapons; (4) a collective, group mystique; (5) the pressure of a unique and extraordinary duty to perform; (6) the negligence, cowardice, conflicting interests or outright hypocrisy of politicians and judges who first encouraged and protected but then abandoned interrogators; and (7) isolation from society, and misrepresentation by the media and alleged 'human rights' organisations exercising one-sided judgment.
2. Torture is the **measured and professional use of violence** in order to obtain information. It is not only a legitimate resource – because the enemy also uses it – but an essential one.
3. **Gratuitous suffering** is different than necessary suffering. Specifically, gratuitous suffering defines torture. Since suffering inflicted on the detainees is *motivated* (it seeks *only* to obtain information, nothing more), it isn't considered torture (see also Gil, 1999).
4. To torture someone it is **enough to keep them standing, naked and without food for five days.** After that, if offered something as simple as cup of coffee, most people will talk.
5. There are three kinds of torturers: (a) those who only seek information; (b) those who use power to punish the other, or whatever the other represents; and (c) sadists, who enjoy torture.
6. Torture is not an individual phenomenon or isolated action, but a comprehensive **state policy** that requires to a greater or lesser extent the action, omission, connivance and covering-up of multiple actors at different levels of power including, of course, the highest ones. It must be understood as part of a global machinery that encompasses both the tortured individual and the effects of such torture on a societal level (Viñar and Ulriksen, 1990). In this sense we can speak of a global system that imposes agonising fear and terror through the random infliction of torture on a significant part of the population, sometimes against activists but in many cases against everyday people.

Ex-colonel Gilberto Vazquez – *Interview with a torturer*

Responsible for the torture and disappearance of hundreds of political prisoners, the former colonel has always openly declared that he tortured, that torture was necessary and that in the same circumstances he would torture again. He has been interviewed for national newspapers and radio and television programs on several occasions. Below, we quote from one of these interviews[3] (Frias, 2011).

The usefulness of torture.

'Why did torturing begin?' *'It was useful. It changed things because the reality was that at first I could not turn to anyone . . . I could not do anything . . . there was no way.'*

'Did the torture make them stop?' *'When we started to crack down on them and the guys began to talk, they taught us how the MLN [Movimiento de Liberación Nacional] worked and where* *everyone was. In one year they came down. We went from being overpowered to overpowering them. They were confused. We captured one guy and he came to the barracks thinking, "They're going to beat me up." So many of them said, "Let's talk calmly" and there was no need for lots of torture.'*

'But even then you tortured. . .' *'Yes. We did what it took to get information because on the other side there was the life of our soldiers and the peace of the Republic. We lived in a state of permanent unease.'*

'Did you regret what happened?' *'No, on the contrary. I am proud of having been involved in the salvation of the country. Can you imagine Uruguay becoming communist in the middle of the Cold War? Did you see what happened in Vietnam? It would have been horrible here. It was a practical matter.'*

'Don't you regret of having tortured and disappeared people?' *'There was no choice. The alternative was to enable them to go on killing my soldiers, and by default, I would have been an accomplice. I'd rather be dead. In my jail cell I have pictures of my dead comrades, and young people from the army come to see me and don't know who they are. But they've named streets and plazas for those who died on the other side; they are national heroes. I wasn't going to allow them to continue being killed, even if I did have to get my hands dirty. It hurt me in my soul, and it still hurts, but there was no other option. Unfortunately, war, violence, and brutality are part of life. When it's your turn, you have to choose the lesser evil. I either busted them or left them to continue killing my comrades. We were doing things the best we could. We had to do some unfortunate things. It was like when a surgeon has to amputate a gangrenous leg to save someone's life. He doesn't amputate the leg because he enjoys it. He had to do it. We saved the country and we are proud.'*

Hugo García Rivas – *Confessions of a torturer*

Hugo García Rivas was a Uruguayan interrogator who received training and participated in torture sessions over the course of several years, but after experiencing doubt and guilt he applied for, and was granted, voluntary resignation and transfer. Following threats from ex-comrades who feared he would talk, he chose exile in Norway. He voluntarily collaborated with various inquiry commissions, and his story appears in both a book (Victor, 1980) and a documentary film.[4] He now believes that torture is not useful as a way to get information, and should be abolished.

Fear, shame, and guilt. *'I felt remorse and I know many of my colleagues feel remorse, feel that what they are doing is wrong, but they keep doing it, and feel guilty. I know that happens to many people. Very few decide to leave, I do not know why that is, if it's out of fear that they won't find another job or that they may have a hard time. (. . .) Many of my colleagues had the same problems with their families as I did; they were different people when they went home. (. . .). I even walked down the street sometimes, and suddenly felt fear because a person was looking at me, and I thought: "Could they have been arrested by the Company?" The sense of guilt was pretty big. (. . .). There are many who have this fear, who feel unable to live a civilian life. (. . .) Most people think that they're inside and have a steady income . . . and do not want risk facing a civil life, say, earning a living [where someone could recognize them]. I'm sure these are the reasons'* (pp. 27–28).

'I felt bad knowing that my family knew I was a "milico" [member of the military]. I didn't like that they saw that I had a gun at home, and I tried to hide it. Even when I was working on the street with the gun, sometimes my jacket would bunch up and the gun showed, and I was embarrassed. I felt myself blushing. For me, at least, it left me with a feeling of inferiority, because in Uruguay being a "milico" is equivalent to being a freeloader whose salary is handed down from above, as they say; it amounts to being a robot, a person who follows orders, who is nothing' (p. 29).

Purpose of torture. *'There [in Uruguay], a person is usually detained based on suspicions or because of certain information. Then the security services detain people but without knowing if it's true. The method used to find out if the suspicion is true is interrogation – in other words, torture. Torture is systematic. They say it is necessary to obtain information. I know of one person that was brought to the brink of death during torture, and then died. However they couldn't prove that this person had committed a single crime'* (p. 38). *'It's possible to affirm that everyone who is detained in Uruguay is tortured. No one is not tortured. (. . .) Any person who is arrested is immediately tortured to gain information. (. . .) My wife knows of a case involving her close friends. They went to arrest a person and he was not there, so they arrested the brother, who had nothing to do with anything. And they tortured him just the same, even though he had never been involved in anything. Torture is the norm'* (p. 73).

'I think that everything that is happening, this repression, these violations, have a specific purpose, which is that the military wants to be sure that their position will never be threatened. That absolutely no one will conspire against the regime and the government. They don't want to allow anything, or allow anyone to form an opposition group in Uruguay. It's what they're looking to achieve through continued repression and personal violations. They know that most people don't agree and that's why they are constantly sending [plainclothes agents] to different places where there are concentrations of people, so that they can listen to the atmosphere there, the rumors that spread. Clearly they are afraid that someone might be plotting or that a group might form' (p. 42).

The tacho (also referred to as the 'submarine' or 'waterboarding'). *'I witnessed the interrogation of Rosario P.M. She was tortured in the "tacho," as it is commonly called there. We called it the "tacho" because it is a tank cut in half, with water, with a board attached to it where we would lay a person down so that their head was inside the water. They wore a waterproof hood. That went on for one day. Then she was handcuffed with her hands behind her back, the handcuffs were placed on a hook hanging from the ceiling with her arms raised above her body, pulled away from the body. She was kept naked'* (p. 45).

Interrogation classes.

Interviewer (I):	*'Did you receive training in interrogation and torture?'*
H.R.:	*'Yes, interrogation classes, yes. Now Captain Ramos gives them, back then it was captain Alanís.'*
I:	*'How are interrogation classes given?'*
H.R.:	*'Well, they try to instill in students that torture is necessary, absolutely necessary to obtain information. Otherwise, no information is obtained. But torture must be done in a way that does not endanger the life of the person. Not because of that person's life, but because of the fact that if that person dies they take any information with them. In some cases the student, in his eagerness to show the teacher that he knows how to get information, goes too far while torturing.'*
I:	*'Are "practical" classes of torture carried out?'*
H.R.:	*'Yes. They bring a detainee from the Company, the Company generally has detainees. The "tacho" is brought there, to the school hall, and some of the students proceed to beat the detainee or immerse his head under water while another interrogates him'* (p. 66).
I:	*'Are detainees who are taken to these "practical" classes also being interrogated by the Company?'*
H.R.:	*'Not always. It may be that they are no longer being interrogated by the Company but they're brought in anyway, because it is a practical class. Or, more*

> like it's a class for them to get used to torturing. It's not about the interrogation in itself. That's the end.'

I: 'These [classes] are held with all of the students?'

H.R.: 'All of them, yes. Except the foreigners. These classes are not held in the presence of foreigners, only Uruguayans. Now they rotate the students. Because the training lasts just a few days and they want everyone to participate. It's not always the same detainee. One day they use one, another day another. If there aren't detainees in the Company, they "obtain" them from the 13th Infantry Battalion.'

I: 'Are there other kinds of torture in those classes?'

H.R.: 'There are blows, and hanging is also common. Electric shocks are the most common torture. It's very simple. Two or three wires are connected to the electrical outlet, well-twisted and coated with a thick rubber on the outside; a small piece of wire at the end is left exposed. The other end is plugged into just one of the holes in the outlet. Then the wire has electricity, but not 220 volts. That lays a person down. It passes through them, you could say. If low voltage doesn't do much, you can get them wet. If you get them wet it has a much greater effect. You can put [wires] anywhere on the body. There is not a special place. It's just like anything else, right? Sometimes it's a little bit sadistic; [shocks] can be applied to the testicles, for example, or somewhere like that.'

I: 'Does that happen often?'

H.R.: 'Yes, that often happens. When the sadism starts to kick in. When you have an idea like: "Why not put the wire here to see if he is so macho?" or some similar way of thinking. It's a class that they took to heart.'

I: "Were these kinds of classes an important part of the course?"

H.R.: "Yes. They were. They took almost an entire week, so everyone participated."

I: "Were detainees' lives ever in danger in these classes?"

H.R.: "Yes, they often fainted. In those cases, the detainee is revived, the trainee waits until he revives, and then continues. There is a physician there, Dr. Scarabino. If there is a problem and the detainee is interrogated to the point of being in danger, the doctor is called."

I: "What attitude did the subordinates have during interrogation classes?"

H.R.: "We were told that we had to act firmly. It was our duty. In the beginning the youngest ones, those of us who were new to the Company – almost none of us acted firmly. One day, after we had one of those classes, they punished us for not acting how they wanted us to (. . .). We had to go down to the sewers and roam around. It was nasty, very unpleasant" (p. 66–68).

Elements for a definition of psychological torture based on García Riva's testimony

1. The experience of being a 'milico' involves **shame** (after perceived rejection by relatives and society); guilt (from the awareness of the immorality of the acts performed); and fear (of being recognised on the street, of unemployment or of lost protection if one leaves the army).

2. The person is detained and tortured on the basis of circumstances (being somewhere), relationships (knowing someone) or suspiciousness (appearance), without necessarily

having any evidence of a crime. Torture is used as an **indiscriminate technique** to obtain pieces of potential information ('fishing'). Torture is also a form of **social control** designed to instill fear, control rumors and information, and, hypothetically, to prevent the formation of opposing groups. In rare cases, it is also used as a means of confirming an allegation, or obtaining a confession from a detainee. It is therefore part of a global system of control.

3. Torture, at the elite level where García Rivas worked, is **explicitly taught** through training courses that include both theoretical elements and face-to-face torture of detainees. The techniques and methods of interrogating the detainee are decided upon and modeled for students.

4. Torture is part of a **system**. It can never be an isolated initiative. The system designs torture programs, and trains, supervises and protects those who torture. Politicians publicly deny that torture occurs, but when they are forced to, they will turn in the executioner.

Bruce Moore-King – *Unspeakable Acts, Ordinary People*

Bruce Moore-King was a member of the white minority in Rhodesia when the Zimbabwe National Liberation War began. As the war evolved and the white minority was feeling more and more trapped, he enrolled in a paramilitary group (called Grey's Scouts) and participated in the torture of children, adults and elderly men. Grey's Scouts had better arms and fighting conditions than black guerrillas, but they lacked support from the population, which forced them to resort to torture to get information. When Moore-King finally sought exile, he began to question what had he done and wrote a critical book published upon his return to the country seven years later (Moore-King, 1998). In it, he detailed, among other things, the atrocities he committed and presented himself as the victim of nationalist turmoil. Below, we include excerpts from an interview with him, conducted years after he ceased torturing (Conroy, 2000).

'When the tracks led into a kraal, a small village in the bush, it would be impossible to separate the guerrillas' tracks from those of the local residents, and in that situation, Moore-King would pull a young man from the crowd and ask where the guerrillas had gone. If the man pled ignorance, Moore-King might pull a dynamo from his pack, attach alligator clips to the man's ears, and turn the crank. Moore-King believes that the shocks he administered were minor, equivalent to ones he experienced in boarding school and when working on automobile engines, although he concedes that someone with a weak heart might perhaps have been killed. He thinks the real torture was not in the physical pain, but in the fear (. . .) "What does it feel like to someone who has no concept of electricity?" he asked. "What is the effect on a fairly simple black person in the middle of the bush who has never seen a light switch?"' (p. 89)

'As years passed and the conflict escalated, Grey's Scouts often found themselves in villages populated only by women, children, and elderly men. The usual suspects – young males – were all away with the guerrillas. Moore-King would then search for the village elder. The most efficient method of questioning, he says, was not to torture the elder, but to find the elder's grandson. Once the grandson was in hand, Moore-King would order a soldier to hold the child by the ankles and lower his head into a bucket of water. The boy would be brought up for air just before he drowned and would be set on the ground, where he would spew water, writhe in pain, and weep from fear. The process would be repeated until the old man talked' (pp. 89–92).

'I asked him if he felt any guilt about his performance as a torturer. He acknowledged and showed none. There are two Bruce Moore-Kings, he told me, and the one who so casually tortured children and adults had been dead for a long time' (p. 93).

Elements for a definition of psychological torture based on Moore-King's interview

1. **Threats** to a relative and **fear** of the unknown are more useful than pain. Torture is a psychological game.
2. **Exculpation**. *I reject torture, it was not me who did that, it was a past version of myself that was caught up in a collective turmoil for which I do feel responsible, but not guilty. It could have been anyone in my place.*

Damien Corsetti: *The Monster*

Damien Corsetti was a torturer in the US military base in Bagram, Afghanistan, and Abu Ghraib prison in Iraq (Pardo, 2014; Ruiz, 2011). At age 21 he was sent to Bagram as an intelligence officer, with almost no training. It was soon proposed that he work as an interrogator. He began interrogating after a few sessions of watching others do the job. Four weeks later he was promoted for his achievements and assigned to interrogate 'high value prisoners'. He acknowledges using both physical and psychological torture in a learning process based on trial and error. He was identified by two of the detainees (among the many he interrogated) who later denounced the torture. His name was also associated with the photo scandals in Abu Ghraib. He faced charges of dereliction of duty, maltreatment, assault and performing indecent acts. He was found not guilty in a military trial and released with honours from the army at age 25, deemed permanently psychologically disabled and offered paid retirement for the rest of his life. After that, he began to denounce his past and speak out against the use of torture. He considers torture to be useless as a source of information. The following excerpts are from the book *El Monstruo: Memorias de un Interrogador,*[5] and an interview with Corsetti conducted during the book's press release in Madrid.

Lack of training and strategy. *Corsetti, an intelligence officer, describes how his job description quickly changed: 'In the first months of 2002 the [intelligence] members underwent a rapid transformation from spies to interrogators in Fort Bragg, North Carolina, and Old England, in Louisiana. Classes were often based on a soldier role-playing as an interrogator and another acting as a detainee, under the supervision of the instructors'* (p. 12).

'Casual Cruelty', a model based on psychological torture. *'The model (. . .) was informally referred to as "Casual Cruelty": a system designed to humiliate prisoners and steadily subject them to psychological torture'* (p. 12).

'The main hall of the prison on the ground floor was lit up like a mall, but did not have a single window; the roof, about five feet high, showed off a tangle of wires and tubes. (. . .) About 100 prisoners dressed in orange jumpsuits were piled up in the five large collective cages, made of metal with barbed wire tangled around the bars. (. . .) Detainees were sitting motionless on carpets. (. . .) So many people and so little noise caused a strange feeling, accentuated by the stench coming from the mass of human beings living and defecating together' (pp. 13–15).

'The first contact with Bagram prisoners was in the form of barking dogs. The detainees arrived with their hands tied with plastic straps and hoods on their heads (. . .) which were attached to

their clothes with electrical tape, making it difficult to breathe. They could not see anything, but they heard the animals, and sometimes were so close that they could feel their breath (. . .). You have no name, only a number. (. . .). Everything in the process was done screaming, with naked detainees in front of more than a dozen people (. . .) including women. It was an unthinkable humiliation for an Afghan' (p. 15).

'The screening usually lasted between fifteen minutes and one hour. The objective was to determine the importance and the degree of cooperation of each prisoner. Then the prisoners were moved to a solitary confinement cell, although if none was available they were confined in smaller, individual cages, no more than 2.10 meters high, called "vents" (airlocks).'

Stress positions. *'In this new location, the prisoners were kept awake ("sleep dep" in Bagram slang) from 12 to 48 hours, depending on their behavior (. . .). In the event that the prisoner fell asleep, he would soon come to know, in his bones, the meaning of the expression "stress position" (. . .). [Corsetti's] favorite was to force the prisoner to lean with his back and legs straight, head against the wall, and hands behind his head, at an angle of 60 degrees from the ground. (. . .) After a while, if the inmate shifted position, (. . .) it was enough to place one finger on the handcuffs to force him to raise his arms. More advantages [of this position]: the soldier could use the pocket of the orange prisoner's jumpsuit as an ashtray, just to humiliate him, while he smoked cigarettes or pot, played poker, and even drank alcohol'* (pp. 15–16).

Sleep deprivation. *'Often prisoners were held for days or weeks with four hours of sleep per day during intervals of ten minutes to an hour – they couldn't enter the REM stage of sleep in which the brain rests. The objective (. . .) was that the prisoner wanted to be questioned, because returning to face the soldier's questions meant, in a sense, a relief. (. . .). A long period of "sleep deprivation" even without "sensory deprivation" can make anyone become temporarily insane (. . .). [Especially] when applied not as "capture shock," but as a punishment for failing to cooperate in interrogations (. . .). As always in torture, "sleep deprivation" is useless. After four or five days of "sleep dep," inmates were rendered useless as a source of information, because they suffered from hallucinations and mixed up dates and people. They spent hours screaming, and soldiers sometimes asked translators what they were saying. I remember a prisoner who shouted, calling for his wife, who was dead. Others called for their mothers. I have those cries here in my head'* (p. 17).

Sensory deprivation. *'[In Bagram] each prisoner has a carpet in their cell measuring 1.2m by 2.5m. And they spend 23 hours a day sitting on it, in silence. If they speak, they are chained to the ceiling for 20 minutes and black visors are put on them so they can't see, and their ears are covered so they can't hear. They are taken down to the basement once a week, in groups of five or six, to shower. It's done to drive them crazy. I almost went crazy myself. (. . .) Apart from those normal cells, there are six isolation cells in the basement of the prison, plus two rooms for "special guests"'* (p. 19).

Combined effect. *'After several weeks of fruitless interrogation, Khan Zada was subjected to fourteen days of "sleep deprivation." In the first six days, he was subjected to a strict regime: handcuffed to the ceiling; although they let him sit from time to time to recover physically. In the last eight days, they let him sleep his four regulatory hours a day without interruption. When he came out of "sleep deprivation," Zada Khan was a different person. When the silent Afghan saw Corsetti, the man who had terrified him, he smiled at him and hugged his legs. "How could they want me to treat this guy badly?" [Corsetti] asked himself'* (p. 20).

'There were detainees who did not know what Al Qaeda was (. . .). Ninety-eight percent were innocent and had been sold by leaders of different Afghan militias to Americans for ransom.' (p. 20)

Intoxicated questioning. *'More often than not my breath smelled of alcohol (. . .). I conducted more interrogations drunk than sober. And my case wasn't the only one'* (p. 23).

Arbitrariness and abuse. Finding the detainee's limit. *'The interrogator could choose between insults and threats, such as "do the Guantanamo," the "stress positions," "sleep deprivation," "sensory deprivation," or "monstering." Everything was up to us. We had the freedom to apply the techniques we wanted, when we wanted'* (p. 23). *'Nothing was ever totally clear: who was who, which person was trustworthy, which rules had to be applied. Furthermore, the implementation of those rules was left to inexperienced soldiers'* (p. 26).

Torture as a psychological game. *'The key to this protocol was to combine abuses with sporadic moments of false complicity. It was a psychological game. A person's resistance doesn't break like it does in the movies. Nobody suddenly collapses and starts talking (. . .). It's more like a very flexible sapling, you have to bend it little by little, and it can snap back to its original position at any time (. . .). It was better to treat the prisoner in a relatively friendly way: an angry inmate is always less willing to work (. . .). The "game" of the interrogator and the interrogated was based on generating some trust and even a bit of gratitude towards your interrogator'* (p. 26). *'The key to breaking the psychological resistance of a suspected terrorist is, above all, to surprise him and provoke emotions that he can't control (. . .). It's like a game of chess. You can't win using brute force'* (p. 30).

Brutality and sadism. *'Sessions (. . .) with special interrogators were marked by extreme brutality (. . .). The prisoners were systematically subjected to (. . .) waterboarding, i.e., simulated drowning. (. . .). No one can stand more than two minutes. (. . .) I know that nobody resists longer because once a group of soldiers tried the technique on ourselves. The feeling is terrifying. You think you're drowning. And if you stand more than two minutes, you can feel beyond proud (. . .). I always had the feeling that finding information was not the important issue at these meetings. It was more torture as punishment as a method to get something. (. . .). [It was a process] marked by sadism, without any practical result'* (pp. 27–28).

'The civilians who took part in the interrogations used waterboarding whenever they wanted. They applied it for five or ten minutes and didn't ask anything (. . .). Torture is always sadistically useless, and these sessions prove it in the most compelling way possible. It is questionable whether prisoners had any value as intelligence assets because they were left in a deplorable physical and psychological state (. . .). In Abu Ghraib and Bagram they were tortured to make them suffer, not to get information out of them. (. . .). [At times the torture had no other goal than] to punish them for being terrorists. They tortured them and didn't ask them anything' (pp. 28–29).

Guilt, depression and psychosis. *'It's paradoxical that I received congratulations and good references for doing things that I would now want to forget at any price (. . .). Soon, the first symptoms of psychosis appeared, (. . .) as well as anxiety attacks (. . .) probably exacerbated by Corsetti's massive consumption of ecstasy and cocaine. His guilt complex also played an important role, which began to grow from the time he began replaying in his mind the things he had done and seen in Afghanistan and Iraq'* (p. 56).

Nothing is comparable to torture. *'I firmly believe it was torture, and unfortunately I took part in it. I don't think anyone can capture what happened without being there. It's not just fear of dying. It's not just the carnage you see around you. It is the total mess that you're operating within during the war. You have no plan of action. You have to make split-second decisions. I'm a pretty open-minded guy, but when you're in a war it's "you against me." You may think that's wrong, but you can also save an American life. My basic feeling on the front was fury. But while I was scrubbing floors at Fort Bragg, I realized that everything had been simply monstrous. I realized that there is nothing like seeing a tortured man. I've been to war. I've been shot. I've shot. I've killed people. None of that is as bad as torture"* (p. 56).

In the interview, Corsetti said: *'Look, they leave us alone in this room, they give me a roll of duct tape to tie you to the chair, I turn off the light and in five hours you sign a piece of paper for me saying that you're Osama bin Laden.'*

Cold water. *'I remember one of my prisoners trembling with cold. His teeth wouldn't stop chattering. I put a blanket on him and then another, and another, and his teeth never stopped chattering, never stopped. You could see that the man was going to die of hypothermia. But the doctors are there so that they don't die, to be able to torture them one more day.'*

Psychological torture, administered by psychiatrists. *'They tell them they are going to kill their children, rape their wives. And you see on their faces, in their eyes, the terror that that causes them. Because, of course, we know all about those people. We know the names of their children, where they live. We show them satellite photos of their houses. It is worse than any torture. That is not morally acceptable under any circumstances. Not even with the worst terrorist in the world.'*

'Sometimes, we put one of our women [female US military personnel] in a burqa and we made her walk through the interrogation rooms and we told them, "That is your wife," and the prisoner believed it. Why wouldn't they?'

'Torture doesn't work. One thing is losing your temper and punching a prisoner, another is to commit these acts of brutality.'

Elements for a definition of psychological torture based on Corsetti's interviews

1. Torture is a part of **system** that presses for results, that trains interrogators, permits practices that are officially forbidden, covers up their actions, and offers impunity if they are ever uncovered. Although the system knows that torture is not useful, it always resorts to torture.
2. It is **easy to become involved** in torture. The use of euphemisms, group pressure, an unbreakable chain of command, the idea that one can save the lives of comrades, and the context of secrecy and impunity make it very difficult to resist participating. It is difficult to realise this until one gains distance and perspective.
3. Torture has a **pleasurable side**. It involves a psychological challenge, a sense of heroism and of duty fulfilled, and gives an incredible sense of power.
4. It also involves **negative, unpleasant elements** that are often blocked out with the use of high doses of alcohol and drugs, emotional detachment from the victims, and small gestures of humanity towards certain detainees that allow torturers to maintain a benign, human self-image, or to tell themselves that others would do worse.
5. The price of discovering the pleasing side of torture while being unable to forget some of the unpleasant actions causes deep **guilt and shame**, especially if the torturer is rejected by society and the heroic myth of the freedom fighter falls apart.
6. Torture can be devastating in a very short period of time. It is easy to completely destroy a person. Three days of total sensory deprivation or five days of sleep deprivation can cause a psychotic breakdown and completely destroy a detainee's conscious mind. Interrogators know that they **have the power to destroy a person**. But this is not useful for obtaining information, it is only useful when the interrogator is not interested in information and wants to seek 'revenge' or punish the detainee.
7. Although rules may exist to prevent physical violence, and torture may be designed to be mainly psychological (using fear, terror, confusion, humiliation and manipulation), some amount of **physical violence** is always needed. The context of impersonalisation

and impunity makes it almost impossible to set institutional limits on violence, and brutal and sadistic behaviours will always show up, although they go against the interrogator's best interest and do not help obtain information.

8. The torturer tends to interpret **silence as deception**. No matter how severe treatment becomes, the interrogator will not take 'no' for an answer; silence is seen as equivalent to resistance and lack of cooperation. Innocent people can be tortured for months and nobody will believe them or be sure enough of their innocence as to stop interrogation.

'Harsh interrogation': Behavioral Science Consultation Teams

The Behavioral Science Consultation Teams (BSCTs, pronounced 'biscuits') are groups of medical doctors, psychiatrists and psychologists who studied detainees in American detention sites. They were held responsible for the formulation, implementation and supervision of Enhanced Interrogation Techniques. They guaranteed that interrogations were based on scientific, medical knowledge and ensured that there was no 'permanent' damage to the detainees. Their work was especially well known in Guantanamo and Abu Ghraib, where they formulated protocols (sometimes tailored to specific detainees) and directed interrogations (as many soldiers testified in official commissions, among them Damien Corsetti). Some of these protocols have later been regarded as torture by the Senate Intelligence Committee that investigated them in 2014. John Francis Leso and Larry C. James, the chief psychologists in charge of BSCTs, have always rejected these accusations and firmly denied that their work could be considered torture; they argued that their role was necessary and ethically correct. The Center for Bioethics at the University of Minnesota (2014) has collected and made publicly available most of the evidence of intervention by psychologists in interrogations, revealing that though sometimes psychologists spoke out against interrogators' harsh treatments, in most cases they recommended psychological strategies to break the prisoner.

The following excerpts are from the book *Oath Betrayed* by Steven Miles (2009), who has conducted extensive research on the work of the BSCTs, and an interview with Larry C. James (Simmons, 2008).

'General Miller created Behavioral Science Consultation Teams . . . to work with the Intelligence Committees in Iraq and at Guantanamo. In his Iraq field assessment, he described the BSCTs' purpose thus: "These teams, comprised of operational behavioral psychologists and psychiatrists, are essential in developing integrated interrogation strategies and assessing interrogation intelligence production." This statement must be translated in light of Secretary of Defense Rumsfeld's "counter resistance" interrogation directive: "Interrogations must . . . take into account . . . a detainee's emotional and physical strengths and weaknesses . . .". Interrogation approaches are designed to manipulate the detainee's emotions and weaknesses to gain his willing cooperation (. . .). BSCTs played a central role in designing interrogation plans to exploit prisoners' psychological and physical weaknesses. (. . .). There was no precedent or policy for Miller's interrogational BSCTs.'

'Abu Ghraib and Guantanamo BSCT personnel reviewed medical information relevant to the conduct of interrogations, performed psychological assessments, recommended physically and psychologically coercive interrogation plans, monitored and provided feedback during interrogations, and taught behavioral techniques to interrogators.'

'One of the most controversial of the BSCTs' powers was that of reviewing prisoners' medical records for material useful for selecting interrogation approaches. Under Guantanamo's 2002 policy, medical personnel were obliged to give nonmedical personnel, including members of the BSCT,

medical information relative to the "national security mission" upon request. (. . .). General Miller simply denied to Red Cross officials that medical records were available to intelligence staff. The Red Cross protested the "integration of access to medical care within the system of coercion" to no avail. Medical personnel in Iraq, in Afghanistan, and at Guantanamo confirmed that investigators had access to medical records (. . .). First, clinical examinations were used to "clear" prisoners for harsh interrogation plans. (. . .). An intelligence officer at Camp Na'ma in Iraq complained that "every harsh interrogation was approved by the [commander] and the Medical *prior to its execution*'" (p. 55). *'Second, the BSCTs used medical and psychological information to develop a plan to break a prisoner's resistance to questioning. Clinicians at Guantanamo made records available to intelligence staff or met with BSCT personnel "to provide information about prisoners' mental health and vulnerabilities" (. . .). Such information included phobias (fear of the dark or of being alone) or medical conditions that could be exploited for "Fear Up Harsh," "We Know All," or "Manipulation of Environment" techniques. A military intelligence specialist in Iraq applied her background in psychology in a "special section" responsible for designing approaches to "interrogat[ing] those who could not be broken." She approved coercive interrogation plans involving sleep deprivation, but opposed the use of dogs or nudity, though her protests were in vain. Ultimately she asked to be relieved of interrogation duties. (. . .) Steve Stefanowicz, a civilian "interrogator," testified that he requested interrogation plans that included sleep deprivation (four hours per day for three days, followed by sleeping for twelve hours, then repeating the process), sensory deprivation for up to seventy-two hours, "meal plans," isolating detainees "in the hole" for thirty days with a possible thirty-day extension, and shaving a detainee's beard or hair (to neutralize Muslims in the interrogation setting). (. . .). Behavioral clinicians reportedly micro-managed some interrogations. General Sanchez's policy stated that interrogators should appear to "control all aspects of the interrogation to include the lighting, heating . . . as well as food, clothing and shelter given to security detainee." At Mosul prison, the guards' general orders stated, "Firm control, coupled with mental stress, can greatly weaken a detainee's will . . . . The guard force will take all instructions from the Sergeant of the Guard and interrogation team personnel [for] . . . providing appropriate mental stress on detainees." (. . .). The guards, for example, were allowed to do what was necessary to keep a prisoner awake during sleep management within the approved interrogation plan.'* (pp. 52–53)

'Guantanamo's BSCT included a psychologist and psychiatrist, neither of whom were specialists in criminal investigative psychology. The BSCT's psychologist, Major John Leso, was a counseling psychologist with expertise in assessing pilots' flight fitness' (p. 54). *'In 2002 (. . .) [he] monitored the interrogation of Mohammed al Qahtani. The fifty-day diary gives a detailed chronology of the application of isolation, sleep deprivation, humiliation, masking, head shaving, shackling, and threatening with a dog and so on'* (p. 61).

The American Psychological Association condemned these practices, but still rejected the possibility of a direct indictment of any of the professionals involved for deontological reasons (Soldz, Raymond and Reisner, 2015).[6] In January 2008, the US Army published an official interview with psychologist Larry James on its website. James explained his work, denying any direct involvement in the interrogation of detainees but acknowledging that he helped design interrogation procedures. He didn't believe that his behaviour could be considered 'torture', or unethical:

'From a moral standpoint, it is always good to feel that not only do you have the support of your loved ones when you are deployed forward, but you also have the support of your professional peers around the country. (. . .) It's clear given the vote at the APA convention that there is overwhelming support for psychologists who wear the uniform all around the world in defense of this nation.'

'James said his team works with the JDG [Joint Detention Group] to help ensure that Troopers have the knowledge and skills necessary to properly manage difficult detainees. By walking through the camps

and observing interactions between guards and detainees, the BSCT is able to make suggestions on how to further improve the communication process. In addition, the BSCT works with interrogators assigned to the Joint Intelligence Group by monitoring their interactions with detainees and providing feedback on how they can strengthen their repertoire-building techniques.'

'Although the BSCT team has gone through several iterations since its inception in summer 2002, James said its objectives remain the same – to read behavior, look for clues on how to improve communi- cation, and to teach techniques on how to manage uncooperative detainees.'

'"The BSCT does not have any command authority over the interrogators or the guards. However, we work with them on a consulting basis where they will come to me and ask my opinion." (. . .). James said his team educates Troopers on the importance of operational security and how sharing information with detain- ees, family members, and shipmates can be detrimental to the mission. (. . .). "We help them understand a lot of the detainee dynamics, and we give them examples of how a detainee can manipulate them, or how detainees can work to pit one guard against another." (. . .). "Many of these detainees have been here for five and six years now, and they have had the opportunity to hone their skills. We teach Troopers how to avoid some of the traps that detainees will try to lure them into" (. . .). Since the guards here are so well trained and motivated before they arrive in Guantanamo Bay, James said BSCT training serves as a refresher for skills already ingrained in many of these Troopers (. . .). "During my time here, I am proud to say that I have not seen a guard or interrogator abuse anyone in any shape or form" (. . .). "These young men and women go out of their way well beyond the call of duty to make sure that detainees are treated safely and humanely at all times" (. . .). "It has been a great mission, and I am happy to be here. It is great to be on the tip of the spear working with these young Troopers in the battle to defeat terrorism."'

Elements for a definition of psychological torture from the point of view of interrogators

- The basis for a **successful interrogation** is (1) the manipulation of physical and emotional strengths and weaknesses, and (2) designing interrogation plans tailored to these weaknesses with the support of medical and psychological personnel with the final purpose of (3) 'breaking' the subject (*'interrogate those who could not be broken'*). This included (4) the manipulation of all environmental factors known to attack the structure of a subject's identity.
- In the most complicated cases, psychologists or psychiatrists directed the interrogations. The **detainee's mind was the ultimate target** of the process.
- This is seen as a necessary and **professional task** in the best interests of the country. Psychology is the cornerstone of a successful interrogation of resistant detainees.

Summary and conclusions: a definition of psychological torture in the experience of harsh interrogators and torturers

Torture as the art of seeking limits

The analysis of the testimonies of interrogators and torturers is consistent with the testimony of the tortured discussed in the previous chapter. It shows that:

a. Certain procedures are considered 'routine' parts of a normal interrogation without any further connotations. Interrogators think:
   - Detainee nakedness is part of the normal process of strip-searching in prisons or police stations, so it is not considered abuse. The law authorises this and permits the

search of clothing and belongings and the inspection of body cavities. Nakedness is treated as a safety measure for the interrogators.

- Sight deprivation (using hoods, masks, etc.) is part of normal security measures for the interrogators and protects their right to safety and anonymity in a very complex and risky occupation.

- Sleep, food, drink and access to sanitary facilities are needs of the detainee, and thus secondary to the demands of the interrogation. This is an exceptional situation in which any needs outside of the interrogation should not be given priority.

Such treatment is seen as causing only minor discomfort, which is justifiable because of the severity of the context; only when treatment exceeds very obvious limits (e.g. several days without food or water) could it be considered a form of constraint or hypothetical torture.

This is so both from the point of view of Uruguayan torturers, and from those who conduct 'scientific' interrogations at Bagram, Abu Ghraib and Guantanamo. Such routinisation is what allowed the chief of the BSCT unit in Guantanamo to claim (as reported in his interview with Simmonds, 2008) that 'he has not seen [torture] nor does he believe it exists where he has worked'. This concept does not seem to have changed much in 40 years.

b. The success of the interrogation has nothing to do with the specific technique used (in Uruguay, the 'tacho', 'picana' or other methods; in the US, sleep deprivation, stress positions, humiliation, etc.) or the amount of physical or mental suffering inflicted on the prisoner, but rather in *finding the limit of physical and mental suffering that a particular detainee is capable of withstanding*. In one case (Uruguay), this limit is found via the interrogator's intuition, and in the other (Guantanamo) with the help of a medical team and a unit of behavioural scientists. In both cases, interrogators believe that torture occurs when the professional gratuitously breaches that limit. That is, he or she does not remain in the area of psychologically breaking the detainee, but crosses into in the area of breaking the detainee's mind.

From this perspective, there is no need to define a line marking the limit between coercive interrogation and torture, because that limit is specific to each detainee (physical condition, age, tolerance, etc.) and the expert (an Uruguayan torturer, or a psychologist–interrogator in Guantanamo) is in the best position to 'sense' when the detainee is close to this point. This implies that there is a 'safety zone' that can be identified by the interrogator between what we will refer to as the Breaking Point of Resistance to Cooperation and the Breaking Point of Physical or Psychological Damage.

c. For Uruguayan interrogators, torture occurs when the limit of 'unnecessary suffering' is breached and an ethical component of professionalism is broken. Corsetti expressed this when he distinguished between sessions at Bagram which – though extremely violent – sought information, and those that were uselessly sadistic, vengeful or humiliating, or when 'inhuman' acts were performed. However, he acknowledged that in the places where he worked, rapid habituation quickly built tolerance to inhumane actions and abuse was normalised as part of 'standard procedure', though the same person who accepted such practices would later recognise them as 'obvious torture'. To Corsetti, the best indicator of what 'inhuman' meant was when he saw people destroyed from a psychological point of view: infantilised, regressive. Torture, in this view, included anything exceeding the normal violence of a coercive interrogation of a source that would not cooperate otherwise, including gratuitously sadistic violence, 'inhuman' procedures driven by the interrogator's intuition, and procedures that permanently destroyed the person. James Miller, the expert from the BSCT, pointed to similar ideas: he believed that the key was to help the interrogator find each detainee's limit, and he trusted that behavioural psychologists intuitively knew what that limit was.

d.   Torture as an 'art'. One of the interrogators interviewed by Tróccoli said, *'I always wondered where the boundary is between what's considered torture and what isn't. Because I've seen people after three, four days of constant standing, of being on "plantón." Their feet were extremely swollen, and they could not go more than five days without water because they could get dangerously dehydrated'* (p. 63). In a private conversation, Professor Marcelo Viñar explained that he was continuously tortured for three months, and the torture stopped when he fainted and someone said, 'Leave him, because with these doctors you never know, he could die on us.'

In other words, the torturer practices something he or she considers an 'art' rather than a 'science' (as was the case in Uruguay), or a science that involves a lot of art (in the examples from US torturers). This means: (1) knowing the limits of the detainee in order to push the detainee to that limit by physical or psychological methods (2) repeatedly and as often as necessary, (3) and when, in the torturer's 'expert' opinion, the detainee has reached the breaking point, the torturer decides to stop the interrogation because he or she is sure that it is not possible to obtain any more information.

From the perspective of the interrogators, every detainee has a limit; finding that limit is a technical problem that requires several fundamental elements: one is (1) having the longest amount of time possible (ideally unlimited). (2) Any method is valid to push the person to the limit of his or her mental or physical resistance. All strategies to manipulate the physical environment, bodily functions or the detainee's ability to think or reason can be used. All instincts (e.g. survival, protection), and principles (e.g. consistency, dignity or ideological or identity-based principles) can be pushed to the limit. Everything depends on the imagination and experience of the interrogator. (3) A true professional knows when to stop a coercive interrogation. (4) Knowledge of various techniques is preferable, but ideally interrogators are especially excellent in one or two methods, and come to know the precise level of pain and suffering produced by these methods in order to bring detainees to their limits (in Uruguay, they sought the limits of physical resistance; US torturers sought the limits of psychological resistance). (5) The final, and fundamental, element involves establishing a 'trusting' relationship with the detainee by using terror, fear and the dependency that is created through the use of these techniques together with some minimal gestures of kindness. Success has much to do with seniority, communication skills and the general ability of the interrogator.

A person usually 'talks' long before reaching their limit of suffering (though not necessarily before reaching the limit of permanent damage). For some people this is not so, and the interrogator observes that he or she is still uncooperative or maintains active resistance. The professional challenge is, then, how to overcome such resistance.

These testimonies reveal the interrogators' belief that torture occurs when interrogators are:

1.   Unprofessional due to lack of qualification or negligence. This applies to interrogators (or their immediate superiors in the chain of command) who know that they have

reached the limits of what the detainee could tolerate, but, after failing to obtain the information they want (or are ordered to get), decide to cross those limits, thus disrespecting the 'tacit agreement' to act within a framework of 'no lethal harm' (in the case of Uruguay). Torture can also occur if inadequate techniques are applied to the person, unnecessarily disabling him or her as a source of actionable information (from in the US perspective).

2. Unprofessional due to exceeding the mandate. Those interrogators who go beyond the goal pursued (getting information) and act out of a desire for punishment (against specific individuals or against the detainee as a representative of an 'enemy' group) with purely punitive and vindictive motives (because of things that happened to the interrogator, to people close to him or her, or to the institution or group that the interrogator represents).

3. Unprofessional because of sadistic attitudes. Those who manifest pleasure or sadistic enjoyment in hurting others, in the use of absolute power or sexual gratification derived from such acts. They are an exception and are well known by their own comrades and often rejected (both in Uruguay and the United States).

From the point of view of the interrogation team, interrogators can be understood in the first case (because of arrogance, lack of sufficient preparation or misinterpretation of orders), and in the second case (because of stress, fear, the risk they assume and difficulties of the job). Interrogations in the third situation, however, must be discreetly relieved of duty because they are a problem for the institution. If their behaviour becomes known to the public, they should be judged for their actions, while taking into account the above attenuating circumstances. A sadistic interviewer gets poor quality information and 'ruins' the detainees if he or she is not under the control of a professional interviewer who can balance out the violence.

What is considered physical torture and what is considered psychological torture from the point of view of interrogators?

In reality, it is not possible to establish a catalog of torture techniques because *what defines the limits of torture from the perspective of the interrogator depends on the resistance of the specific individual being interrogated.* Some people will endure weeks of isolation, confrontation, physical pain or psychological coercion and pressure. And the interrogator will continue to escalate the abuse. Other detainees will break under the pressure of threats, at the first blow. Tróccoli claimed that after a few days of being 'softened up', a coffee and a friendly chat is usually enough to make someone talk. Marcelo Viñar revealed that a torturer confessed to him that after a few days of uncertainty and fear, all it took was tracing a pen across the skin of a hooded detainee for the detainee to talk, with no need for beatings. For Corsetti, shouting at a precise moment was enough for some prisoners (part of the 'Fear Up Harsh' method), or knowing how to handle the specific fears or feelings of humiliation detected in that particular detainee.

Implicit throughout the testimonies of torturers are two ideas that are antagonistic only in appearance: first, psychological torture does not exist, or is an irrelevant element (Uruguay), and second, that psychology is the core of the entire information-obtaining process (United States). In both cases, the interrogators express that physical and the psychological methods are absolutely intertwined and inseparable.

Both Tróccoli and the BSCTs understand interrogations as a confrontation between two human beings who are perfectly prepared and trained for the encounter. From this point of view, interrogations are seen as an intimate space of intellectual exchange (in the case of Uruguay), or a battle with rules and strategies of coercion that are pre-determined and studied before each session (in the case of the United States).

From interrogators' perspectives, speaking of psychological harm is almost always an exaggeration, and in many cases it is a media strategy launched by the detainees as part of their collusion with human rights groups. Years after he was relieved, Corsetti came to disagree with this idea. The responses of interrogators in the above interviews reveal that they all ultimately agree that just as in every battle, everyone involved in an interrogation is psychologically damaged – both the interrogator and the detainee.

Implications for a definition

Based on their testimonies, we propose that the following is how harsh interrogators and torturers would define torture: torture is a loaded term that should not be used to refer to these procedures. Coercive interrogation is the art of obtaining information from otherwise uncooperative sources (those who do not comply with normal interrogation procedures) by finding detainees' emotional and psychological weak points and pushing them to their limits and beyond, so that cooperating and providing information is their best – and only – choice. This is achieved by (1) creating a situation of strong unease and discomfort; (2) using specific psychological pressure techniques tailored to each detainee; and (3) conducting a skillful interrogation that helps uncover the information even against the active resistance of the subject. In short, coercive interrogation is a legitimate resource. Interrogation amounts to torture when the interrogator uses techniques that are 'inhuman'; acts unprofessionally; produces severe, permanent physical damage to the person; or when interrogations are conducted for purposes other than those mentioned above (e.g. sadistic pleasure, punishment or revenge).

This definition is summarised in the three interrogator mindsets outlined below.

Mindset 1 (see Figure 3.1) represents a cognitive map with two hypothetical conflicting selves in the centre: the self of the hero who is working on an essential and invaluable task, and the self who fights against remorse and shame – conscious that certain things should not be happening while attempting to resolve cognitive dissonance in the best possible way. The first self dominates during the years of professional work. The second, which was probably always present, may not emerge until years later, if at all.

In this exchange of conflicting selves, two topics are at the heart of defining the interrogator's task: (1) 'torture' is not seen as the appropriate word for their own behaviour because it is a term that should be reserved for unprofessional behaviour (such as punishment and humiliation); and (2) their actions (to obtain information) are necessary in wartime: those who condemn them are hypocritical.

In practice, the interrogator's task is conceptualised as knowing how to find the limit of each detainee. This is seen as an art. It requires skills acquired through experiential or vicarious training, and trial and error.

Mindset 2 (see Figure 3.2) further develops this idea. Interrogators believe that some aspects of an interrogation are unavoidable and part of standard procedures and routines:

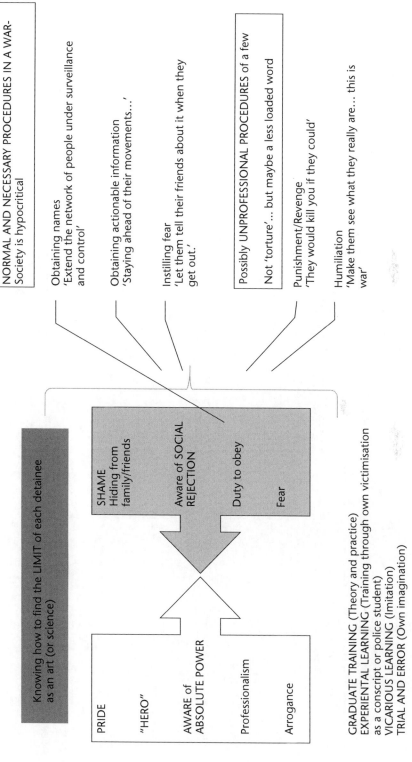

FIGURE 3.1 Mindsets of psychological torture based on torturer's accounts: the role of the wider context.

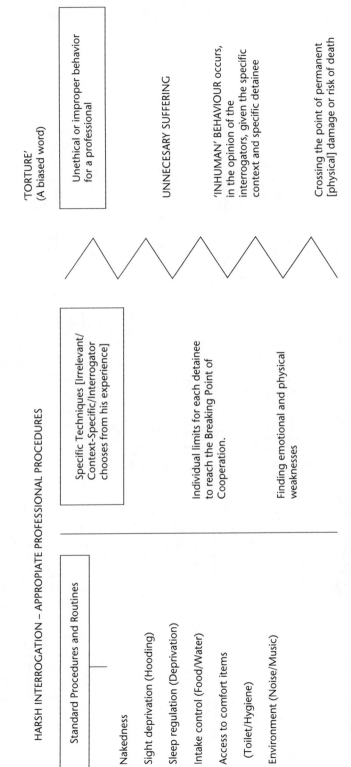

FIGURE 3.2 Difference between harsh interrogation and torture from the point of view of interrogators.

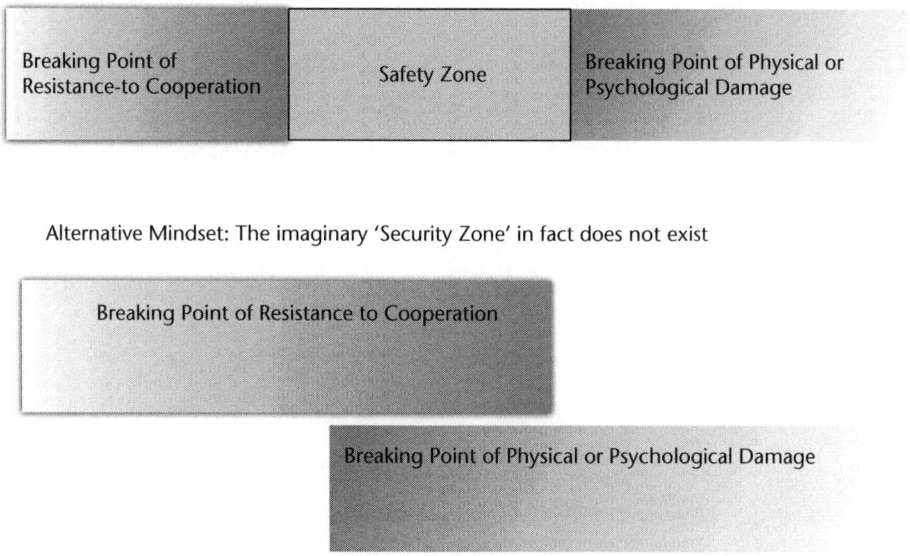

FIGURE 3.3 Working with the safety zone.

(1) those related to strip searches, sleep regulation, intake control and others. No one can pretend that being detained is a comfortable situation. The detainee must adapt to basic security measures and the interrogation timetable. This cannot be considered ill-treatment, although outside observers might wrongly think so. (2) Specific techniques. It is irrelevant which methods the interrogator chooses, as long as they help find the detainee's Breaking Point of Resistance to Cooperation without crossing the line of unethical or improper professional behaviour.

Mindset 3 (see Figure 3.3) continues to build on these ideas. The professional plays with two 'breaking points' (an art learned only through experience and a 'clinical eye'). The first one we shall call Breaking Resistance to Cooperation (when the detainee 'surrenders' and starts to 'confess'); the second is Breaking Psychic Equilibrium or Breaking the Mind (when the barrier of transient or reversible damage is crossed and permanent damage commences, which is unavoidable in wartime). The second breaking point may involve losing a source of information and eventually encountering legal problems. Both breaking points have blurry boundaries, and the interrogator sees him or herself as the judge who simultaneously controls life and death. The interrogator seeks to reach the point of Breaking Resistance to Cooperation without going so far as to (irreversibly) Break the Mind.

Notes

1 Tupa: The Tupamaros National Liberation Movement was a guerrilla group in Uruguay.
2 'Castrense', meaning part of the military in Spanish, has no direct English equivalent. It comes from the word 'castrar', or 'to castrate', in the sense of suppressing personal desires.
3 http://focoblanco.com.uy/2011/01/gilberto-vazquez-coronel-retirado-entrevista-de-maria-jose-frias-ultimas-noticias/
4 www.youtube.com/watch?v=sSu-FyajacMas retrieved in March 2015

5 *The Monster, Memories of an Interrogator.* Published in Spanish; there is no published English translation currently available.
6 In 2015 it was revealed that members of the APA held secret meetings with high-ranking officials from the US Army, in which they received instructions on how to justify the involvement of psychologists in the torture of prisoners (Soldz, S., Raymond N. and Reisner S. (2015). All the president's psychologists: The American Psychological Association's Secret Complicity with the White House and US Intelligence Community in Support of the CIA's "Enhanced" Interrogation Program. Available at https://s3.amazonaws.com/s3.documentcloud.org/documents/2069718/report.pdf).

SECTION 3
Current legal perspectives

4

PSYCHOLOGICAL TORTURE IN INTERNATIONAL LAW

An analysis of jurisprudence

A number of sentences have recognised 'psychological torture' as an entity in itself. The most cited in international case law is the case of Miguel Angel Estrella, an Argentinian pianist detained and tortured in Uruguay. In their comment, the Human Rights Committee (HRC) (1980)[1] quoted him describing psychological torture as occurring in:

> threats of torture or violence to relatives or friends, or of extradition to Argentina to be executed, in threats of making us witness the torture of friends, and in inducing in us a state of hallucination in which we thought we could see and hear things which were not real. In my own case, their point of concentration was my hands. For hours upon end, they put me through a mock amputation with an electric saw, telling me, 'We are going to do the same to you as Victor Jara.' Amongst the effects from which I suffered as a result were a loss of sensitivity in both arms and hands for eleven months, discomfort that persists in the right thumb, and severe pain in the knees. I reported the fact to a number of military medical officers in the barracks and in the 'Libertad' prison. (para 1.6)

This was considered torture by the HRC. Estrella was later imprisoned, where, the HRC writes,

> a policy of arbitrary sanctions is continually applied for the purpose of generating moments of hope followed by frustration. He alleges that the whole system at Libertad is aimed at destroying the detainees' physical and psychological balance, that detainees are continuously kept in a state of anxiety, uncertainty and tension and that they are not allowed to express any feeling of friendship or solidarity among themselves. (para 1.12)

The HRC goes on to quote Estrella's claim that 'many detainees are psychologically ill and that the present psychologist, Mr. Britos, is largely responsible for the policy of repression prevailing at Libertad prison' (HRC, 1980, para 1.12). The Committee considered the conditions of this imprisonment 'inhuman'. The Human Rights Committee stated that Mr. Estrella was subjected to inhuman conditions of detention and severe 'physical and psychological torture, including the threat that the author's hands would be cut off by an electric saw, in an effort to force him to admit subversive activities' (para 8.3).

Other Uruguayan cases were also found to include psychological torture. In *Cariboni v. Uruguay*, the HRC (1988) identified torture in detentions in which the victim was 'blindfolded, hooded, forced to sit up straight, day and night, for a week, in the presence of continuous screams apparently coming from others being tortured, and threatened with torture himself' (para 23). And in *Gilboa v. Uruguay* (HRC, 1985), cruel and degrading treatment was found in a case in which a victim 'had to remain naked in front of the guards and torturers. She was insulted and threatened with further acts of cruelty'. It seems that in order for the HRC to find that psychological torture has occurred, there must be a certain degree of severity in combination with other factors that increase the vulnerability of the victim.

European Court of Human Rights

As mentioned in Chapter 1, the European Court's decision in *Ireland v. UK* (1978) adopted restrictive criteria and considered the 'five techniques' to constitute CIDT but not torture. The votes of three judges deserve special mention because they argue that mental suffering by itself can amount to torture. Judge O'Donoghue of Ireland stated in his separate, dissenting opinion:

> One is not bound to regard torture as only present in a medieval dungeon where the appliances of rack and thumbscrew or similar devices were employed. Indeed, in the present-day world there can be little doubt that torture may be inflicted in the mental sphere. (. . .) Accordingly, I conclude that the combined use of the five techniques constituted a practice of inhuman treatment and torture in breach of Article 3. (ECHR, 1978b)

Judge Dimitrios Evrigenis of Greece expressed a similar opinion:

> The Court's interpretation in this case seems also to be directed to a conception of torture based on methods of inflicting suffering which have already been overtaken by the ingenuity of modern techniques of oppression. Torture no longer presupposes violence, a notion to which the judgment refers expressly and generically. Torture can be practiced – and indeed is practiced – by using subtle techniques developed in multidisciplinary laboratories that claim to be scientific. By means of new forms of suffering that have little in common with the physical pain caused by conventional torture it aims to bring about, even if only temporarily, the disintegration of an individual's personality, the shattering of his mental and psychological equilibrium and the crushing of his will. I should very much regret it if the definition of torture that emerges from the judgment could not cover these various forms of technologically sophisticated torture. Such an interpretation would overlook the current situation and the historical prospects in which the European Convention on Human Rights should be implemented (. . .). I am sure that the use of these [five] carefully chosen and measured techniques must have caused those who underwent them extremely intense physical, mental and psychological suffering, inevitably covered by even the strictest

definition of torture. The evidence which, despite a wall of absolute silence put up by the respondent Government, the Commission was able to gather about the short- or long-term psychiatric effects which the practice in question caused to the victims (paragraph 167 of the judgment) confirms this conclusion (pp. 125–126).

Finally, Judge Matscher of Austria expressed that 'the modern methods of torture which in their outward aspects differ markedly from the primitive, brutal methods employed in former times are well known. In this sense torture is in no way a higher degree of inhuman treatment' (pp. 124–125).

Subsequent sentences after the *Selmouni v. France* (1999) case clearly follow this line of thinking (Neziroglu, 2007). For instance, in *Elçi and Others v. Turkey* (ECHR, 2003a), the ECHR defines torture following clear psychological criteria as 'being in dire conditions of detention – cold, dark and damp, with inadequate bedding, food and sanitary facilities, being insulted, assaulted, stripped naked and hosed down with freezing cold water' (para 641). In *Ilascu and Others v. Moldova and Russia* (ECHR, 2004), the ECHR ruled, based on psychological criteria alone, that torture had occurred in a case that involved 'a long period of detention with the constant threat of execution of an unlawfully imposed death sentence, beatings, death threats and mock executions, denial of food, light, and medical assistance, isolation from other prisoners and the outside world' (paras 434–40). A second case, in the same sentence, also found that 'blows, denial of food, warmth, light and medical assistance and isolation from other prisoners . . . with the aim of punishing [the victim]' (paras 443–7) constituted torture.

In *Akkoç v. Turkey* (ECHR, 2000a), the Court also applied psychological criteria and ruled that torture had occurred because the female victim was blindfolded, stripped and forced to walk naked between officers who touched her and abused her verbally. Photographs were taken of her when she was naked. She was handcuffed to a door, forced to listen to the sounds of other people who were being ill-treated and was told that her children had been brought into detention and were being tortured. The ill-treatment included playing loud music and physical methods. The Court especially emphasised the threats concerning her children and stated that it caused intense fear and apprehension for the plaintiff. In *Aydin v. Turkey* (1997), a 17-year-old girl alleged that in addition to physical ill-treatment, a soldier had forcibly removed her clothes and raped her. The victim asserted that she suffered debasement and long-term psychological damage. The Commission accepted that the treatment was an attack on her physical and moral integrity. The Court also noted the deep psychological effects of rape, as well as mental anguish and physical and emotional suffering, and decided that considered together, the victim's experience amounted to torture.

The comprehensive jurisprudence of the Inter-American Court of Human Rights

The Inter-American Convention to Prevent and Punish Torture states that the degree of suffering is not a condition for torture, and explicitly says that torture also includes 'the use of methods upon a person intended to obliterate the personality of the victim or to diminish his physical or mental capacities, even if they do not cause physical pain or mental anguish' (see Chapter 1). The Inter-American Court of Human Rights has developed the most advanced jurisprudence in this regard.

In *Cantoral-Benavides v. Peru* (2000) the Court established that the ultimate purpose of physical and psychological torture is psychological, namely: 'wear[ing] down [the victim's] psychological resistance and forc[ing] him to incriminate himself or to confess to certain illegal activities' (para 104). In the sentence the court took into account the conditions of detention, pressure to self-incriminate and public exposure in humiliating conditions, and stated that 'according to international standards for protection, torture can be inflicted not only via physical violence, but also through acts that produce severe psychological or moral suffering in the victim' (para 100).

The position sustained in *Tibi v. Ecuador* (IACHR, 2004b, para 148) found that 'the aim of repetitive execution of these violent acts was to diminish [the] physical and mental abilities [of the victim] and annul his personality [and] for him to plead guilty of a crime'. The sentence also reaffirms the Court's previous criteria and states that these kinds of acts 'can be classified as physical and psychological torture'.

Fear and threats constituting torture in international law

Many sentences from the European and the Inter-American Courts, as well as communiqués from the Human Rights Committee, acknowledge that actions that produce overwhelming fear and terror on their own (including the threat of torture when perceived to be immediate and real) can be considered inhuman treatment or even torture. As mentioned above, the case of *Estrella v. Uruguay* (1980) in the HRC primarily dealt with *threats* of torture and mutilation as a form of psychological torture.

In 1982, the ECHR was faced with the case of two Scottish women, Mrs. Campbell and Mrs. Cosans, who denounced a public school for its use of corporal punishment as a disciplinary measure, arguing that their sons Gordon and Jeffrey were 'victims of torture'. The principal of the school had repeatedly threatened the two boys with the use of a tawse (a leather whip applied to the palms), causing them to be frightened. However, they were not actually beaten. The case was considered inadmissible, although the sentence established that 'provided it is sufficiently real and immediate, a mere threat of conduct . . . may itself be in conflict with that provision' (the Convention) (ECHR, 1982). This sentence has been repeatedly cited in other cases in which fear and threats were involved, and is seen as a precedent that threatening someone with torture might constitute inhuman treatment in certain circumstances. In subsequent sentences the same tribunal has decided that not only physical suffering, but also moral anguish, must be taken into account.

The Inter-American Court has been extremely sensitive to psychological factors in allegations of ill-treatment and torture, especially in their recommendations for reparations, and has repeatedly affirmed that fear and terror are sufficient elements to show that torture occurred. In *Maritza Urrutia v. Guatemala* (IACHR, 2003, para 92) the Court stated that 'the threat or real danger of subjecting a person to physical harm produces, under determined circumstances, such a degree of moral anguish that it may be considered "psychological torture"'. In *Baldeón García v. Peru* (2006) the Court found that 'threats and real danger of physical harm causes, in certain circumstances, such a degree of moral anguish that they may be considered psychological torture' (para 118).

Collective terror as a form of torture

Different sentences of the Inter-American Court of Human Rights (IACHR) in connection with collective cases (especially cases regarding massacres perpetrated in Guatemala and Colombia) have widely acknowledged the importance of psychological factors in general, and terror in particular. To cite just some of the many examples: in

Gómez-Paquiyauri Brothers v. Peru (IACHR, 2004a, para 118), the Court stated that in situations of massive human rights violations, 'the purpose of the systematic use of torture is to intimidate the population', bringing all such cases within the scope of the Convention. In the collective cases of *Villagran-Morales v. Guatemala* (IACHR, 1999), *19 Tradesmen v. Colombia* (IACHR, 2004c), the *Rochela Massacre v. Colombia* (IACHR, 2007) and others, the Inter-American Court repeatedly stated that witnessing the torture and execution of other people, and the desperation and realistic fear of being immediately tortured with extreme violence and executed, should be recognised in itself as torture. The Inter-American Court considered the 'intense psychological suffering of the survivors' to be a form of torture.

The International Criminal Court for former Yugoslavia (ICTY) had more restrictive criteria when judging the massacre perpetrated on April 16, 1993 in the small village of Ahmisi in central Bosnia. In a matter of hours, 116 inhabitants (including women and children) were killed and about 24 were wounded; 169 houses and two mosques were destroyed at the hands of the Bosnian-Croatian army (*Prosecutor v. Kupreškić and Others* (ICTY, 2000)). The sentence describes the events and how military and paramilitary members of the army went from house to house killing people:

> The primary purpose of the massacre was to expel the Muslims from the village, by killing many of them, by burning their houses and their livestock, and by illegally detaining and deporting the survivors to another area. The ultimate goal of these acts was to spread terror among the population so as to deter the members of that particular ethnic group from ever returning to their homes. (para 456)

The sentence quotes one of the witnesses as saying: 'I do not fear the shells and bombs that may fall on my house. (. . .). They do not ask for my name. I fear the foot soldiers who break into my house and kill and wound in a very personal way and commit atrocities in front of the children' (para 752). Five of the six men judged were convicted of persecution, murder, and cruel and inhuman treatment toward the victims (paras 784–785 and beyond). In the words of the sentence, 'the main target of these attacks was the very identity – the very humanity – of the victim' (para 752).

Rape as a special case of physical and psychological torture

There is strong case law to support considering rape as torture based on the psychological and psychosocial consequences for the victim.

The Inter-American Commission became the first international body to recognise rape as torture in *Raquel Martí de Mejía v. Peru* (IACHR, 1996). In a groundbreaking sentence, the Commission affirmed that rape is a method of psychological torture and detailed the unique psychological and psychosocial components it entails:

> the Commission considers that rape is a physical and mental abuse that is perpetrated as a result of an act of violence. (. . .) Rape is considered to be a method of psychological torture because its objective, in many cases, is not just to humiliate the victim but also her family or community.

Particularly in Peru,

rape would appear to be a weapon used to punish, intimidate and humiliate (. . .). The fact of being made the subject of abuse of this nature also causes a psychological trauma that results, on the one hand, from having been humiliated and victimised, and on the other, from suffering the condemnation of the members of their community if they report what has been done to them.

Raquel Mejía was a victim of rape, an act of violence that caused her 'physical and mental pain and suffering'. As she states in her testimony, after being raped she 'was in a state of shock, sitting there alone' in her room. She was in no hurry to file the appropriate complaint for fear of suffering 'public ostracism'. The Commission emphasised that

> the victims of sexual abuse do not report the matter because they feel humiliated. In addition, no woman wants to publicly announce that she has been raped. She does not know how her husband will react. [Moreover], the integrity of the family is at stake, the children might feel humiliated if they know what has happened to their mother.

The ICTY has clearly stated that it considers rape to be torture because it involves psychological suffering. Here we examine two particularly significant cases. In *Prosecutor v. Anto Furundžija* (ICTY, 1998a), the accused was a commander of a special unit of volunteers of the Croatian Defense Council (called the 'Jokers') who interrogated Bosnian Muslims in Nadioci (Bosnia and Herzegovina) in May 1993. He was convicted by the ICTY of torture and outrages upon personal dignity for the interrogation of a naked woman that included humiliation and attacks on human dignity. After the interrogation, the woman was raped in an adjacent room. The sentence stressed that the extreme humiliation and lack of action to stop the rape by men under his command was enough to qualify the offense as torture.[2]

In *Prosecutor v. Delic* (ICTY, 2008), part of the Čelebići Camp hearing,[3] the ICTY found Hazim Delic guilty of torture for the rape of Grozdana Cecez. She was personally interrogated by Delic and then taken to another room where three men, including Delic, raped her. The Court found that these rapes constituted torture. In the sentence, the Chamber emphasised that in considering whether rape gives rise to pain and suffering, one 'must not only look at the physical consequences, but also at the psychological and social consequences of rape' (para 486).

In Strasbourg in 1997, the ECHR issued its first sentence in which rape was recognised as torture, and emphasised psychological damage as one of the key elements of rape. In *Aydin v. Turkey* (1997), a 17-year-old woman was raped by a member of the Turkish security forces. Sukran Aydin had been taken into custody as part of a security operation to obtain information from her and other members of her family about supposed terrorist activities or sympathies. Her detention lasted three days, and during that time she was repeatedly beaten, sprayed with water while naked and raped while blindfolded. This was the first time that Aydin had had sexual intercourse and, following her experiences, she suffered long-term psychological sequelae. The rape was intended to cause humiliation and deliberate destruction of Aydin's identity as a member of a targeted ethnic group. The tribunal found that Article 3 of the European Convention was violated because of the purpose of both the physical and psychological suffering inflicted, and stated that either criteria would have been enough to rule that torture had occurred (McGlynn, 2009). The Court confirmed in *Dikme v. Turkey* (ECHR, 2000) that assaults causing mental suffering (including, but not limited to, rape) may fall within the scope of Article 3 of the European Convention, even if they do not leave medically certifiable physical or psychological scars.[4]

Sentences from the ICC, the International Criminal Tribunal for Rwanda and other courts define rape as torture based on the psychological suffering of the victim (Amnesty International, 2011; Office of the High Commisioner for Human Rights, 2010; Peel, 2004).

In sum, since the 1990s many international courts have found that rape clearly constitutes torture based on the physical, and especially on the psychological and psychosocial, impacts of rape on the victim.

Detention conditions

Where suffering is sufficiently severe and the purposive element is met, conditions of detention may also amount to CIDT or even torture. In *Prosecutor v. Krnojelac* (ICTY, 2002), the ICTY accused the Chief Commander of the KP Dom Detention Camp from April 1992 to August 1993 where non-Serb people were held, and found him guilty of committing inhuman treatment but *not* torture. The sentence found CIDT to have occurred because

> the non-Serb detainees were subjected to harrowing psychological abuse during their period of detention at the KP Dom. The detainees were exposed to the sounds of torture and beatings [of other detainees] over a period of months, in particular in June and July 1992. They became nervous and panicky as a result of these sounds, and they could not sleep at night. They could not identify the criteria for the selection for beatings, and they constantly feared that they would be the next to be selected. Some wrote farewell letters to their family fearing they would not survive. Some witnessed family members being taken out and heard them being subjected to severe beatings. (para 56)

The physical and psychological health of many non-Serb detainees deteriorated or was destroyed as a result of the living conditions at KP Dom. Surprisingly, in spite of such treatment and widespread starvation within the camp, the president of the Tribunal (a judge from the US) ruled that the detention conditions did *not* amount to torture because severe physical pain was not caused. He convicted the accused of torture based only on the beatings they inflicted on some prisoners, alleging that 'the infliction of severe pain in pursuance of a given prohibited purpose must be established beyond reasonable doubt and cannot be presumed' (para 188).

This extremely low criterion was not shared by any other judge in the ICTY. In the Čelebići Trial cited above, it was stated – contrary to the Krnojelac case – that severe pain was not considered a necessary requirement, and that *humiliation and outrages to dignity* amounted to torture (para 470). Another relevant ruling was the concurrent opinion of the judges of *Prosecutor v. Kvocka* (ICTY, 1998b), who asserted that the inhuman conditions at the Omarska Detention Camp (for which the accused was responsible) should be considered torture. These conditions included 'interrogating detainees and acts of humiliation and psychological abuses' and 'virtually all acts of intentionally inflicting physical and mental violence were committed with an intent to intimidate, humiliate, and discriminate against non-Serb detainees' (para 157).

The KP Dom and the Omarska sites were concentration camps. Many sentences have recognised torture in detention centres with far better conditions. In the most cited sentence, *Mukong v. Cameron* (HRC, 1991), the United Nations Human Rights Committee ruled that detention in an overcrowded cell with no sanitary conditions or access to food and water for extended periods of time amounted to CIDT. The ECHR has ruled that CIDT occurred in detention conditions with poor and often non-private sanitary facilities, vermin or insects in detention cells, overcrowding and lack of movement; see *Peers v. Greece* (ECHR, 2001b), and *Kalashnikov v. Russia* (ECHR, 2002).

Other conditions amounting to cruel or inhuman treatment based on psychological suffering

The ECHR has also recognised CIDT in situations not directly linked to detention or interrogation procedures. In 1978, in a pioneering and widely cited case, the Court ruled that the spanking of a 15-year-old boy by a policeman (in the presence of his father) constituted degrading treatment. They took into consideration the fact that he was treated as an object in the power of the authorities, as well as the boy's anguish while anticipating punishment. The Court found that Article 3 was violated and an attack to the person's dignity and physical integrity had occurred (ECHR, 1978c); this was considered 'degrading' but not 'inhuman' treatment. What the Court found important in this case was not the pain or cruelty in itself, but the *symbolic* (psychological) component of the punishment and its effects on the child. The Court used this same line of reasoning when it found that punishing a detainee for his private writings (which criticised the police and judicial system) with isolation, lack of food, light and hygiene, and the shaving of his head was 'degrading' (*Yankov v. Bulgaria* (ECHR, 2003b)).

In their reviews of the most significant cases in which the ECHR identified degrading or inhuman treatment, Neziroglu and Webster find that a wide range of situations were included (Neziroglu 2007; Webster 2011):

- Victims who watched the burning of their homes and most of their property by security forces. The sentence specifically mentioned the victims' feelings of upheaval and insecurity, and the inadequacy of precautions taken to secure their safety (*Bilgin v. Turkey*).
- A male victim who was strip-searched in the presence of a woman, and whose sexual organs and food were touched with others' bare hands (*Valasinas v. Lithuania*).
- The plaintiff's compulsory migration to another city, where he faced extreme hardship with almost no state assistance (*Akdivar and others v. Turkey*).
- Unwarranted physical force by state agents, with no serious physical injuries to the victim (*Barbu Anghelescu v. Romania*).
- Relatives of disappeared people who suffered deep anguish when they were denied information – or received false or distorted information – from state authorities (*Timurtas v. Turkey, Kurt v. Turkey, Taş v. Turkey, Cakici v. Turkey*, and others).
- The failure to receive adequate medical care in detention (*Nevmerzhitsky v. Ukraine*).

In most of these cases it was the particular context of each situation, the repetition or the duration in time, the characteristics of the claimant (age, sex and state of health of the individual) and the impact of the wrongdoing on the person, that caused the Court to find that Article 3 had been violated.

Considered together, the aforementioned rulings reveal that a true international system prohibiting all forms of torture is taking form. The Inter-American Court has played a decisive, leading role, and other international tribunals increasingly include a broader view of the concept of torture, one that seriously considers the importance of psychological suffering.

Indicators of psychological torture in international human rights law

Daniel Crampton (2013), working jointly with Nigel Rodley, proposed a set of indicators of psychological torture that stem from the analysis of sentences in international human rights law. As lawyers, the purpose of their review was not to make a comprehensive analysis of the phenomenon of psychological torture to derive measurement methods, but rather to propose broad criteria that signaled the presence of psychological torture to a tribunal. Such a legal approach assumes that cases create jurisprudence; Crampton deducted the underlying concept of psychological torture in international human rights law (IHRL) and proposed indicators for future cases by reviewing sentences that took into account the psychological component of torture. The results were highly convincing because most of the sentences cited drew their conclusions, at least in part, from psychologists and psychiatrists who spoke as expert witnesses. Additionally, the authors offered a brief review of psychological literature that complements their proposal.

The authors' approach is to treat circumstances as indicators 'signaling the potential existence of something, which in order to be proven may necessitate corroboration through other information' (p. 29). Indicators, they said, are not evidence (the opposite is also true: absence of the indicator does not mean there is no psychological torture). Though their review did not include all possible circumstances, it is worth examining the four indicators that they proposed:

1. **Actions that prevent the detainee from maintaining stable mental health.** They use the concept of homeostasis as proposed by Jacobs (2008): in detention the person has different sources of imbalance (sleep deprivation, changes of temperature, hunger, temporal disorientation, etc.) that are unavoidable. Usually the person reacts and tries to regain control using corporal and mental homeostatic mechanisms; Jacobs argued that psychological torture consists in preventing him or her from regaining such control. Crampton and Rodley found that it is irrelevant if the guards achieve this through stress positions, sleep deprivation, sensory over- or understimulation, or other methods, in that specific instance because the indicator focuses on the effect rather than the method. This approach helps distinguish cases in which such occurrences are incidental to detention and interrogation, from those in which destabilisation is intentionally inflicted.

2. A second indicator, in their proposal, is the **significance of the psychological maltreatment.** For instance, in the *Estrella v. Uruguay* case mentioned above, the authors suggested that the threat that the torturer would damage the hands of the victim had special relevance because he was a famous pianist. Rape in the context of ethnic cleansing clearly takes on additional, unique and severe psychological connotations. Torture that attacks the victim's identity fulfils the criterion of 'significance' as defined by Crampton and Rodley.

   Methods that target the core values and principles of the detainee qualify as provoking 'severe psychological suffering', and therefore as torture. These kinds of attacks can also affect the victim's ability to form and maintain relationships, the retention of some form of fundamental agency, and the maintenance of a somewhat safe future, which are also important elements to take into consideration.

3. **Design and planning of the torture.** The third indicator (closely connected and sometimes difficult to distinguish from the second) is when the torment was planned as a **personalised process.** This means that the torturer designed torture methods to have

a special impact on the person or group of persons. Because of the severity of suffering this causes, cases in which this indicator is present may more easily be found to violate the prohibition of torture. The criteria here relate to the *purposive* element of the conditions of detention and treatment.

4.   The fourth indicator is **the Next of Kin criteria** and relates to **the use of loved ones in the course of psychological torture**. The torturer uses affective bonds as a way to pressure the victim to act against his or her will. Cases of relatives of people detained or disappeared are of special importance.

The authors reviewed sentences in IHRL that found psychological aspects to be nuclear or adjunctive elements in the delimitation of torture; their proposal did not seek to be inclusive of all cases of psychological torture but rather to direct attention towards certain circumstances that could act as useful indicators.

Conclusion: psychological torture slowly gains recognition

Since the *Estrella v. Uruguay* case (1980) there has been increasing jurisprudence from the Human Rights Committee of United Nations, the European Court of Human Rights, and especially the Inter-American Court, that supports the concept of psychological torture as a defined entity. In particular, many sentences from these three bodies acknowledge that actions that produce overwhelming fear and terror on their own (including the threat of torture when perceived to be immediate and real) can be considered inhuman treatment or even torture. The Inter-American Court has been extremely sensitive and has repeatedly affirmed that fear and terror are sufficient elements to show that torture occurred. The Inter-American Court has also ruled that torture occurred in cases of massacres and collective terror, in situations where the victim was forced to witness the torture and execution of other persons, or in which they experienced the terror of anticipating impending torture. In addition, there is strong case law from the Inter-American, the former Yugoslavian, the Rwandan, and the European Courts to consider rape as a form of physical and psychological torture. The sentences are based on the stigma, intense psychological suffering and often long-lasting fear suffered by the victim; the use of rape as an ethnic attack; and the humiliation that rape inflicts not only upon the person but also, in certain cultures, the impact on his or her family and community. Conditions of detention may also amount to CIDT or torture if suffering is sufficiently severe and the purposive element is met, according to different sentences from the ICTY and the ECHR. All courts have found a wide range of situations in which degrading or inhuman treatment was identified based on psychological elements alone. Considered together, all of the above reveals that the concept of psychological torture is slowly gaining recognition in case law. To that end, the Inter-American Court has played a leading role in broadening the concept of torture and building a more modern concept in which psychological suffering has a decisive place.

Notes

1   Miguel Angel Estrella v. Uruguay, Communication No. 74/1980, U.N. Doc. Supp. No. 40 (A/38/40) at 150 (1983). The HRC found a violation of Article 7 of the International Covenant on Civil and Political Rights, and ruled that he was subjected to torture during the first days of his detention in 1977.

2 For a detailed analysis see C.G. Marzen, 'The Furundzija Judgment and its Continued Vitality in International Law,' Creighton Law Review, 2010, Vol. 43, pp. 505–27.
3 The Čelebići prison camp, which was operational from May to December 1992, was used to detain 700 Bosnian Serb prisoners during the Bosnian war. Detainees at the camp were subjected to torture, sexual assaults and beatings that sometimes resulted in death. The Čelebići Trial lasted 20 months, with the presentation of 691 exhibits, 122 witnesses and 28,000 pages of court transcripts. It was the first case decided using the legal principle of superior responsibility; the defendant was found guilty based on responsibility for acts of persons who committed crimes while under his command or authority.
4 *Dikme v. Turkey* (2000) ECHR 366, para 80.

5

FROM DIGNITY TO IDENTITY: HUMILIATION AS A PARADIGM OF THE DIFFERENCES BETWEEN LEGAL AND MENTAL HEALTH PERSPECTIVES

The authorities have also used animals to sexually abuse detainees. One male former political prisoner describes his interrogation: '. . . I was then made to assume a position similar to the "Semigwa dance," while pins were placed underneath my elbows and knees. I was stripped of all my clothes. There were four guards in the police station, all drunk, and they found a large dog, which they made mount my back. They then used their hands to arouse the dog's penis and placed it against my anus. The dog ran away, as such a thing is not natural, but the authorities brought it back and continued with the abuse. This did not last long, but it was deeply humiliating . . . I can forgive my torturers for everything but the sexual abuse. No religion permits such an act. It has destroyed my self-esteem, my dignity. (Assistance Association for Political Prisioners, Burma, The Darkness We See, 2005, p. 55)

Dignity is often cited as the foundation of all human rights. We saw in Chapters 2 and 3 that humiliation was one of the most relevant elements in survivor's subjective experiences of torture, but this clearly contrasts with case law regarding the status of humiliation in jurisprudence. For many victims and experts in forensic mental health, attacks against dignity *are* torture (in the symbolic sense of the term), but in the legal world, humiliation ranks lowest on the torture scale because it does not involve physical pain. Nevertheless, it is increasingly common for sentences to question this assumption by ruling that the judicial system cannot evaluate psychological torture using the same parameters as physical torture, and finding that pain should not be the ultimate foundation for defining the illegality of an act.

This is a controversial issue that is paradigmatic of other contexts in which legal and mental health perspectives collide, and criteria among different legal institutions diverge. This chapter delves into the definition of the concept of dignity and related emotions, and explores what happens when both legal and psychological points of view are taken into account.

Torture as an attack on human dignity

The Universal Declaration of Human Rights (UDHR) is built upon the concept of *human dignity*, and in its first substantive article it states that 'all human beings are born free and equal in dignity and rights'. This equality of dignity is a cornerstone of the human rights regime.

A similar position is held in the UN charter and other key documents in international human rights law (IHRL).

For example, the African Charter on Human and People's Rights states in Article 5: 'Every individual shall have the right to the respect of the dignity inherent in a human being and to the recognition of his legal status. All forms of exploitation and degradation of man, particularly slavery, slave trade, torture, cruel, inhuman or degrading punishment and treatment shall be prohibited" (Organization of African Unity, 1981). The Article affirms a direct relationship between dignity and torture.

Absolute prohibition of torture is based, for most jurists, on the essential and inherent value of human dignity (Castresana, 2012). Dignity is one of the hallmarks of democratic societies, and is the very basis of the modern social contract. The classical argument would say that to accept the practice of torture (even in its less severe CIDT modalities), or partially remove its ban, threatens the collapse of our entire social and legal system. In a democratic society, human dignity cannot be negotiated.

The juridical world employs a definition of the concept of dignity that assumes it is a metaphysical property inherent to each and every human being. However, not all authors agree with this assumption. The concept of dignity has a long tradition in the fields of philosophy, neurobiology and psychology.

The concept of dignity: a positive definition

Dignity as a social concept. Contrary to legal perspectives on dignity, philosophy considers dignity not as an immanent quality of human beings, but rather as a relational one (Baumann, 2007; Luban, 2009; McClelland, 2011). In other words, dignity is not a 'given', inherent to human beings, something acquired at birth. Instead, it is relational in the sense that it has to do with the considerations of others in our social group. It represents the basic human need for **recognition** and **respect** from others. Respect is one of the principle human rights in traditional societies, and providing respect is inherent to the relationships among humans in all cultures.

The concept of **reciprocity** includes both of these components. In traditional societies, reciprocity is the inherent moral obligation to respond with material elements (e.g. wealth) and immaterial elements (e.g. recognition, respect, work or time) within the group to maintain cohesion and social balance. The very act of recognising and respecting the other as an individual with dignity implies that they deserve such recognition and respect. McClelland (2011) states that reciprocity has ethological grounds and it is probably linked to the neural circuits of empathy and gratitude.

Stoecker (2011) adds that respect should be understood not only in relation to others, but also to the self. He believes that a key aspect of dignity is **self-respect**: how one *relates to oneself*. Self-respect is an evaluative attitude we have towards our individual dignity and the way we care about our identities. A related concept is **self-worth** (Kuch, 2011): the way one *values oneself*. Self-worth is related to **pride**. Both dignity and pride are key components of **identity**, and are part of the perception we have of ourselves.

In short, dignity is a relational, not an immanent, property that requires receiving adequate recognition and respect from others and from oneself.

When it relates to status within a group, dignity is closely connected with **honour**, the need for other members of the group to act according to the status that one thinks one has or deserves within the group. The concept of honour reflects the need to maintain rank and status in a group.

TABLE 5.1 Dignity in modern and traditional societies

	Dignity: The way we are valued and treated by others	
	Modern societies	Traditional societies
Basis	Non-discrimination	Honor
Threatened value	The right to be treated as equal to other members of society, to have equal recognition and respect. Worth and status is based on being considered human with full rights without suffering any prejudices.	The right to be treated as different from other members of society according to a perceived quality of worthiness and respectability that affects both the social standing and the self-evaluation of an individual and the groups to which he or she belongs (e.g. family, nation). Worth and status are based on respect for tradition and moral codes.
Related quality	Being equal is important.	Being different is important.

Dignity and social institutions. As a relational property, Düwell (2011) writes that dignity also includes the relationship of the subject to collective entities (such as the state or social and political institutions). Each citizen is also entitled to recognition and respect, and deserves to be treated with dignity.

The relationship between dignity and human rights. A corollary of seeing dignity as a relational property is that it is not an inherent characteristic of human beings (that is, one *has* dignity simply because one is a human being), but that dignity is a *possibility, and depends on one's relationships with others.* As Pollman (2011) points out, dignity is a precarious *possibility* that needs to be protected in the definition of human rights. It is precisely because *human beings do not have equal human dignity* from the start that they all have equal human rights, including the right to dignity.

The negative side: humiliation and related concepts

With these definitions of dignity in mind, we turn to the negative side of human relations to define **humiliation** as acting towards others in a way that deprives them of the social respect and recognition entailed in the idea of dignity (see Figure 5.1). Hartling and Lucheta (1999) define humiliation as 'the internal experience associated with being, or perceiving oneself as being, unjustly degraded, ridiculed, or put down – in particular, when one's identity has been demeaned or devalued' (p. 7).

Shame is another important emotion to define when studying psychological torture. Feelings of shame are related to the negative opinions (whether real or perceived) others have about oneself and one's actions. The difference between humiliation and shame is that humiliation is the feeling associated with being deprived of dignity by others. It occurs in a specific context and is therefore directly relational and interactive. Someone *humiliates* us.

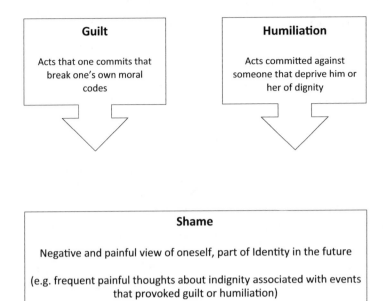

FIGURE 5.1 Guilt, humiliation and shame as related to torture.

Shame is a long-lasting, self-focused negative feeling of being unworthy and without dignity in the eyes of others. Shame is a negative component of self and identity. Not all humiliation leads to shame.

There are different pathways to shame. One is humiliation. The other is **guilt**. While humiliation involves something being done to us, guilt is the negative feeling associated with our own acts when they are considered to violate our moral principles:

A relational definition of torture

If we assume that torture is a violation of human dignity and we accept that dignity is relational, it's clear that what makes torture a violation of dignity is the relationship between perpetrator and victim that torture establishes. The relationship itself is where dignity is attacked through the absolute lack of recognition and respect as a human being.

Maier (2011) proposed a relational definition of torture: 'torture is the infliction of physical and mental suffering on a person by another person (action-level conditions) with the intention to enforce the perpetrator's will on the victim (attitudinal conditions) performed in a social setting in which [the] perpetrator can fully determine everything that happens while the victim is completely helpless and fully exposed (contextual conditions)' (p. 105).

While the UNCAT states that what defines torture is severe suffering, motivation (confession, self-incrimination, punishment, etc.) and context (inflicted by a representative of the state), the relational definition proposed based on the philosophical concept of dignity emphasises the absolute power of the perpetrator and the absolute powerlessness of the victim.

Even within proponents of a relational definition, there is debate among philosophers about which properties in the relationship are central to the definition of torture. For instance,

William Tunning (1978) writes that torture is defined by the act that provokes the suffering of the victim; the motivation of the perpetrator only adds to the determination of responsibility. This means that there could be involuntary torture. Sussman (2005) assumes that what makes torture essentially wrong is the fact that the tortured person is forced to play an active role in his or her own suffering. The person is not only forced to act against his or her will, but also to betray him or herself. Henry Shue (1978) holds that what makes torture morally wrong is the fact that the victim is put in a situation of helplessness where he or she is completely exposed to the torturer.

Absolute control

Manfred Nowak writes: 'In my opinion, it is the experience of absolute powerlessness which creates the feeling among the victims of certain gross human rights violations to have lost their dignity and humanity' (Nowak and McArthur, 2006; Nowak, 2011). As a 'spectacle of power', torture is not just about inflicting pain, but also a demonstration in inflicting pain (Scarry, 1985). Humiliation is related to the absolute loss of one's power. In torture there is not only an absence of recognition as a human being, but also a total stripping of agency: that is its humiliating core (Kuch, 2011).

During torture, the victim is deprived of his or her human condition, and forced to sink back into his or her own bodily existence as a piece of flesh, an animal, a number. The victim is excluded from humankind. This is why a small gift (a cigarette, a smile, a touch) or even the simple act of being listened to, can have incredible power – not because of the value of the gift in itself or the two minutes a cigarette can last, but because of the impact of recognising the victim as a member of the human community, someone who deserves to be given a cigarette or listened to for a while.

The efficacy of humiliation in torture settings

Short-term efficacy: producing dependency

When someone debases us, it generates rage. But there is also a tendency to question ourselves, to try to adapt and search for acceptance. We all have a need to feel acceptance and belonging within the group – if possible, the group of the majority. There is a cognitive tendency to adopt the position of those in power, who are perceived as successful or brilliant. Humiliation is very effective in changing opinions and creating dependency because it takes advantage of the unconscious tendency to resolve cognitive dissonance by adjusting one's reasoning to fit one's new reality.

Respect is one of the most basic assumptions in normal human relationships. Everyone knows they should 'treat others as they would like to be treated', and that they should expect approximately the same in return. We are taught to respect others, especially certain groups, like teachers and elders. Showing absolute and radical disrespect without any logic breaks this human assumption and confuses and blocks the person. The victim reasons, often in an unconscious manner, *What can I do to make the world logical again and be recognised (and treated) as a human being?* This is, for some people, the basis for dependency. There is a tendency to question oneself instead of questioning the other, to attribute rejection to one's own characteristics or errors, and to try to gain affection by changing in the ways that the other (e.g. the torturer) desires.

Long-term efficacy: producing shame and breaking identity

Torture creates environments that foster permanent feelings of humiliation, with the ultimate goal of creating shame, breaking self-worth, destroying willpower and obtaining submission. Torture is not always about pain, as we saw in Chapters 1 and 2. Torture techniques are acts that include humiliation and guilt as their keystones, with the ultimate aim of producing permanent feelings of shame. The psychological pain will then be inscripted on the body and mind and integrated into the identity of the victim.

The origins of shame are not self-evident. What we do know is that shame involves the unconscious mind, relates present experiences to the past and calls upon hidden norms and values introjected in infancy (as well as previous shaming experiences in one's life). Shame occurs when we imagine how others might be judging us, and includes our perception of their invisible gaze.

In terms of resilience, dignity can be seen by the survivor as a vulnerability which stems from the need for recognition, as discussed above (Kuch, 2011). The subjective perception of oneself (identity) might be seen by the victim as immune to the torturer's opinion; victims can distance themselves psychologically from the situation to the point that they no longer recognise themselves as being a part of what is happening. Though this challenges attempts at humiliation, it is by no means easy and requires a great deal of control. Shame, however, is beyond the victim's control. The experience has connected with relevant elements of his or her previous psychological life and his or her identity is shattered. The experience, both difficult to communicate and profoundly shaming, can alienate the person from others for the rest of his or her life; it affects self-worth and the capacity to interact with and relate to others.

From theory to data: clinical and research-based studies

Humiliation has long-lasting and devastating effects when used in the context of torture; some even deem its effects to be more important than the effects of physical torture (Vorbrüggen and Baer, 2007). When perpetrators destroy the victim's ability to experience his or her own identity, humiliation takes hold. In Abu Ghraib, prison guards threatened male detainees with rape, forced detainees into certain sexually explicit poses and told them to masturbate (Ahuja, 2011; Jaffer and Singh, 2006). The prisoners had no other option than to comply with acts that caused them deep shame, and which aimed to impose submission and destroy their personal integrity, self-esteem and pride. In these situations, prisoners are forced to feel deep shame and degradation, especially when they come from a culture in which public nudity and sexuality are highly stigmatised. On a clinical level this damages a person deeply, making recuperation a long process for survivors. Although bodily scars may heal, mental scars remain forever: the trauma of this type of dehumanisation can last a lifetime.

Alexa Koenig (2013) provides empirical support for the role of humiliation and shame in torture. In her doctoral dissertation, she interviewed 78 ex-detainees in Guantanamo from around the world. She conducted semi-structured interviews asking, among other questions, 'What was the worst in Gitmo?' Then she ran a software-aided content analysis of the answers. Koenig found that 'the worst' treatment for many prisoners was not physical cruelty, as is often assumed, but treatment that could be categorised as 'inhuman and/or degrading'. She was surprised to find that almost ten per cent of interviewees described being naked in front of soldiers as among the very worst treatment at Guantanamo (worse than beatings, worse than isolation). In almost every interview, forced nudity was mentioned as a particularly upsetting practice.

'You are forcefully being naked in front of twenty, thirty people, standing there, watching you, you are naked, and that is the worst feeling ever, you, you feel like you want to die, but you can't die, and they . . . you feel like nothing, you just feel so lost, so small, so terrible' (p. 27). One man from an Arab country cited being naked around other men in the showers as his worst experience at Guantanamo: 'Maybe for Europeans and Westerners it's fine, but for us Arabs and Muslims, we are not used to that . . . it just did not cross my mind before, that I will be in such a situation' (p. 32). He explained that such practices constitute 'complete humiliation . . . to our religion, traditions, and things that are related to our ideology and values' (p. 32). This contrasts with comments from an interviewee from Western Europe who stated, 'the physical abuse was probably the worst. Physical, you know. Because obviously if someone humiliates you, he's not really causing you pain except for, you know, you're just embarrassed, you know. But when someone's like, if I had a choice to be humiliated or beaten up to hell, then I rather get humiliated rather than getting beaten to death. That's the option I would choose, you know' (p. 32). Thus, while disrespect for gender norms, including nudity in front of the opposite sex, may have been experienced as relatively benign by many European or American male victims, such practices may have been experienced as torture by those prisoners who adhered to particularly stringent rules about such interactions.

Koenig introduces three important ideas from these results:

a.   She quotes Waldron (2008) to point out that a key issue in law is ascertaining whether each prohibition is perpetrator- or victim-oriented. 'Inhuman', for example, has typically been perceived by courts as a term used to describe acts of the perpetrator, not the experiences of the victim. A proper definition of humiliation requires standards of reference. But what are these standards? Koenig asks, 'On what basis is the judgment made as to whether specific acts are cruel, inhuman or degrading? Judges' gut instincts?' (p. 4). In order to fully understand the wrong done, the idea of 'humiliation' must include the experiences and subjective perspectives of the victims themselves.

This brings us to the question of whether to approach humiliation and degrading treatment as an objective or subjective experience from a legal point of view. In a legal study on the jurisprudence of the ECHR, Webster (2011) analyses the question of the significance of the individual experience of degradation for judges. She begins by arguing that what one woman might find degrading another might find mildly irritating, or even gratifying. If a person *feels* degraded, does this imply that she has *been* degraded? Or if she does not feel degraded, does this imply that she has not been degraded? Is degradation dependent on context?

Given the large number of sentences in which degradation was *not* taken into account, two things about the European Court become evident: first, it uses different criteria than those employed by the ICTY in the Furundžija and Kvocka cases, and second, it finds that the subjective emotional experience of humiliation per se is not sufficient as the sole basis for a conviction. Webster's analysis reveals that the *feeling* of humiliation appears to be implicit in the plaint: if the person claims to have been humiliated, it is assumed he or she *feels* humiliated. The European Court analyses whether or not the person has *strong and objective reasons* to feel humiliated given the particular context and circumstances. This could hypothetically include cases in which a person does not *feel* degraded but the Court considers he or she has been subjected to a *degrading treatment* (unnecessary nakedness in detention is one example). In other words, sentencing is an interpretive process in which judges generally apply their own social and moral standards, traditions, and political convictions when ruling whether a person has been degraded (see Webster, 2011).

b. It is important to think about the cultural contexts of each case when assessing proposed standards for identifying inhuman and degrading treatment and torture. Judges from one culture may face difficulties perceiving the psychological impacts of CIDT and torture on victims from a different cultural background.

The central conclusion of Koenig's work is that cruel, inhuman and degrading treatment should be treated as three independent categories, and the qualification of a wrongdoing in each category must be based on the *victim's point of view*. In this regard, forensic psychological assessments are essential to understanding the subjective effects of torture.

c. *Attacks on dignity* and *humiliation* could be considered the 'worst' form of torture by a group of victims despite the fact that they do not entail pain or physical injury. The associated psychological damage to victims may be permanent. The idea that this is the 'lightest' possible form of wrongdoing on a progressive scale that begins with humiliation, intensifies to ill-treatment and finally reaches torture (see Chapter 1) makes no sense for a mental health forensic expert. Humiliation per se can fully amount to torture.

Conclusion: dignity and humiliation from legal and mental health perspectives

Because the definition of torture in the Convention undervalues psychological factors, we can conclude that it was heavily influenced by at least three factors: the European and American origins of most of its members; the kind of torture that prevailed in the 1980s (mainly physical and pain-based); and culturally biased preconceptions about what factors were most relevant to the victim when judging whether torture has occurred.

The classical definition introduced in 1969 by the ECHR named three levels of severity of ill-treatment (torture, cruel and inhuman treatment and degrading treatment), and was based on the idea that humiliation was a minor form of aggression not on par with torture. This definition ignored the authority's intentions, as seen in the *Ireland v. UK* case. The idea was successfully incorporated into the criteria adopted by most subsequent cases – with some exceptions. The ECHR explicitly named humiliation as a relevant factor in the Selmouni sentence (see Chapter 1). In that case, the plaintiff, an Arab man detained and accused by the French police for drug dealing, was forced to kneel down in front of a young woman and was insulted. One police officer then showed him his sexual organs, vexing him, and finally urinated on him. The police also threatened him with a blowtorch and then a syringe. The Court defined this kind of treatment as 'humiliating' and found that it constituted torture when combined with other elements. Being naked has been considered degrading treatment in itself, and CIDT if combined with other elements (see *Akkoç v. Turkey*, and *Aydin v. Turkey*, among others, in Chapter 4).

One example of a broad view of 'humiliation' is the *Hurtado v. Switzerland* case examined by the European Commission. In addition to physical injuries, the police action caused the plaintiff to defecate in his trousers. The police did not provide him with clean clothes on the day of his arrest. The Commission concluded that this was humiliating and debasing for the complainant.

Former UN Special Rapporteur Manfred Nowak considers that, in practice, any use of physical or mental force with the purpose of humiliation constitutes degrading treatment, and any infliction of severe pain or suffering for a specific purpose (as specified in the Convention) constitutes torture (Nowak and McArthur, 2006). But this perspective is misleading. According to our findings, and the results of both philosophical and mental health studies, humiliation is more complex, and may be employed in two distinct ways: humiliation as an end in itself (degrading treatment) and humiliation as a means to torture (which should be qualified as torture). The testimonies from Abu Ghraib show that humiliation was not an end in itself but a means to provoke helplessness and submissive and compliant behaviours, which is at the core of a definition of torture. This was achieved by dehumanising the victim through inducing feelings of shame and guilt and provoking intense mental suffering. As we have seen, experiences such as these have long-lasting, often permanent, effects. An important question remains: will tribunals agree to consider this emotional suffering a form of torture?

6

THE PERPETRATOR'S PSYCHOLOGICAL AND LEGAL RATIONALE: MOTIVATION, INTENTION AND PURPOSE

In Chapter 1 we outlined the three key problems in the UNCAT definition of torture: assessment of the 'severity of suffering', determination of 'intentionality' and 'motivational criteria'.

In order for an act to be considered torture, it must be inflicted for certain specific intentional *purposes* (obtaining a confession, intimidation, coercion . . .). This opens broad subjectivity in the definition that we will analyse here.

The debate on motives, intentions and purposes straddles psychology and law.

1. Motivation refers to the reasons for people's actions, desires and needs. A motive is what prompts the person to act in a certain way. Motivations may be internal (i.e. ideological commitment, feeling proud of oneself, expecting others admiration . . .) or external (monetary reward, promotion, avoiding punishment). Motivation is related to human needs: hunger is the motivation for eating. Safety, a sense of belonging, or exploring feelings of power may be motivations for becoming a torturer. This is the field that most interests social and cognitive psychologists and the avenue to the prevention of torture.

2. Intention refers to one's willingness to perform an act. An act is intentional when the person has committed it on purpose and the person consciously factored in its consequences. While intentionality is not relevant as a concept in psychology, it is a key notion in the legal world.

3. Purpose is the pursued goal, the effects (either physical, emotional, cognitive or behavioural) that are expected to produce in the victim. Purpose, as related to accountability, is also highly relevant in the legal world.

   A person can torture someone to feel proud (motivation), receive specific training and thus carefully plan the torture (intentionality) and aim to humiliate the opponent and exact a confession (purpose).

TABLE 6.1 Motivation, intention and purpose in evil-doing

MOTIVATION (Why)	INTENTION (Knowing and willing)	PURPOSE (What for)
INNER MOTIVATION Psychology of good and evil Psychology of moral decisions [Studied by Cognitive Psychology]	INTENTIONALITY [Studied by Law]	PURPOSE [Formulated in Laws and Penal Code]
EXTERNAL MOTIVATION Social psychology of good and evil Social psychology of moral decisions [Studied by Social Psychology]		

Intentionality: knowingness and willingness

Definition: wilful misconduct and criteria indicating intent

While psychology takes an interest in the underlying reasons for a person to perpetrate evil, generally speaking, law ignores these aspects and in determining liability or a sentence it considers them irrelevant. Law has, however, made great strides in outlining and nuancing the degree of a person's direct responsibility in committing a crime in order to make distinctions between the punishment for those who do so irresponsibly or involuntarily without aiming to, and those who, fully aware that their actions constituted a crime deliberately intended to do so (wilful misconduct). If additionally the person prepared the crime and its outcome, one speaks of malice aforethought.

Therefore, we speak of intentionality or wilful misconduct as the degree of wilfulness or lack thereof, with which a person engages in a conduct that perpetrates evil. In the definition of torture, this criterion is considered essential and stands as the barrier that most jurists consider separates torture and ill-treatment (degrees 1 and 2) from cruel and degrading treatment (degree 3).[1]

Two factors must concur in order for there to be wilful misconduct. The person committing the crime of ill-treatment or torture must:

1. Know that the fact he or she is committing it constitutes that crime (an intellectual element). This obviously does not mean that the person must necessarily have detailed knowledge of the articles in the law, but merely have a profane, rough knowledge of the fact that what he or she is doing may constitute a crime.
2. Intend to commit it (an element of volition), which means there is a *decision* on the part of the person to commit the crime.

This implies that, hypothetically, a civil servant who obeys instructions regarding the treatment of a detainee who *honestly believes it does not constitute ill-treatment or torture* could potentially be exonerated by a judicial official. In other words, when in Chapter 3 the Uruguayan torturers stated that keeping a prisoner permanently naked and hooded was a standard security procedure and that restricting feeding was inevitable to suit the police station's working hours, the person judging the case would need to decide whether this is indeed so and it could potentially be considered that it is merely degrading treatment, that is, unintentional. The very testimony of Damian Corsetti and others shows that this is a complex terrain in that there is a tendency for civil servants in charge of detainees to normalise any practice, as brutal as it may be, and consider it 'standard treatment'. This is a murky and certainly tautological criterion, and ruling a person *guilty* cannot be left to merely evaluating *intentionality* of committing acts of ill-treatment or torture. From that standpoint, a civil servant committing torture could be acquitted if the judge interprets that he did not know what he was doing or honestly believed that he was not wrong in his actions. The issue is whether intentionality should be interpreted vis-à-vis the facts, i.e. whether or not severe suffering was inflicted, or vis-à-vis how the facts are defined by law.

Degrees of intentionality

Generally speaking, justice has examined these aspects in great detail, although in the field of torture they are generally unexplored. Though they vary depending on the jurisdiction, most legal systems normally determine several degrees of intentionality.

Degree 1. The person wants to do exactly what he or she did. A civil servant repeatedly uses ill-treatment on a detainee and consciously endeavours to do so causing grave psychological consequences. This would be considered *direct wilful misconduct*.

Degree 2. The person does not want to do so, but it is a necessary result. For instance, a civil servant who detains a person violently decides to also detain those accompanying him, who witnessed the fact. He does not subject them to ill-treatment directly, but the detention has a terrorising effect that particularly impacts one of them. This would be considered *indirect wilful misconduct*.

Degree 3. The person does not want to do so, but it is a plausible result. The person decides to take that risk and goes ahead. For instance, a police officer who does not intend to cause grave harm in a detainee but who, knowing that the person has epilepsy, intimidates him with several shots of a Taser gun to confess and causes status epilepticus. Legally speaking, this would be considered *potential wilful misconduct*.

Degree 4. The person does not want to cause harm and does not believe it can occur, but unforeseen events cause it nonetheless. For instance, a civil servant watches a detainee who he intends to treat properly. During the detention, unknowingly, he gives the detainee water that is unsuitable for consumption and causes an illness triggering very severe suffering and permanent intestinal consequences. The prison physician evaluates a detainee considering that his complaints of depression and suicidal ideas are unfounded and that he is simulating them to obtain benefits and therefore decides to uphold solitary confinement in his cell. That same day the prisoner hangs himself by his sheet. Legally speaking, both of these cases could be dealt with as *imprudence* resulting in injury and *imprudence* resulting in death.

In the vast majority of juridical literature, the tendency is to consider crimes of torture, as set forth in the United Nations definition, to be 'wilful crimes', in other words, crimes committed with a clear intention. Of the previously mentioned examples, the vast majority of the time we would be looking at direct wilful misconduct, i.e. clear intention to commit a crime. There would be situations where the perpetrators may not have sought to directly injure and used ostensibly less harmful methods, but the harm was done nonetheless. In other words, the risk was present but not avoided (potential wilful misconduct). In either case there would be intentionality and therefore liability for the crime.[2]

A legal analysis of whether intentionality is really a prerequisite for torture

Intentionality is explicitly mentioned in the United Nations Convention against Torture definition as well as the definitions used by the European Court of Human Rights and the

Inter-American Court of Human Rights (ICHR) and is generally used to separate torture and inhuman treatment from degrading treatment (see Chapter 1).

In the Inter-American Court case *Bueno Alves vs. Argentina*[3] the judgement states that '*The evidence attached to the record of the case proves that the acts committed were deliberately inflicted upon the victim and not the result of negligent conduct, an accident or force majeure*' without defining how this conclusion was reached. It does, however, rule out an act of negligence constituting torture. In 2009, in an individual vote on the *González and others v. México* case, also known as the 'Campo Algodonero' case,[4] and in what is actually the only mention in the Court's jurisprudence addressing intentionality per se, the magistrate states that 'intentionally refers to the subject's awareness that s/he is performing an act that will cause suffering or a feeling of humiliation and aim refers to the reasons for which it was performed: domination, discrimination, sadism, bringing about a given action or lack thereof on the part of the victim or others. Both of these elements may exist in cruel, inhuman or degrading treatment. Therefore, what actually distinguishes torture from other treatment, in the terms formulated by the Court in the Bueno Alves case, is the severity of physical or mental suffering.' The European Court of Human Rights and the Inter-American Court agree on the substance, that is, the true line of demarcation is the degree of suffering. However, the great step forward taken by the Inter-American Court with respect to the ECHR comes when considering that when the state is clearly involved, there is no need to know the 'intentionality' of the perpetrator, as this is sometimes impossible to elucidate. In the *Velásquez Rodríguez v. Honduras* cases (later cited in other judgments) it was specified that: '*Violations of the Convention cannot be founded upon rules that take psychological factors into account in establishing individual culpability. For the purposes of analysis, the intent or motivation of the agent who has violated the rights recognized by the Convention is irrelevant – the violation can be established even if the identity of the individual perpetrator is unknown. What is decisive is whether a violation of the rights recognized by the Convention has occurred with the support or the acquiescence of the government, or whether the state has allowed the act to take place without taking measures to prevent it or to punish those responsible.*'[5]

The irrelevance of intentionality with respect to degrading treatment is manifest, for instance, in the ECHR case *Cyprus v. Turkey*[6] where the Court sustained that the denounced State was responsible for having violated article 3 of the European Convention[7] for not providing water, food and medical assistance to several persons who were detained in the custody of Turkish troops. This was considered 'degrading treatment', irrespective of the intention behind the treatment, and this was upheld in subsequent judgments: *Whether the purpose of the treatment was to humiliate or debase the victim is a factor to be taken into account, the absence of any such purpose cannot conclusively rule out a finding of violation of Article 3.*[8] The United Nations Human Rights Committee made a pronouncement along these same lines[9] in a case against Finland.

Can the intentionality of wilful misconduct in a perpetrator be determined?

There are certain criteria for wilful misconduct than can be used to help determine a perpetrator's intentionality and establish acts to ill-treatment or torture.

Intent may be established through (a) indicators related to the overall context of detention and (b) indicators related to the specific interaction between victim and alleged perpetrator. We have set both of these indicators out on a scale (see Chapter 6 and Appendix 7) not for the purpose of scoring, but rather to put forward a qualitative auxiliary tool for judicial officials to establish perpetrator intentionality.

Overall context indicators include:

1. A situation and context analysis determining whether the sum of elements a person is subject to during detention constitutes a *torturing environment* (see Chapter 18 and the Torturing Environment Scale in Appendix 5).
2. A *plan*, understood as a planned sequence of events where each event is designed to cause a specific result or final consequence (malice aforethought).
3. A *pattern*, reflected by repeated actions against the same person, or against different people (that shows similarity in procedures indicating both a behavioural pattern and a strategy or plan).
4. *Plausibility*, based on the history and social roles of the persons involved.

Specific interaction indicators include:

1. Analysis of the pattern of interaction between the victim and alleged perpetrator, drawing on the idea that torture is relational, related to absolute suppression of the victim's will.
2. Continuation of the actions despite the observation of the damage inflicted and the victim's defencelessness (overkill or viciousness).
3. Knowledge of the final result. The judge evaluates whether the person would have acted the same way or acted otherwise if s/he were absolutely certain of the final result. Wilful misconduct would be established in those that would have continued 'no matter what'.
4. Whether or not the person was informed of the potential consequences that the acts performed could have and decided to continue. An associated variant involves evaluating the extent to which the person, knowing what could happen, did not take any measure to prevent it. Certain jurists address the individual's representation of risk. In other words, they judge whether s/he had a realistic expectation of the likelihood that his/her actions would lead to negative consequences or knowingly thought that these negative consequences to be irrelevant. Or, the extent to which the person thought that harm could occur, accepted it as a necessary evil but believed it would be a lesser evil than what finally occurred. Attempts to establish this place one in an unacceptably speculative terrain.
5. An evaluation of feelings or attitudes. Here, certain judges would appraise the coldness or indifference of the accused party vis-à-vis the facts or their results. This is generally a subjective criterion and most jurists usually reject it as a way of establishing wilful misconduct.
6. Proof or indicators of planning or premeditation of specific *sub-judice* action, i.e. the result was 'sought'.
7. Indications of wilfulness:
    *   Intensity of the aggression or severity of the techniques used
    *   Reiteration, prolongation over time
    *   Persistence despite the perception of the adverse consequences in the detainee

It is important to highlight two aspects of this checklist:

*   Its objective is to determine the alleged perpetrator's degree of intentionality and not whether or not torture occurred. When discussing the 'severity' of suffering criterion and the demarcation between torture and ill-treatment, the intensity of pain and reiteration criteria used by certain judges are highly questionable. Research indicates that psychological torture with no extreme physical pain may be far more devastating then purely physical torture (Başoğlu, 2009). An ostensibly harmless act, such as keeping a (male) detainee permanently nude before a woman, can be the most devastating type of torture

for those from a given cultural background, such as orthodox Muslim, where nudity is a taboo as of childhood (Koenig, 2013). Here the criteria of reiteration, viciousness and intensity are used as indicators of *intentionality*. Intentionality may or may not be associated with torture.

While some criteria are very weak and subjective and can never sustain intentionality by themselves (i.e. plausibility), others are stronger and provide a solid basis for building an opinion (i.e. overkill or reiteration).

TABLE 6.2 Intentionality Assessment Checklist

		Intentionality Assessment Checklist (IAC)			
			1. Consistent **2. Not present, unknown or irrelevant** **3. Inconsistent**		
		OVERALL INDICATORS			
1	Torturing Environment	Situation and context analysis. The overall detention context constitutes a torturing environment.			
2	Plan – Malice	There is a plan, understood as a planned sequence of events designed to produce a specific result or consequence (malice aforethought).			
3	Pattern or strategy	There is a similar pattern of strategies, behaviours or procedures taken against different people.			
		SPECIFIC INDICATORS			
4	Social role	The social role of the people involved is compatible with an alleged intentionality			
5	Interaction	Absolute suppression of the victim's will. The victim is maintained at the mercy of others.			
6	Intensity	The aggression is particularly intensive or the techniques used are particularly grave.			
7	Prolongation or reiteration	The acts are prolonged or repeated over time, particularly when this occurs even when perceiving the consequences.			
8	Viciousness	Harm is sustained despite the victim's defencelessness.			
9	Attitude (the end justifies the means)	The person knows the adverse consequences but would have continued even in the knowledge that the final result would be the worst possible.			
10	Objective	A functionality or clear objective can be established.			

Purpose

Another issue is purpose. According to the UNCAT definition, torture occurs: '*For such purposes as obtaining from him or a third person information or a confession, punishing him for an act he or a third person has committed or is suspected of having committed, or intimidating or coercing him or a third person, or for any reason based on discrimination of any kind.*'

While the Convention cites four purposes, it does so as an example ('such as') and ends with "*any reason based on discrimination of any kind*". The Inter-American Convention adds a masterful criterion:"*Torture shall also be understood to be the use of methods upon a person intended to obliterate the personality of the victim or to diminish his physical or mental capacities, even if they do not cause physical pain or mental anguish.*'

UN Special Rapporteurs have established doctrine by using this broader understanding of purpose to consider situations that do not clearly fall under the four examples provided by the Convention as torture. In fact, Manfred Nowak put forward that, in the event of powerlessness, provided all other criteria are fulfilled, any infliction of severe pain or suffering constitutes torture (Nowak and McArthur, 2006). In health care settings, when analysing whether suffering inflicted can be considered torture, Juan Méndez states, 'There is a general acceptance that the stated purposes explicitly named in Article 1 of CAT, for which pain and suffering amounting to torture is inflicted, are only of an indicative nature and not exhaustive. At the same time, only purposes which have "something in common with the purposes expressly listed" are sufficient'[10] (Center for Human Rights and Humanitarian Law, 2014, p. 17). In short, the trend is for torture rapporteurs to consider new definitions and contexts in addition to those explicitly cited as examples in the Convention definition.

Likewise, debate on purpose also deals with who the perpetrator is. The Convention clearly establishes that torture is committed by States, either directly or by those representing them. It textually states,'. . . *when such pain or suffering is inflicted by or at the instigation of or with the consent or acquiescence of a public official or other person acting in an official capacity*'. What must be established here are the limitations of the terms 'instigation, consent and acquiescence' and how they can be proven. While this is straightforward in certain cases where policing or law and order functions are subcontracted to private security companies, in others where para-State or paramilitary forces are involved in certain countries, it is more complex. While they require the State's support or consent in order to train, bear arms, circulate freely and commit intimidating or violent acts, this is something that the State will always refuse to accredit and that will generate public controversy. Qualifying massacres perpetrated by the so-called *Autodefensas Unidas de Colombia* (AUC) and other Columbian paramilitary groups as acts of torture stands as an example. This problem can sometimes be circumvented by invoking States' obligation to protect their citizens from torture and by asserting that any type of armed group may commit torture[11] and particularly those who control territory and act as shadow or de facto States. Even broader is the position of those who consider that criminal groups, mafias or other types of strictly private actors should be included based on the grounds that the State is negligent in its duty to protect.[12,13] Lastly, domestic legislation permitting, there are certain judgments that have considered violence between private parties, particularly cases of gender violence, to be torture.[14]

Subjectivity in establishing purpose

The purpose of torture is often self-evident. And determining the exact purpose of the perpetrator is relevant, which is why a single slap can be considered ill-treatment, provided the actor is associated with the State. But at the same time, this determination opens the door to the judge's discretion, and often, in State-perpetrated torture, the judge decides based on his/her personal ideological position, weighing the individual's right to not be tortured against society's right to national security. The elucidation of the accused party's purpose can thus become the gateway for some judges to avoid prosecuting public officials who mistreated or tortured detainees. The judges might argue that there is a distinction between dishonest, oppressive or corrupt purposes (e.g. a sadistic police officer who causes unnecessary suffering), and reasonable purposes (e.g. use of the minimum force required to perform security tasks). But, as explained in Chapter 3, this rationale mirrors the torturer's in that it focuses on the *justification* not of the purpose itself (i.e. extracting information), the nature of the acts (i.e. inflicting harm) or the impact on the victim, but of the rightness of the purpose. This parallelism between the reasoning of certain torturers and certain judges calls into question the ethics in decision-making processes regarding whether or not torture has occurred, and it highlights the need for a definition as free as possible from this type of ideological biases.

The idea of wilful misconduct is therefore useful here. When there is conscious or intentional disregard for the rights or safety of others and the individual is doing what he or she intends to do, when it is neither accidental or due to negligence, there is ill-treatment or torture. This was suggested in the *Peers v. Greece* case mentioned above and in the separate opinion of Judge Fitzmaurice in *Ireland v. UK* where he accepts sheer sadism as the motive, excluding any other end.[15]

Motivation

While they are the least relevant aspect for the jurist, motivations are probably the aspect that most interests mental health professionals and that has generated the greatest amount of research.

Knowing what motivates a person's perpetrating evil-doing is a field that has been researched since psychology has attained the status of a science and there are some excellent reviews (i.e. Bandura, 1999; Miller, 2004; Staub, 2003). An entire book could be written on this subject alone.

In Chapter 3 we reviewed the definition of psychological torture through the testimonies of harsh interrogators and torturers, thereby deriving their cognitive map of torture (see Figures 3.1 to 3.3) and showing how contextual and cognitive factors interact in the structuring of a torturer's motivations. What can be seen at first glance are the justifications given to defend the use of torture as ethically legitimate and necessary in order to transfer the responsibility over to the victim. This is what we could call *self-justification*, which Bandura describes very well through his moral disengagement (Bandura, 2002) model.

Yet this is only a part of the tremendously complex weave of threads that configure the moral decision to inflict harm on another person. Figure 6.1 offers a comprehensive view of only some of the most significant threads. It also attempts to place concepts and constructs from various different and sometimes overlapping fields together. For instance, ideology, part of a vision of the world and a value system, is determined by a personality's cognitive structure and to a large extent depends on one's moral motivations. The elements in the figure are not separate compartments but rather models of thought on moral conduct, or, so to speak different lamps shining against the same background in different tones.

Moral decisions: preliminary considerations on ethics, morality and justice

Jurists, philosophers, psychiatrists, social psychologists, anthropologists and educators alike take an interest in the relationship between ethics, morality, justice and feelings of shame or guilt.

One of the most interesting avenues is perhaps what has been called experimental philosophy, which analyses Plato's and Aristotle's classical theories of virtuosity in the light of social psychology to conclude, generally speaking, that classical philosophy had a static notion of morality as a virtue towards which human beings tended (Anthony, 2008; Doris, 2010). This dovetails with psychology based on *static personality traits* that most contemporary authors distance themselves from (Doris, 2010). As of the 1980s, social psychology began to take the opposite view, considering environment to be the main if not the only factor behind a person's moral decisions and that therefore any person could become a potentially resistant (Sagarin, Cialdini, Rice and Serna, 2002) hero or a perpetrator (Zimbardo, 2004). For certain authors, Zimbardo and Milgram's studies meant the end of Aristotle and classical ethics involving moral traits. In defence of Aristotle, it can be said that over the last few years, neuropsychology has progressed towards a definition of certain value-traits that may have a universal neuro-biological basis (currently, empathy and compassion are cited based on so-called 'mirror neurons' (Rizzolatti and Craighero, 2004)). This interesting development could potentially prove whether or not biological differences, understood vis-à-vis one's disposition, exist.[16]

Moral habits versus moral decisions

Certain preliminary distinctions may be useful in understanding the rationale behind moral decisions. First, most day-to-day decisions do not require deliberate thought, but can rather be ascribed to what could be called 'moral habits' understood as intuitive principles acquired through one's upbringing. These habits are 'automated'. Not stealing, giving up one's seat on the bus for a pregnant woman or standing on a queue for the cinema do not require complex thought processes. Minor, everyday guilt or shame has to do with these micro-transgressions and the importance one attaches to 'doing the right thing' as a central element in his or her structure of identity and in the way s/he perceives him or herself (Blasi, 1980; Caton et al., 2005). A distinction must be made between this and critical judgments or complex dilemmas for which there is no available 'automated' response. These highly complex dilemmas, i.e. regarding abortion, euthanasia, letting a person die so that others can be saved . . . in other words legitimacy versus legality dilemmas, are not included in the normal childhood *scripts*. In much evil-doing, the perpetrator has undergone *habituation* where, through a process of training or de-sensitisation, a person goes, sometimes in an extremely brief period of time, from making a moral decision to harm others to acquiring a mere habit.

Factors that explain the decision to cause harm to others

A host of factors explain, to varying degrees, a human being's moral decisions in the light of experimental psychology and help understand how, from a strictly psychological standpoint, there can be perpetrators. Without aiming to be exhaustive, the following stands as a synopsis.

Identity. Every person has an image of him or herself as related to the others and the surrounding world. Several elements of this identity are considered particularly pertinent, considered by the person to be at the 'core' of his or her manner of being. These elements belong to the narrative the person builds around him or herself, which could be called a moral identity.

Moral identity. From an ethical standpoint, it is relevant to examine the extent to which *morality and the congruity between moral ideas and actions* is important in a given person's identity structure. In other words, to what extent is it important for the person to *act correctly morally* speaking? Does the person conceive him/herself and the world around him/her in moral terms? These questions include both the degree to which the persons are concerned and devote energy to being and being perceived as moral persons and the extent to which they tend to code the social world in terms of morals (Syed et al., 2006). For those who consider morals to be a key value in their identity, other values, such as safety or comfort or convenience, may take a back seat and these persons may have heroic attitudes. Conversely, persons for whom success, triumph or personal promotion are more important may tend to act as perpetrators.

Attaching a great deal of importance to morality does not necessarily mean having a high concept of oneself as a moral being. That is to say, one thing is how much importance is attached to morals and another is the perception one has of him/herself, or one's 'moral self-regard' which is there to defend (Bushman and Baumeister, 1998). As we will see, many perpetrators, for instance, need to prove they conduct themselves with high morals and devote a great deal of energy to seek reasons to back these ideas, or develop cognitive mechanisms to morally distance themselves from their victims or their actions (Bandura, 1999). This need for moral self-regard explains many curious situations. For instance, in a series of experiments on moral decisions, participants who displayed highly ethical attitudes generated admiration among neutral observers and hostility and rejection among those that had done the experiment before and had not taken the same type of decisions (Syed et al., 2006). Rather than being seen as examples, they were perceived as threats to their moral self-regard (this is known as 'moral resentment') and this led to a reassertion of these participants of their perpetration in a quest to bolster their own moral self-regard.

Several studies have analysed the relationship between self-esteem, narcissism and moral decision-making. Perhaps the most highly elaborated model is *Threatened Egotism* (Bushman BJ and Baumeister RJ, 1998) based on a distinction between narcissism, understood as the intensity of affective and libidinal feelings towards oneself and self-esteem, understood as the positive or negative conception a person has of him or herself. In Threatened Egotism experimental models, people must take decisions after having had their self-esteem attacked (or not) by, for instance, receiving very negative comments about themselves in a previous task. Those with a high profile of Threatened Egotism (high narcissism and low, fragile self-esteem) perform aggressive actions when they feel called into question (Crocker, Lee and Park, 2004). What is important is not the task, but rather one's value in that task. In the scope of affection, relationships and so forth, life is perceived to be a zero sum game, i.e. what someone else gains, I lose. Negative information, not verified with others, is accumulated, meaning that that other person becomes larger vis-à-vis oneself, etc. In his autobiography Rudolf Hoss, an Auschwitz commander who sent tens of thousands of persons to the gas chambers, remembers memories from his childhood and describes, for instance, several situations where he extols himself with plethoric self-esteem which is then called into question by minimal threats to his ego (such as a letter of reprobation from a superior), where his melancholic, violent and disproportionate (Hoss, 2009) response fell upon his subordinates and victims.

Structure of norms and moral system. We govern ourselves as human beings by a generally succinct and concrete set of rules for functioning that we acquire in our infancy either directly or vicariously from examples and advice from adults that act as our moral references. These automatic moral responses are acquired, to a large extent, by what we hear and see when we are children. If in one's childhood someone attached an extremely great weight to group loyalty (i.e. the family), the approval of a group leader as opposed to other members of the group (perhaps an overbearing father as opposed to one's brothers) or an upbringing where what is important are the results irrespective of the efforts (high grades at any price), then we can find the value structure of a perpetrator (loyalty, competition, efficiency). This structure of norms, together with other factors, may make an adult, in the right context, place effectively obeying orders seamlessly over the respect for the physical integrity and life of others. Nothing enables us to assume that there is a universal hierarchy of norms and that the respect for physical integrity of another person will be the first universal rule. Undoubtedly, when perpetrating evil-doing, the attachment bonds in one's childhood and the ability to provide empathy and care for others that one has acquired play a very significant role in the moral decisions to perpetrate certain acts as an adult (Roccato, 2008).

A **cognitive personality structure** encompasses a complex weave of dimensions that determine one's predisposition to respond to certain patterns or schemes in certain standard situations. Millon's theory of *personality styles* assumes that a person's psychological structure is configured into motivational goals, cognitive modes and interpersonal behaviour and puts forward various dimensions for each.

Various levels can be established in the hierarchy of perpetrating evil-doing: the ideo-logue or person who provides the justifying structure, the primary executor who plans and issues orders and often avoids contact with the victims, the material executor who obeys these orders to different degrees of acquiescence shielded by the duty to obey and delegation of responsibility and lastly the passive observer or bystander who prefers not to know what is occurring or if s/he knows, does not interfere. Models of personality style may be what best explain why different people may place themselves at any given one of these four levels in the hierarchy of perpetrating evil-doing. The variables involved include leaning towards optimism versus pessimism, independence versus acquiescence, submission versus resistance, internal versus external causal attributions (locus of control), etc.

But we still lack specific models to accurate predict who will be an ideologue, primary executor, secondary executor, or bystander.

Worldview and belief system. When taking the moral decision to cause harm, a person will also be influenced by his or her belief system, understood as the view the person has of his or her surrounding world. Of the many facets in a belief system, safety, predictability and controllability are particularly pertinent here. Goodness, communicability, trust and so forth are encompassed by one's vision of human beings (Pérez-Sales, 2006; Pérez-Sales et al., 2012). A person who perceives the world to be unsafe and threatening and where rigid control must be exercised over one's surroundings is more likely to be a perpetrator, as is someone who perceives human beings to be intrinsically selfish, evil, dangerous, or to be mistrusted.

In any event, subconscious perception will influence automatic moral decision-making (a boy in an underprivileged neighbourhood who believes he will be attacked will kill before thinking), while reflexive, conscious perception will influence deliberative decision-making (a soldier who is forced to remain in a firing squad thinks about whether s/he should actually withdraw). But the distinction between the two is not always clear.

Ideology and a person's position in the group straddle belief systems and cognitive structures. They are more sociological or group cognitive structures particularly pertinent to the field of moral decisions to perpetrate harm, such as authoritarianism (Altemeyer, 2006), social dominance (Pratto, Sidanius, Stallworth and Malle, 1994), the belief in a just world (Lerner, 1980) or the degree to which one tends to justify the social and economic system in which one lives (Jost, Krochik, Gaucher and Hennes, 2009). Common sense points to those with a higher tendency towards authoritarianism, social dominance, and justification of the system and with a low tendency to believe in a just world being most inclined to decide to perpetrate harm, though there are not experimental studies that back this hypothesis.

Lastly, one can speak of a **value structure** for which there are also several different paradigms and models that have been linked to moral decision-making (Cohrs, Maes, Moschner and Kielmann, 2007, 2010).

Staub, one of the main researchers in altruistic conduct and explanatory models of bystanders, hinges his model around **moral motives** (Staub, 1999, 2003) which are comparable to the notion of beliefs. Moral motives, then, are a person's set of needs. From a highly functionalist point of view, Staub speaks of human beings' having basic needs, and of their moral decisions, i.e. to help or perpetrate harm, being made based on the degree to which they fulfil these needs. This idea is very similar to Aristotle's Nichomachean ethics. Staub considers eight basic needs that human beings have in the field of morality: safety (preventing physical and psychological harm, having food and shelter . . .), the feeling of efficiency and control (being able to protect ourselves and others, achieving our goals in life . . .), maintaining positive connections with those around us, living in a world with meaning (meaningfulness) which he relates to religion and ideology, having a positive identity (a positive perception of who one is, what one does and who one wants to be), perceiving oneself as independent and autonomous, having long-term satisfaction (what we would call a feeling of fulfilment) and having a feeling of connection (connection with nature, the universe, superior forces, values of altruism or social change . . .). If we turn around Staub's model, we can hypothesise that those who would perpetrate harm are those who would gain safety, efficiency and control over their environment and would positively connect with relevant others who share their view of the world. By causing harm, they would also give meaning and purpose to their lives (i.e. through their religion or ideology . . .), feel fulfilled and transcend.

It could be argued that a human being's basic needs are these or others, but what Staub puts forward through a host of experimental studies is that decisions are not a product of deliberation or moral reasoning, but rather a functional product of one's basic needs (Staub, 2003).

These interwoven factors, i.e. one's beliefs regarding the world, identity, and value system and the structure of one's motivations or attitudes, serve as a matrix for fighting the battle of moral decision-making.

The moral decision to perpetrate harm

Deliberative moral decisions (those that are not automatic and require thought) are considered in the form of **dilemmas**, that is to say situations where one can consciously choose between different actions.

Here again, a host of virtually unpredictable factors may intervene in decision-making, including:

1. So-called **moral level of development**. Kohlberg's well known theory (Kohlberg, Levine and Hewer, 1983) which is not the only one but undeniably serves as the major point of reference, affords several decision-making archetypes that conjugate these factors. Kohlberg speaks of those with pre-conventional morals as those who guide their decisions by expectations of immediate punishment or reward, like a child who acts to avoid punishment or gain favour from his or her parents without aiming to understand

the rationale behind the rules. On Kohlberg's second level, persons act according conventional morals where they understand the rules and the reasons for punishment or reward and inserted them into a sort of catalogue of 'right' and 'wrong'. What is important is abiding by law and order, without considering questioning it. The last category includes those who act with post-conventional morals, that is, those who put their own system of ethics first, as opposed to rules or norms, in order to guide them in their decisions. These people place legitimacy before legality and are able to question the status quo. In experimental studies, most of the population adopts conventional moral systems, i.e. their moral is the same as the law. This helps understand the rationale behind much of the evil-doing perpetrated under dictatorial regimes where laws or certain states of emergency allow for, incite or harbour the abuse of power, arbitrary detention, ill-treatment or the death penalty.

2. **Feelings**. Decisions about our actions take place against an emotional backdrop. It is not the same to act or decide in a state of sadness as it is in a state of happiness, in a state of anger or in a state of shame. This has to do not only with the timing and specific circumstances in which the decision is made, but also a person's disposition as we saw previously (for instance, those with a greater tendency to perceive the world as a threatening place will make decisions driven be the core emotion of fear). Anderson goes beyond this and speaks of **internal states** and considers one's level of arousal, cognition and affect (Anderson and Carnegey, 2004).[17] In Chapter 2, Carlos Liscano detailed the emotional fight between perpetrator and victim, and in Chapter 3 Damian Corsetti explained the interrogators' intense feelings of fear, rage and pride and their relationship with heavy alcohol and marihuana use.

3. **Costs and benefits**. Any decision entails some kind of cost-benefit analysis (Staub, 2003), be it more or less elaborate. The costs and benefits or moral actions are not limited to one personal sphere but extend to others close to oneself or to society at large (the concept of a higher good). This, for instance, is behind creating climates of impunity where perpetrators are convinced that no matter what they do, nothing will happen to them, or environments that incentivise perpetration of harm. A torturer always requires a torturing system. Ultimately, violence is perpetuated when it achieves its objective, i.e. domination, survival, attention, and so forth.

4. **Critical evaluation**. After many moral decisions, there is a dilemma between what one *should* do and what one actually *wants* to do. There are several mechanisms that enable a person to change his or her moral decision based on what s/he *should* do and turn it into what s/he *wants* to do. Several authors have worked on moral justifications for anti-ethical decisions. Perhaps Bandura's writings have provided the most comprehensive view (Bandura, Barbaranelli, Caprara and Pastorelli, 1996; Bandura, 1999, 2002) due to their clarity and congruousness. Bandura refers to *moral disengagement* and describes four major patterns of justification of reprehensible actions, summarised in Table 6.3.

Aristotle contended that once a moral decision was made, the person would tend to always decide in that same way thereinafter and 'consolidate' a given moral action. This, he said, is how wisdom is built. And perpetration of harm as well, one could add. Contemporary experimental psychology has confirmed that even the most morally complex decisions can become automatic through practice and become decisions made without the least bit of effort (Anderson and Carnegey, 2004). The training of torturers follows this same rationale. Texts for training torturers or military elites, such as the Kaibiles in Guatemala to cite one example, show how candidates are gradually forced into a dynamic of increasingly reprehensible and inhuman decisions where the person no longer has time to think and face the moral dilemmas. In a short period of time they are led to justify harm that they have *already* perpetrated, leaving a headlong path towards even higher levels of harm as the only escape.

By putting both together, a circle can actually be configured where stereotypes and mindsets can be developed, i.e. 'all Muslims are potential terrorists', which justify torture (for instance 'they are trained to cheat, conceal and resist'). This facilitates subsequent moral detachment, i.e. 'that scum doesn't deserve to be treated as a person'. These become founded, objective reasons for making a given decision. Naturally, if this is repeated once and again, it will become increasingly automatic and the person will feel more confident that these immoral actions are moral.

TABLE 6.3 Bandura's model of moral disengagement

Mechanism	Description	Example
Altering the perception one has of reprehensible conduct	Giving oneself a supposedly higher moral justification Posing a false dilemma between two equally moral options	*'It has to be done for the good of the Homeland'* *'We have to save our countrymen'* *'It's them versus us'*
	Making mitigating comparisons about what could happen in the same circumstances elsewhere	*'They were lucky because if they were in X's hands they would know what being hit hard means . . .'* *'In their country they would have. . . .'*
	Using euphemistic expressions for one's conduct	*'Corrective or enhanced interrogation techniques'* *'Legitimate use of the minimum force necessary'*
Altering the perception of its consequences	Minimisation	*'Nothing ever happened to anybody because of a few slaps. Tomorrow they won't even remember'* *'Women love to make a huge deal about nothing . . .'*
Altering the perception of reprehensible conduct and its effects	Diffusing responsibility Due obedience	*'I just obey orders'* *'Ask the one who manufactured this . . . I'm just using what they gave me . . .'* *'You're here to obey orders' 'I just did my duty'*
Altering the perception of others adversely affected	Dehumanisation	*'They're all dogs that would kill you if they could'* *'If he treads where he shouldn't, he knows what's going to happen'* *'They were looking for it . . . they were looking for it because if they didn't get into these messes nothing would happen . . .'*

5. **How am I going to feel? Expected consequences and associated self-evaluated feelings**. In the process, not only does one's feeling at the time matter, but also how one will feel afterwards, i.e. pride, anger, dignity, shame. . . . Certain authors consider that certain subsequent emotions can be *cognitively regulated*.

6. **Self-regulation**. Bandura integrates this into a social moral decision-making model hinging around self-regulation included in his overall theory of the self (Bandura, 1991; Benight and Bandura, 2004). He contends that cognitive mechanisms of moral disengagement, emotions associated with decisions made, perception of the consequences of our actions, and so forth are constantly re-evaluated thereby affording a person the opportunity to change course. In other words, the person can decide, see and feel the consequences, and shape new responses. Whether or not one does so will depend primarily on whether s/he believes 'that's the way s/he is' and cannot be changed or 's/he is who s/he wants to be'. Bandura terms this 'self-efficacy'. In his model, the perpetrators, or at least those materially responsible, will have a low perception of self-efficacy. Bandura considers self-efficacy to be a social variable developed through interaction with one's environment.

7. **Group pressure**. Lastly, moral decisions are made under a group's watch. Pride, guilt and shame are emotions that require either real or imaginary observation by others. Training of torturers usually takes place in groups, and several ethnographic descriptions attest to how groups can foster massacres or genocides (Browning, 1992; Gourevitch, 1998). Several experiments with juries show how some members can subscribe to unfair guilty sentences so as not to feel themselves different from the rest (Saks, 1992).

All of the previous factors may determine moral action and depend both on the person him/herself and his/her environment. This renders the maximalist idea put forward by Zimbardo (2006) and others that any human being, including the reader, is a potential perpetrator given the right circumstances, unsustainable (Haslam and Reicher, 2006; Packer, 2008). A host of factors come into play when perpetrating harm.

If, for instance, based on what has just been explained we attempted to define the profile of an 'altruist' or a 'rebel', and conversely an amoral person tending to inflict harm on other human beings, we could presume altruists or rebels to be those with (1) moral motives lying at the heart of their identity system; (2) solid conventional rules coupled with critical principles enabling a sense of justice going beyond a given system of mainstream rules and the status quo; (3) behaviour placing benefit for others and for the common good above personal costs and benefits; (4) a tendency towards intense feelings (of pride, shame or guilt) when evaluating their own decisions; (5) the ability to identify moral justifications and avoid using them in dilemmas between what ought to and what one wants to do; and (6) a great ability to self-regulate their own conduct and belief themselves. These people's proper moral conduct would be even more likely in a favourable group setting.

Figure 6.1 points towards several avenues for preventive action in training those exposed to the potential risk of evil-doing.

It seems that Aristotle's trait theories inherited by Adorno (1950) and those in experimental psychology and philosophy who studied the authoritarian personality as a seed to perpetrating evil-doing have progressed towards complex, diffuse and dynamic models for understanding human behaviour. Although these constructs often may overlap or provide only a partial view, overall, they do help us to understand that a certain degree of free will does exist, that there are a host of complex yet isolatable factors that determine behaviour, and that one can become aware of this. While there are concurring factors that help explain certain behaviour, there are also clear decision-making processes competing within a given person.

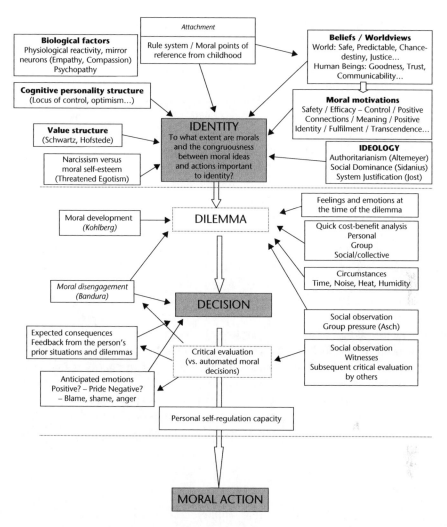

FIGURE 6.1 Cognitive processes in moral action.

When jurists partake in the complex exercise of examining psychological mechanisms that may have a bearing on a decision – and these include factors ranging from those linked to biology to others related to upbringing, moral development, learning and experiences, an ideological system and worldview, emotions and thoughts before and after decisions are made – they cannot infer that a person is merely a victim of this complex web. This brief review indeed shows that *decisions* are actually made through *conscious deliberative* processes. Zimbardo, the director of the well-known experiment at the Stanford prison, always remarked that *all* of the students who had to play the role of prison warden participated in acts of evil-doing against those who played the role of prisoners. Subsequent replicas showed how easy it was for resistant or rebellious persons to appear among the wardens (Packer, 2008; Reicher and Haslam, 2006). In Milgram's classical experiment where electric shocks were administrated to actors, allegedly in order to help them learn pairs of words, 60 per cent of those in that role in the experiment administered lethal shocks. But this means that 40 per cent did not (Blass, 1991; Packer, 2008; Rochat and Modigliani, 1995).

The perpetrator's internal and external motivations

All of this information taken together maps out the psychological processes that may be involved in making a decision to perpetrate evil-doing.

It can therefore be inferred that a torturer can act for many different reasons. Sometimes these actions may be based on positive motives (such as ideological commitment, personal gain, promotion, financial benefit, the feeling of belonging to a group, a sense of self-efficacy, etc.) while others may be based on negative ones (such as avoiding punishment or sanctions, feeling excluded, or shunning feelings of guilt or shame by reinforcing previous decisions to perpetrate harm).

Among the positive motives, a torturer's maximum efficacy arises when a positive identity is developed hinging around perpetrating harm in which the person is identified with what s/he considers positive values. Associating torturing or decapitating someone with having the strength, conviction, decisiveness, clarity and valour to do what *must be done*, with being one of the few who *can do it* stands as an example. This certain mythomaniac or heroic dimension based on a self-image built around the valour and power conferred by the destruction of others is far from the image of a mild-mannered civil servant that has repeatedly been put forward (Berkowitz, 1999) and which certainly does exist. Osvaldo Romo, perhaps the most sadistic torturer of the Pinochet dictatorship, gave an interview shortly before he died in which he confessed he was proud of everything he did and asserted that he would undoubtedly do it again (Guzmán, 2000). A recent doctoral thesis in which torturers from seven different countries were interviewed concluded that most of them did not regret their actions and even vindicated them years later (Payne, 2009).

In light of this, it is not hard to understand that there are people whose moral decision-making systems and internal and external motivations are powerful enough to outweigh the moral duty to protect life and not inflict harm to anyone else, even more so if that person is not perceived as one's equal.

Conclusions

The United Nations definition of torture requires *intentionality* on the part of the perpetrator for his or her acts to be considered torture. As we have analysed over this chapter, in the clearest of situations, the person must have *known* that what he or she did was ill-treatment or torture and must have *intended* to perpetrate it. Jurisprudence refers to these situations as those of *direct wilful misconduct*. However, there are also other situations considered to be *indirect* and *potential wilful misconduct*. Some jurists consider that if the State is responsible, it makes no sense to get into a legal debate over the intentionality of the specific perpetrator since it is the system that acts through that person.

When asserting that establishing the State's responsibility is criterion enough to establish intentionality, what is being said from a more general standpoint is that intentionality can be inferred by indicators of environment and interaction between the person(s) exercising control and those being controlled. The Intentionality Assessment Checklist (see Appendix 7) includes ten intentionality criteria on the part of the alleged perpetrator and aims to help establish this.

One step further is to determine purpose. Intent and purpose come hand in hand, and so if a purpose can be proven, then intentionality is proven with it. Conversely, it is hard to infer purpose if there is no evidence of intentionality. The Convention recognises four purposes explicitly, although it leaves the door open to others ('*such as . . .*'). Here, it worth adding that perhaps it makes no sense either to establish a list of *purposes* for torturing. Other criteria such as those put forward by Manfred Nowak on defencelessness (Nowak and McArthur, 2006) or by the Inter-American Convention when it speaks of 'obliterating one's personality' seem highly pertinent here. We utilised this idea in putting forward some of the items on the Torturing Environment Scale, described in Chapter 18 and Appendix 5.

Finally, the most complex step is to discern not intentionality or purpose but motivation. We have briefly dealt with some moral decision-making processes. This brief outline is more than sufficient to understand discerning the individual and group processes involved leading a specific person to perpetrate harm is complex and subjective, making them relatively impertinent legally speaking.[18] Yet these are precisely the decisive elements for developing pedagogical material to educate youth in values and design training programmes for State police forces and armies. Analysing individuals' motivations and group influence sets the groundwork for preventing torture in the future.

Notes

1 What is established here is not whether alleging ignorance would exonerate one from the crime (something which nearly no criminal system includes and which is described by the well-known Latin expression *Ignorantia juris non excusat*), but that the elements enable the legal official to establish that there is a component of *intentionality* (wilful misconduct). In cases of torture, a crime is considered to have wilful misconduct *de facto* to the extent that intentionality is built into the definition. Rather than aggravating the crime, wilful misconduct must be present, otherwise torture would be ruled out according to the United Nations definition.
2 The debate as to whether the wilful misconduct is direct or potential actually only serves to establish the degree of liability (it may be an attenuating or aggravating factor). And these degrees of liability are not established in most national criminal codes or in the jurisprudence of international courts. The implications of considering wilful conduct to be direct or potential is pertinent in any event philosophically and psychologically speaking.
3 CIDH, *Bueno Alves v. Argentina*. Judgment of 11 May 2007.
4 CIDH, *González and others* ("Campo Algodonero") *v. Mexico*. Judgment of 16 November 2009, separate opinion of Justice Cecilia Medina Quiroga.
5 *Velásquez-Rodríguez v. Honduras*, IACHR (Series A) No. 4, judgment of 29 July 1982, §173; *Godínez-Cruz v. Honduras*, IACHR (Series C) No. 5, judgment of 20 January 20 1989, §183.
6 *Cyprus v. Turkey*, 6780/74 y 6950/75 (first and second claims), 2 D and R 125, pp. 136–7 (1975).
7 Article 3 of the European Convention on Human Rights: 'No one shall be subjected to torture or to inhuman or degrading treatment or punishment.'
8 European Court H.R., *Case Peers v. Greece*, 19 April 2001, Judgement, para 74.
9 UN Human Rights Committee: Communication no. 265/1987: Finland. 02/05/89. General CCPR/C/35/D/265/1987, 2 May 1989. Spanish Original: English, § 9.2.
10 Therefore, he considers that: 'As for the State's core obligations under the prohibition of torture and ill-treatment, I have noted that under CAT "each State party should prohibit, prevent and redress torture and ill-treatment in all contexts of custody or control, for example, in prisons, hospitals, schools, institutions that engage in the care of children, the aged, the mentally ill or disabled, in military service, and other institutions as well as contexts where the failure of the State to intervene encourages and enhances the danger of privately inflicted harm."' Therefore 'medical treatments of an intrusive and irreversible nature, if they lack a therapeutic purpose, constitute torture or ill-treatment when enforced or administered without the free and informed consent of the person concerned (. . .) specially on patients from marginalised groups, such as persons with disabilities, notwithstanding claims of good intentions or medical necessity' (Center for Human Rights and Humanitarian Law, 2014).

11 They are defined by the NGO Geneva Call (2005) as: '*armed actors with a basic management structure operating outside the control of the State and using force to obtain their political or presumably political objectives* (Armed Non-State Actors and Landmines, p. 10) and by the OCHA as '*groups with the potential to use arms in using force to obtain political, ideological or economic objectives; they are not within the formal military structure of a State or alliances between States or intergovernmental organizations and are not under the control of the State(s) in which they operate.*' (Hugh & Bessler, 2006, p. 87).

12 For instance, Judge Cecilia Medina Quiroga in a separate opinion in the judgement of the *González and others v. México* case[12] stated '*It is the duty of the State party to afford everyone protection through legislative and other measures as may be necessary against the acts prohibited by Article 7, whether inflicted by people acting in their official capacity, outside their official capacity or in a private capacity*'. The European Court in the recent case *Opuz v. Turkey* also invoked '*the obligation of State to secure that individuals within their jurisdiction are not subjected to torture or inhuman or degrading treatment or punishment, including such ill-treatment administered by private individuals*' (www.corteidh.or.cr/docs/casos/articulos/seriec_205_ing.pdf).

13 Particularly pertinent here is the request by the *Asociaciones de Familiares de Desaparecidos de México* through a popular initiative for Enforced Disappearance and Extrajudicial Execution at the hands of private individuals to be defined as a crime in the criminal code. Similar requests have been made in El Salvador.

14 Columbian legislation, for instance, does not explicitly define the actors that can commit crimes of torture. On 11 March 2015, a Medellin court (in Colombia), for the first time in the country, sentenced 56-year-old AJR for a crime of *psychological torture* of his former partner E.L.G., aged 48, due to harassment and both physical and verbal aggression that he subjected her to in her home after the two separated.

15 ECHR, *Ireland v. UK*, cit., separate opinion of Judge Fitzamaurice.

16 Along these same lines would come studies on psychopathy, understood from a classical perspective in its most biological sense, i.e. persons with low emotional reactance in situations of stress and threat who are unable to anticipate the positive or negative consequences of their actions, and persons with low empathy or emotional synch with others. Sadism, whose structure seems more literary than real, would be excluded. We are unaware of research confirming that sadism (experiencing pleasure in someone else's pain) exists. Reality is far more complex and mechanisms that allow us to understand the conduct of 'sadists' reach far beyond the simplicity of the term.

17 Another host of ecological and circumstantial factors related to physical discomfort or well-being such as noise, heat, humidity and pain must be added to this (Anderson and Carnegey, 2004).

18 In extreme cases, psychology can be used to construe the perpetrator as being actually a victim, and this was attempted in a trial against one of the United States torturers in Iraq (Zimbardo, 2007). The torturer could be exonerated in the very rare event that s/he acted due to *force majeure*. (One example is the context of violence within paramilitary groups where certain members who were or are tortured must torture others or die . . .). But these external determining factors act as elements coercing one's free will, and not intrapsychic determining factors or external determining factors acting upon the intrapsychic system without altering one's final decision-making capacity.

SECTION 4

Scientific approaches to defining psychological torture

7

CATALOGUING TORTURE METHODS

Over the years there have been many efforts to classify torture methods. The most ambitious work to date is the 825-page *Torture and Democracy* by Darius Rejali (2007). Survivors have taught us that the torture method itself is inconsequential and simply represents the symbolic space in which the interaction takes place (see, for example, the testimonies of Villani and Liscano in Chapter 2). From their point of view, the method represents the way in which pain is produced, but does not encapsulate the full experience or impact of torture. Nevertheless, it is clearly important to study and understand torture methods, and to classify them as part of the process of defining psychological torture.

Torture research formally began in the 1970s with the pioneering work of several small human rights groups working under harsh conditions in Latin America, and continued in the 1980s with the work of the Amnesty International Medical Group in Denmark, which later developed into the International Rehabilitation Center for Torture Victims (IRCT) network. The research done at that time and during the 1990s was mostly clinical and epidemiological, and there were several attempts to classify torture methods either theoretically or through statistical analysis of records from rehabilitation centres for torture victims. These preliminary works provide a useful picture of a specific moment and context – the dictatorships in Latin America in the 1980s and 1990s — but new theoretical debates have emerged in the 21st century. We will review these contributions below.

We begin by looking at the efforts to build scales of measure, then proceed to classifications based on epidemiological studies, and finally review several new theory-driven classifications.

Psychometric tools for measuring torture

Torture method checklists

There have been different attempts to create checklists of torture methods, including the Exposure to Torture Scale (Başoğlu, 1999), the Allodi Torture Scale (Allodi, 1991) and the Torture Checklist (Rasmussen, Crager, Keatley, Keller and Rosenfeld, 2011). A recent review (Green, Rasmussen, and Rosenfeld, 2010) collected up to 48 different checklists of war-related events (including torture) ranging in length from 8 to 164 items. None of these checklists have been validated (Green et al., 2010; Hollifield et al., 2002), nor have their psychometric properties been published; they are useful insofar as they provide a structured recollection of data during therapy or as part of the documentation of torture. These checklists are mostly designed as semi-structured interviews for use in rapid assessments in refugee camps, as an aid to clinical histories in rehabilitation centres, or for forensic assessments of asylum claims.

A first step: creating an item bank. Common sense dictates that creating an exhaustive list of torture methods is impossible. The number of techniques described in reports is enormous and only limited by the circumstances and the imagination of torturers (Costanzo and Gerrity, 2009). One step in the right direction would be to develop a bank of items from all of the available checklists and collate them under *conceptual* categories through consensus (using a methodology similar to that employed by Del Vecchio et al. (2011) to develop a meaningful item bank for measuring PTSD from all of the available self-reporting scales).

Checklist versus single query. A study of a group of African refugees (n=1134) compared the prevalence of torture revealed by two different methods: asking one question (the item on torture in the Harvard Trauma Questionnaire: presence-versus-absence of torture), versus going through a checklist of torture methods (the Torture Checklist – see Appendix 4). In general there was not much difference between the efficacy of the two forms of questioning (Jaranson et al., 2004). On the checklist, only 14 per cent of those checking a torture method answered 'No' in the single torture question, and 9 per cent of those who answered 'Yes' to the single question were unable to identify any specific torture method from the checklist. The authors conclude that a single question can be a useful and reliable measuring tool for correlational studies of torture against other factors without resorting to lengthy questionnaires.

Cultural validity. This does not mean that a universal tool can be built. The same torture technique can be understood in many different ways depending on the context in which it is applied. Checklists should be adapted to the characteristics of each cultural group and situation. Traumatic events, as well as the meanings attributed to them, vary according to the specific historical, political and social context in which the trauma occurred (Elsass, Carlsson, Jespersen and Phuntsok, 2009; Shoeb, Weinstein and Mollica, 2007), and a process of tailoring the tool will always be necessary.

Assessing the legal definition: Torture Screening Checklist

One of the problems with checklists is that they do not allow clinical researchers to evaluate whether a person has been tortured in legal terms or not, because 'torture' is not only an ethical or clinical concept (Rasmussen et al., 2011). A clinician filing a forensic report can recognise and affirm that a person has been tortured, but that same victim's legal claims may still be dismissed in court or judged as falling under a different category. Jaranson et al. (2004) posits that *if a survivor has gone through one of the experiences* in the Torture Checklist, he or she *is* a torture survivor and can be classified accordingly for research and forensic purposes. One alternative is the Torture Screening Checklist (TSCL). The TSCL is a narrative coding tool that classifies survivors' history as involving torture (or not), as specified by the legal definitions of the United Nations, the World Medical Association and domestic legislation from the United States. The TSCL is not a self-reporting questionnaire (i.e. filled out by the survivor) or a structured interview, but rather a checklist to be used by the clinician as an aid to establish the potential legal status of the survivor. Each criterion of the definition of torture was split into items that were checked off after the interview. Fourteen different mental health professionals were involved in the validation of the scale.

The Torture Screening Checklist was supposed to help clinicians evaluate patients in terms that would have more weight in the legal sphere. The results, however, were disappointing because the majority of cases qualified as torture: 132 out of 160 patients fulfilled the 'abuse by official authority' criteria; 131 (99.2 per cent) met criteria for the WMA definition of torture; 128 (97.0 per cent) met criteria for UNCAT; and 124 (93.9 per cent) met criteria for the US definition. Overall, the three definitions clearly overlapped and almost all patients fulfilled criteria for the legal definition of torture according to the clinicians, a result with which tribunals would probably disagree.

Clinicians focus on the experiences and narratives of the survivor, while a judge focuses on whether acts committed by the perpetrator qualify as torture. In other words, a clinician can say that *a survivor has suffered torture* based on a legal definition and his or her forensic assessment, while a judge might say that *the facts* as they stand do not amount to torture in the context of a trial in which the claimant seeks compensation or status claims (such as asylum), or that the alleged perpetrator *has not committed torture* according to the defendant's views, the investigation and the description of the acts in context (in the case of trials denouncing torturers). It would be a fascinating exercise to gather a panel of clinicians and judges and analyse the sources of their differences.

Torture severity measurements

A checklist gives equal weight to each torture method, but does not give an idea of the *severity* of a given method's impact. Taking severity into account is a first and necessary step for research. Half of the studies in Green's review derived scores by simply summing the number of different types of abuse suffered (whether or not they were considered to be torture). A small number of studies also took into account the frequency and duration of techniques. None of these measures includes the subjective perception of the impact of each torture method. Only Başoğlu's Semi-Structured Interview for Survivors of Torture operationalises torture severity in a comprehensive way by calculating the total number of types of torture (from a list of 44 events), frequency of exposure to torture, duration of detention and perceived severity of each type of experienced torture (i.e. distress) rated along a 5-point Likert scale (see Appendix 4).

Classification based on mathematical procedures

There have been different attempts to classify torture techniques by applying statistical methods using the above-mentioned scales or other semi-structured methods of information collection. We will briefly review them here, focusing our reflections on how these classifications help define psychological torture.

Most data come from factor analytic studies of small samples of survivors in rehabilitation centres. The results have limited value for two reasons: (1) the results of the statistical procedure depend on the psychometric tools used in the interview (pre-existing categories), and (2) the small sample size causes outcomes to be conditioned by the age and country of origin of the survivors attended at a given moment. Only finding strong commonalities across studies could produce more universally applicable results. In the following selection of six studies we excluded studies which explore general wartime 'traumatic experiences' using tools too broad in scope to specifically explore torture, like the Harvard Trauma Questionnaire (i.e., Silove, Steel, McGorry, Miles, and Drobny, 2002).

In Study 1, Cunningham and Cunningham (1997) used a principal components factor analysis to classify torture methods in a group of 191 survivors under treatment in the STARTTS centre in Australia. They identified six factors, although it was difficult to label four of them, and impossible to label the remaining two. They described the factors as: (1) *common torture* (beating, isolation, threats and bondage); (2) *torture of family members*; (3) *fear of death* (mock executions, near-drowning) and (4) *passive torture* (blindfolding, forced standing and sleep and water deprivation).

In Study 2, The IAN Center for Rehabilitation of Torture Victims in Belgrade developed an ad-hoc questionnaire to analyse methods of torture in people detained in concentration camps in former Yugoslavia. They listed 81 methods of torture and published results from a sample of 322 survivors (Jovic and Opacic, 2004). The analysis yielded three factors: (1) forms of torture that *respect physical integrity*: threats to the victim or to relatives; forcing victims to perform humiliating acts; watching others being tortured; deprivation of food and water; or physical ill-treatment that usually does not lead to severe bodily injuries (such as slapping, kicking or beating, pulling of hair, hitting or beating with rifle butt, whip, belt, stick, or tying with rope); (2) torture methods aimed at *inflicting serious injuries* (hanging by limbs; plunging into water; burning with cigarettes, open flame, or boiling water; forced extraction of teeth; throwing from high altitude; electrocution; and amputation of body parts, among other methods); (3) torture methods linked to *sexual humiliation and abuse, including rape*. The authors conclude that their data points to two types of torture methods: (1) torture methods in which the victim still recognises him or herself as a subject and as an independent, living person; (2) torture that treats the detainee's body as an object over which full and ruthless control has been established. Dividing methods into these two categories makes sense, and would undoubtedly have great significance if the authors could show a correlation with clinical elements or a differential psychological impact.

In a similar study in the Bellevue Center for Survivors of Torture in New York (Hooberman, Rosenfeld, Lhewa, Rasmussen and Keller, 2007), data for 325 survivors was obtained through a retrospective review of records (Study 3). The authors used HURIDOCS, the international standard for the classification of human right violations, and summarised torture methods in 20 categories. A factor analysis generated a model with five factors corresponding to: (1) *witnessing torture of others* (experiences in which the participant saw someone else who had experienced torture and violence); (2) *torture of family members* (traumas involving a family member, such as witnessing the torture of family, or family being harassed); (3) *physical beating* (physical assault of any type); (4) *rape or sexual assault*; and (5) *deprivation*, or passive torture (deprivation of food or water, sensory deprivation). They tried to validate the results by correlating the factors with clinical data, but psychological distress (PTSD, anxiety and symptoms of depression) was significantly correlated only with the fifth factor, rape or sexual assault.

A new study in the Balkans (Study 4) analysed the severity and psychological impact of captivity stressors in 432 torture survivors from Turkey and countries formerly part of Yugoslavia (Başoğlu, 2009). A principal components analysis of 46 captivity stressors revealed seven underlying factors: (1) *sexual torture* (rape, genital manipulation); (2) *physical torture* (beating, burning); (3) *psychological manipulation* (threats of torture, witnessing torture); (4) *humiliating treatment* (forced nudity, feces in food); (5) *forced stress positions* (forced standing for long periods of time, binding the body to restrict movement); (6) *sensory discomfort* (extreme cold, blindfolding); and (7) *deprivation of basic needs* (sleep, food). Among the many important findings of this study is the fact that non-physical torture was more strongly associated with perceived torture severity and lasting psychological damage than was physical torture. Based on this analysis, Başoğlu argues for an inclusive, contextual definition of torture that goes beyond specific techniques and takes into account the loss of control, terror, feelings of helplessness and lasting psychological damage experienced by victims of torture.

In Study 5, Punamäki, Quota and Sarraj (2010), looked at data from a sample of 275 Palestinian men who reported torture experiences in detention and imprisonment in Israel using a principal component analysis. The authors used a clinical interview, the Harvard Trauma Questionnaire (HTQ), and the Torture Experience Survey (which checks for the presence and frequency of techniques used from a list of 30 torture techniques). The results show four factors: (1) *physical torture*: rape attempts, electrical torture, acid burns, injection of chemicals, burning parts of the body, falaqa; (2) *psychological torture*: humiliation through attacks on the detainee's national identity, sham executions, forced confessions, death threats, threats against family, religious humiliation, false accusations, threats to rape sisters or wives, family members' humiliation, naming friends, personal humiliation; (3) *sensory discomfort and deprivation*: water deprivation, cold showers, starvation, jumping on the body, beating of genitals, crucifixion, isolation and solitary confinement, strong light, sexual harassment; and (4) *beatings*: beating with sticks, standing under direct sunlight, beating with guns, breaking bones. The results clearly show that what the authors call Sensory Discomfort and Deprivation falls under a different category than Psychological Torture, which includes techniques linked to threats, humiliation and cognitive manipulation of the victim. Interestingly enough, both physical and psychological methods were associated with increased PTSD symptoms, *especially when combined*. And psychological torture – but not physical torture – was also associated with increased somatic symptoms, showing a specific contribution to mental health damage independent of sensory manipulation and physical torture.

A recent study (Phillips, 2011) analysed methods of torture in a sample of 181 cases of kidnapping for ransom from 32 countries through a SSA multidimensional scaling procedure that distributed torture techniques in conceptual maps (Study 6). The aim was to understand the degree of intensity of each torture method, its pattern, and its function during the kidnapping. The study analysed the presence or absence of 34 different torture methods and grouped them. The results show four patterns that also correspond with different stages of the kidnapping: (1) *social isolation*: the person is left alone and deprived of any human contact (even with the kidnapper). This includes being put in a cage or a small space, drugged and blindfolded, as well as different levels of sensory deprivation. (2) *Physical and psychological manipulation of the victim*: in this second stage, the perpetrator wants to ensure full control over the victim. This includes all of the mistreatment of the first stage in addition to threats, beatings and the deprivation of hygiene, food and water. Physical violence appears spontaneous and shows high hostility. The purpose of both physical and psychological violence is fear and, through fear, the feelings of uncertainty, permanent danger, loss of control and, ultimately, cooperation. (3) *Sadistic interactions*: if the person is not released, in around 15 per cent of the overall sample of victims, this stage involves sadistic interactions (harsh interrogation, mock executions, rape, mutilations of fingers or ears and other abuses). Violence becomes more carefully calculated to meet specific aims. (4) *Positive interactions and rewards*: at different stages, but especially when the kidnapping is close to the end, there is a pattern of positive personal interaction when the kidnapper presents him or herself as human, tries to create conversation and establish a positive rapport, and provides small gifts or privileges. A high percentage of victims undergoing this latter stage of techniques feel grateful to their kidnappers and decline to denounce their aggressors.

This final study shows the difficulty of analysing data from the static picture that classical factorial analysis offers, and the usefulness of more complex, dynamic analyses. It introduces the idea of psychological manipulation of the victim, including positive interaction and rewards, something never included in any previous study nor regularly investigated in work with torture survivors.

Table 7.1 summarises the studies. The results provide useful information:

1. In general, we can conclude that the two studies conducted with survivors of the Balkans war (Başoğlu, 2009; Jovic and Opacic, 2004) and the study with survivors of kidnapping by ransom (Phillips, 2011) obtained strikingly similar results. The seven categories proposed by Başoğlu are a useful point of departure for classifying torture methods.
2. A closer look at the details of these studies reveals that their theoretical proposals and categories do not always coincide. For instance, Study 1 emphasises the distinction between the *active* production of pain by the torturer, and *passive* torture methods in which (using the KUBARK concept) the person fights against his or her own pain. In Study 2 the emphasis is on whether boundaries of identity are respected, or violated through brutality. The study only partially overlaps with the 'fear of death' category in Study 1. But there are also interesting commonalities: Studies 1 and 2 both use very broad categories that share the distinction between primarily physical and primarily psychological methods. Studies 3 and 4 share a category for techniques that use physical force against the person (3.3 and 4.2), and separate it from deprivation or manipulation of environment (1.4, 3.5, 4.6, 4.7). Threats to family appear in two studies (1.2, 2.2). Rape and sexual abuse always appear as a distinct category (1.5, 2.3, 3.4, 4.1) except in Study 5, which spreads sexual abuse across three factors, and Study 6, which includes it under 'sadistic interactions'. We can conclude that:
    *   There are techniques aimed at manipulating the victim's environment and basic needs, which differ from techniques aimed at producing pain. Although pain can always appear, the ultimate aim of these techniques is control.
    *   All of the studies clearly differentiate between physical torture and psychological torture (which aim to instill fear and obedience).
    *   Psychological techniques all attack identity and try to foster compliance and cooperation, and threats to family and humiliation are both common and central elements of these techniques.
    *   Rape and sexual violence is a distinct category that should be analysed separately from others.
3. There are strong and consistent results indicating that *there is no correlation between methods (whether psychological or physical) and psychopathology* in any of the studies, with the notable exception of rape. The psychological methods produce at least the same amount of psychological distress as physical methods (even the more brutal ones), indicating that – as Başoğlu et al. (2007), Punamaki et al. (2010) and others have found – there are no grounds for differentiating between more and less severe forms of ill-treatment or between CIDT and torture. Rape is a different kind of torture in which it is not unusual to find strong self-conscious emotions of rage and guilt, and a direct threat to identity and worldview.

TABLE 7.1 Factor analytic studies of torture methods

Study	Sample (S) and Methods (M)	Results
[1] Cunningham and Cunningham (1997)	S: Multicultural mixed sample of torture survivors receiving treatment at the STARTTS Center in Australia (n=191)	1. Common torture (e.g. beating, isolation, threats) 2. Torture of family members 3. Fear of death (e.g. mock executions, asphyxia) 4. Passive torture (e.g. blindfolding, forced standing, sleep and water deprivation)
	M: Semi-structured interview	Two additional factors were too mixed to be labeled.
[2] Jovic and Opacic (2004)	S: Survivors of concentration camps in Croatia, Bosnia and Serbia (n=322) M: Exposure to Torture Scale	1. Torture that respects physical integrity/the other as a person (e.g. deprivation of food and water, threats, humiliation, witnessing torture, beatings) 2. Torture inflicting serious injuries/the other as an object – full control (e.g. asphyxia, electricity, burning, amputations) 3. Sexual torture
[3] Hooberman et al. (2007)	S: Multicultural mixed sample of torture survivors receiving treatment at the Bellevue Center in New York (n=325) M: HURIDOCS	1. Witnessing torture of others 2. Harassment or torture of relatives 3. Physical beatings 4. Rape/sexual assault 5. Deprivation/passive torture
[4] Başoğlu (2009)	S: Torture survivors in former Yugoslavian countries and Turkey (n=432) M: Exposure to Torture Scale	1. Sexual torture (e.g. rape, genital manipulation) 2. Physical torture (e.g. beating, burning) 3. Psychological manipulations (e.g. threats of torture, witnessing torture) 4. Humiliating treatment (e.g. forced nudity, feces in food) 5. Forced stress positions (e.g. forced standing for long periods, binding the body to restrict movement) 6. Sensory discomfort (e.g. extreme cold, blindfolding) 7. Deprivation of basic needs (e.g. sleep, food)
[5] Punamäki, Quota and Sarraj (2010)	S: Palestinian men who reported their experiences in detention and imprisonment (N = 275) M: Exposure to Torture Scale	1. Physical torture 2. Psychological torture (e.g. humiliating attacks on national identity, sham executions, forced confessions, death threats, threats to family, religious humiliation, false accusations, threats to rape sister/wife, family members' humiliation, naming friends, personal humiliation) 3. Sensory discomfort and deprivation 4. Beatings

Study	Sample (S) and Methods (M)	Results
[6] Phillips (2011)	S: Victims of torture during kidnapping for ransom (n=181 from 32 countries) M: Ad-hoc scale	1. Social isolation 2. Physical and psychological manipulation of the victim (fear) 3. Sadistic behavior 4. Positive rewards/social interactions

Consensus groups

Istanbul Protocol

The Istanbul Protocol (IP) adopted a classification based on experts' consensus on broad categories that combine methods and effects. The main purpose of the protocol was to guide systematic interviewing in forensic procedures to document torture (see Appendix 1 and Chapter 18). As we will discuss in Chapter 19, the IP categories include physical, psychological and mixed methods. Methods of psychological torture are grouped in seven categories, which are undefined and partially overlap. The main category is *psychological techniques to break down the individual*, which is not defined – indeed, it is difficult to know what, exactly, it means.

Chapter 19 is dedicated to these shortcomings and the possibilities for improving the IP's classification of psychological torture.

HURIDOCS

In 1981 an international task force was created, spurring a process of consensus on a taxonomy of torture methods among experts from around the world. As a result, HURIDOCS was built. HURIDOCS is an international system of cataloguing human rights violations (http://www.huridocs.org). It is updated regularly, and provides different software solutions and a detailed system of codes for creating databases of human rights violations with a special focus on litigation. The Event Standard Format and the Micro-Thesaurus in their last revised version (Dueck, Guzman and Verstappen, 2009) roughly follow the IP and put a strong emphasis on physical torture. While there are 18 codes and 37 subcodes detailing ways of producing physical pain, and 5 codes and 13 subcodes for manipulation of the environment, there is only one self-defined catch-all code (03.20, without subcodes) called Psychological Torture and Ill-treatment (see Appendix 1). Additional codes include degradation (3.21), threats (3.22), and witnessing torture of others (3.24).

Theory-driven classifications

Almerindo Ojeda

Ojeda, professor of Linguistics at the University of California, committed himself to trying to define psychological torture (Ojeda, 2008). He begins by saying that a perfect definition is impossible, and, as we saw in Chapter 1, he suggested that the best definition may simply be that PT is 'the intentional infliction of suffering without resorting to direct physical violence' (p. 5). He proposes working with what he calls an *extensive definition* (a comprehensive list of every technique that has been described as 'psychological' in the torture literature), and saying: *if you do this, you are inflicting psychological torture.* He then proposes a theoretical model with thirteen categories that include, in his view, all of the PT techniques. The list is a theory-driven, personal proposal that he cross-checks with different sources to produce a table that intends to show that every technique has a place in his proposal.

The idea was groundbreaking, and the categories proposed by Ojeda are logical (see Table 7.2).

Ojeda's proposal is highly advanced. Unfortunately it has several shortcomings:

1. The model is essentially derived from the experience of the author as director of the Guantanamo Testimonials Project. It begins with the work of Biderman in the US (Biderman and Zimmer, 1961), the KUBARK Manual (Central Intelligence Agency, 1963), and different US Army Field Manuals, and concludes with the different memos and official documents issued by the US government authorising or denying certain

TABLE 7.2 Extensional definition of psychological torture

A1. Isolation: solitary confinement (no human contact whatsoever) or semi-solitary confinement (contact only with interrogators, guards and other personnel ancillary to the detention).

A2. Psychological Debilitation: the effect of deprivation of food, water, clothes or sleep; the disruption of sleep cycles; prolonged standing, crouching or kneeling; forced physical exertion; exposure to temperatures leading to stifling or hypothermia.

A3. Spatial Disorientation: confinement in small spaces; small, darkened or otherwise nonfunctional windows.

A4. Temporal Disorientation: denial of natural light; nighttime recreation; erratic scheduling of meals, showers or other regular activities.

A5. Sensory Disorientation: use of magic rooms, i.e. holding facilities or interrogation chambers that induce misperceptions of sensory failure, narcosis or hypnosis.

A6. Sensory Deprivation: use of hooding, blindfolding, opaque goggles, darkness, sound proofing/canceling headsets, nasal masks (possibly deodorised), gloves, arm covers, sensory deprivation tanks or vaults.

A7. Sensory Assault (Overstimulation): use of bright or stroboscopic lights; loud noise or music; shouting or using public address equipment at close range.

A8. Induced Desperation: arbitrary arrest; indefinite detention; random punishment or reward; forced feeding; implanting sense of guilt, abandonment, or 'learned helplessness'.

A9. Threats: to self or to others; threats of death, physical torture or rendition; mock executions; forced witnessing of torture (visually or aurally).

A10. Feral Treatment: berating victim to the subhuman level of wild animals; forced nakedness; denial of personal hygiene; overcrowding; forced interaction with pests; contact with blood or excreta; bestialism; incest.

A11. Sexual Humiliation: forcing the victim to witness or carry out masturbation, copulation or other forms of sexual behavior.

A12. Desecration: forcing victims to witness or engage in the violation of religious practices (irreverence, blasphemy, profanity, defilement, sacrilege, incest, Satanism).

A13. Pharmacological Manipulation: non-therapeutic use of drugs or placebos.

Adapted from Ojeda (2008).

techniques. In other words, it traces the history of US torture. Though it goes without saying that torture is essentially the same in most contemporary democracies, and torturers often learn from quite similar models, Ojeda's sources may not be sufficient to build an entire model.

2.   More importantly, the model lacks a theoretical background that would give coherence to the categories (Why these categories and not others?). It is a list. If we added theory (What is each technique useful for? What is its psychological/neurobiological basis? How does it combine with other techniques? etc.), the final result might be drastically different.

3.   Some categories are very narrow (e.g. Feral Treatment), while others are extremely broad (e.g. Psychological Debilitation); some define a technique (e.g. Sensory Assault), and others an output (e.g. Temporal Disorientation).

4.   Each category lacks a definition. One might wonder, for example, why 'forced nakedness' is included in the Feral Treatment category and not in the Sexual Humiliation category.

5.   It does not include purely cognitive techniques (e.g. interview and interrogation procedures, deception, forced betrayal and prisoner's dilemma), which are essential for an understanding of contemporary psychological torture.

Despite these shortcomings, Ojeda's model is a good starting point, and it is groundbreaking at a time when very few people are working on similar ideas; it should be considered part of any discussion on the issue.

Christopher Behan

Three years after Ojeda, Christopher Behan, Assistant Professor at the Southern Illinois University School of Law, made a similar attempt to classify torture methods (although seemingly without being familiar with Ojeda's work). He conducted a similar exercise, this time comparing several sources: Albert Biderman's proposal; the description of torture and interrogation by Alexander Solzhenistin in Archipelago Gulag; the methods used in the Korean War against US prisoners and later incorporated in the SERE training manuals; and the techniques described in the KUBARK manual, with additional techniques from known practices in Guantanamo and Abu Ghraib. He was not attempting to build a global classification of torture methods, but rather to demonstrate that the methods used in Guantanamo were the same as the ones used in the communist era to torture dissidents or torture American prisoners; he wanted to show how unacceptable it was that a democracy would repeat these methods 50 years later. Interestingly, he addressed some of the shortcomings in Ojeda's proposal: (1) he included a column called 'purpose' or 'effect', covering the theoretical background that would give support to the proposal and serving the purpose of a definition; (2) he included cognitive techniques; and (3) he included rewarding techniques. Unfortunately, his proposal is limited to the United States.

Behan argues that the six categories originally proposed by Biderman (1961) more than 50 years ago are still the standard of reference, and he builds upon this schema by adding what he considers to be refinements of the same old techniques. Although he insists that as a lawyer he has no psychological background (and warns the reader to consider this when evaluating his results), his proposal is theoretically sound and a strong step forward for analysing torture in US institutions.

TABLE 7.3 Categorisation of torture methods: Behan's model

Category	Techniques Gulag (1), Korean War/SERE training (2), KUBARK/US Enhanced Interrogation (3)
1. Disruption of Daily Rhythms and Routines	1. Night interrogation 2. Disruption of sleep and biorhythms, manipulation of diet 3. Arresting suspect early in the morning; providing ill-fitting clothing; manipulating diet, sleep patterns and other fundamentals of prisoner's life; removal of all comfort items, including religious items
2. Isolation and Sensory Deprivation	1. Confinement in small 'box' cell; punishment in solitary confinement cells 2. Solitary confinement, complete isolation, semi-isolation, group isolation, confinement in small cell, sensory deprivation 3. Deprivation of sensory stimuli by eliminating lights, sounds, odors, etc.; use of isolation for up to thirty days; hooding of detainees during transportation and questioning
3. Monopolisation of Perception	1. Constant bright light in small, white-walled cell 2. Physical isolation, darkness or bright light, barren environment, restricted movement, monotonous food, sensory overload (lights, noise, etc.) 3. Interrogation in non-standard locations
4. Induced Debilitation; Exhaustion	1. Forcing detainee to repeat everything and speak loudly from a distance, forced sitting on backless stools for hours or days, sleep deprivation, short rations, limiting water consumption, starvation, saltwater-induced thirst, continuous interrogation for several days 2. Semi-starvation; exposure; taking advantage of wounds; induced illness; sleep deprivation; prolonged constraint; prolonged interrogation or forced writing; overexertion; sitting on a pointed, imbalanced block with feet and knees together 3. Threat of debilitation, twenty-hour interrogations
5. Threats	1. Threats, threats against family members 2. Threats of death, threats of non-repatriation, threats of endless isolation and interrogation, vague threats, threats against family, mysterious changes in treatment 3. Threats of inflicting pain, threats to rape family members, threats to rape interrogation subject
6. Lies and Deception	1. Lies regarding evidence against detainee 2. - 3. Use of thick file with subject's name on it, deception techniques, interrogator lies about country of origin, use of falsified documents or reports
7. Occasional Indulgences	1. Psychological contrast (sudden favorable shift in interrogator's attitudes), excellent meal for starving prisoner on condition of signing confession 2. Occasional favors, fluctuations of interrogators' attitudes, promises, rewards for partial compliance, tantalising 3. Multiple-interrogator techniques
8. Demonstrating Omnipotence and Omniscience	1. – 2. Threatening transfer to worse facilities 3. Confrontations, pretending to take cooperation for granted, demonstrating complete control over victim's fate, use of thick file with subject's name on it

Category	Techniques Gulag (1), Korean War/SERE training (2), KUBARK/US Enhanced Interrogation (3)
9. Degradation	1. Use of foul language, preliminary humiliation, confinement 2. Personal hygiene prevented; filthy, infested surroundings; demeaning punishment; insults and taunts; denial of privacy; pouring, flicking or tossing water on subject; immersing the detainee's head in a container with garbage or urine 3. Stripping, removal of clothing, forced grooming
10. Enforcing Trivial Demands	1. (2) Forced writing, enforcement of extremely detailed rules
11. Heightened Suggestibility, Hypnosis and Narcosis	1. (3) Hypnotic techniques (including post-hypnotic suggestion), use of drugs and placebos
12. Self-Induced Physical Pain	1. Forced sitting on edge of chair or stool, forced upright kneeling for 12–48 hours, forced standing for long periods 2. Subject required to hold weighted block with arms extended, stress positions 3. Self-induced, non-severe pain; stress positions
13. Physical Abuse	1. Extinguishing cigarettes on detainee's skin, tickling bound prisoners inside nostrils with a feather, beatings with implements leaving no marks, removing fingernails, breaking backs 2. Facial or abdominal slaps, grabbing detainee's face, blowing thick pipe smoke in detainee's face, waterboarding, shaking and manhandling, forcing subject to the ground 3. Slapping (shoulder, stomach, 'insult slap'), use of mild physical contact such as grabbing, poking in chest, light pushing, waterboarding
14. Exploitation of Phobias	1. (3) Exploiting detainee's individual or religious phobias, such as dogs
15. Sexual Humiliation	1. Female guard striptease to torment detainee, male guards ogling and commenting on naked female detainees 2. – 3. Exploiting religious taboos against contact between men and women

Combined or single methods

There is widespread recognition that analysing torture methods one by one does not make much sense. Most of the time the person is subjected to a combination of methods that have a cumulative effect both in a diachronic and a synchronic way. Diachronic cumulative effects result from 'accumulation over time' (Reyes, 2008): the interrogator uses coercive techniques against a person previously debilitated by sleep and food deprivation and confused by sensory isolation. Synchronic cumulative effects occur when different techniques are applied at the same time, as seen in Marcelo Viñar's testimony of the fear of walking while hooded down a staircase while risking being pushed, possibly to one's death. It is the combination of these elements that terrorises the person.

Not surprisingly, in a review of the torture debate in the United States, the *New York Times* describes how questions posed by CIA interrogators to external assessors did not focus on certain techniques, but on combinations of physical and psychological tactics:

> We were getting asked about combinations – 'Can we do this and this at the same time?' recalled Paul C. Kelbaugh, a veteran intelligence lawyer who was deputy legal counsel at the CIA's Counterterrorist Center from 2001 to 2003. Interrogators were worried that even approved techniques had such a painful, multiplying effect when combined that they might cross the legal line, Mr. Kelbaugh said. He recalled agency officers asking: 'These approved techniques, say, withholding food, and 50-degree temperature – can they be combined?' Or 'Do I have to do the less extreme before the more extreme?' (Shane, Johnston and Risen, 2007)

An example of the complexities of defining and classifying torture methods using lists of methods (a nomothetic approach) is the debate by the International Forensic Expert Group of the IRCT on hooding as a torture method (International Forensic Expert Group, 2011). A panel of 30 experts from 18 different countries reviewed the legal background and concluded that there are conflicting definitions and sentences in International Humanitarian Law, some of which judge hooding as a form of CIDT while others see it as a form of torture. The group reviewed the psychological and medical consequences of hooding (helplessness and extreme fear, disorientation and confusion, asphyxia potentially leading to anoxia and potential brain damage) and concluded that they were dangerous, severe and could lead to permanent damage. Their conclusion shows the difficulty of categorising torture methods in general and, more specifically, of assigning individual techniques to defined categories. The IFEG considers hooding and other equivalent practices to be intentional forms of sensory deprivation that constitute cruel, inhuman and degrading treatment or punishment and should be prohibited in interrogations and detention. When hooding is practiced *in conjunction* with other acts that may be considered cruel, inhuman and degrading treatment or punishment, it may constitute torture. They conclude: 'In our experience, hooding is very often practiced in combination with other methods of abuse and typically, under such circumstances, constitutes Torture.' Their advice can be generalised to many other situations in which there is disagreement over whether methods should be considered ill-treatment or torture: it is the *combination* of techniques that defines torture.

Conclusions: the need to shift from focusing on torture methods to focusing on its objectives

The Istanbul Protocol and the HURIDOCS system (which is mostly based on the IP) are the standards of reference for the international classification of torture methods. Unfortunately, both lack theoretical models or field studies that support their use; they also rely heavily on techniques aimed to produce physical pain, while psychological torture is merely outlined and grouped into a few broad categories.

The results of a factorial analysis (FA) of torture methods heavily depend on the instrument of measure, the context of torture and the characteristics of the sample. FA is simply a mathematical tool to classify what we throw into the mix. It provides a profile of what happens at a certain time and place, but is always limited by the characteristics of the sample. The review of six studies at the beginning of the chapter showed a certain rough agreement around the seven categories proposed by Başoğlu (2009): (1) *sexual torture*; (2) *physical torture*; (3) *psychological manipulation*; (4) *humiliating treatment*; (5) *forced stress positions*; (6) *sensory discomfort;* and (7) *deprivation of basic needs*.

These categories make sense, but they reveal the difficulties of producing a universal classification from statistical procedures without a theoretical background. For example, aren't forced stress positions a kind of physical torture? Why is humiliating treatment a separate category? Would a different context have produced a wider array of categories of 'psychological manipulation'? Research shows, across studies, that the final categories do not predict psychological distress (Başoğlu, 2009; Cunningham and Cunningham, 1997; Hooberman et al., 2007; Jovic and Opacic, 2004). Factor analytic studies are excellent tools for sketching preliminary portraits of ill-treatment and torture in a given context and moment, provided that a broad and homogeneous sample is obtained, the authors use tools which are comprehensive enough to allow for comparison and the data is followed by a qualitative in-depth analysis.

Both Ojeda and Behan attempted to scale up from the local to the global using similar methodology: they compared training manuals or accounts of survivors to look for commonalities, and then tried to organise those commonalities into groups. They relied heavily on Biderman's pioneering ideas on psychological manipulation from the 1960s as well as the KUBARK Manual and other material from the US; in this sense, their focus was quite local. Ojeda did not try to build a classification, but proposed defining psychological torture 'extensively', which, as we saw, entailed its own problems. Behan went one step further and produced a rich proposal with 15 categories that clearly diverged from Başoğlu's model by (1) adding to a similar list of physical techniques (e.g. Disruption of Daily Rhythms and Routines, Self-Induced Physical Pain, Physical Abuse); (2) offering a more refined analysis of the manipulation of environment (e.g. Isolation and Sensory Deprivation, Monopolisation of Perception, Induced Debilitation; Exhaustion, etc.); and (3) including many psychological techniques (e.g. Lies and Deception, Occasional Indulgences, Demonstrating Omnipotence and Omniscience). Başoğlu's analysis comes from the experiences of war survivors in the Balkans, and Behan and Ojeda were informed by the torture lab of Guantanamo.

This chapter has explored the passionate work of scientific researchers who have tried to establish order among the almost infinite array of torture methods used throughout history. There have been great advances and great difficulties. Any meaningful proposal should be applicable independent of context and sample, and should include an analysis of both the purpose of the method in the overall process of torture (*What is this method for?*) and the type of damage inflicted (*What are the consequences?*). This brings us closer to what could be called a teleological approach, which is what we propose in later chapters. We can identify certain common objectives in coercive interrogation and torture, and specific kinds of damage associated with certain torture methods. New ways of harming people could be added to the list of existing forms of CIDT or torture if they sought similar objectives or if they produced a similar kind of physical or mental damage, independently of the mechanics of a given technique.

The teleological approach is a first and necessary step towards classifying torture, but not the only one. As we saw at the end of this chapter, torture methods are almost always used in combination. The next step involves focusing our efforts on the idea of *torturing environments* as part of an alternative theoretical approach to the definition of torture.

We will return to these points when presenting an integrative proposal in Chapters 17 and 18.

8

THE NEUROBIOLOGY OF PSYCHOLOGICAL TORTURE

The neurobiology of trauma includes the neurobiology of psychological torture. There are many different theoretical models in the research on the neurobiology of Post-Traumatic Stress Disorder (PTSD), and reviewing them goes beyond the scope of this chapter. Nearly twenty-five years ago, Saporta and van der Kolk (1992) published a review that integrated clinical, ethological and experimental data that continues to be the main reference text on the subject. Here we choose to focus on two main models of trauma: the fear model and the memory/information processing model.

The fear model views trauma as a conditioned response to an extremely fearful experience that remains inscripted in the amygdala and the limbic system: evoking past situations triggers anxiety. The memory/information processing model emphasises the survivor's difficulties in integrating traumatic events in an ordered and coherent memory sequence (time, space and meaning). The first theory situates the problem in the circuits of fear and startle responses, mainly based in the amygdala, the second in the system of archiving and retrieval of autobiographical memory, based in the hippocampus (Brewin and Holmes, 2003; Ehlers, Maercker and Boos, 2000; Ehring, Ehlers and Glucksman, 2006). Almost all of the research regarding torture survivors follows the fear-based response model. We will briefly review the evidence for each model here.

Fear and loss of controllability

Trauma has traditionally been defined as a **fear-based response** (Cantor, 2009), and fear as the central emotion in PTSD (Silove, 1998). This was, to an extent, the position of the Diagnostic and Statistical Manual of Mental Disorders (DSM-IV). PTSD is seen as a disorder of heightened defense and a fear-conditioned response to an overwhelming aversive stimulus.

Some proponents of the fear model argue that the real clue that explains the impact of a traumatic event is not the fear emotion itself, but the unpredictability of events and lack of control. We sense that reality becomes uncontrollable as events surpass a certain level. This perspective posits that the very **lack of controllability** of events is the best defining and determining element of trauma (Carlson and Dalenberg, 2000; Foa, Hearst-Ikeda and Perry, 1995).

This aligns with testimonies of torture survivors. As we saw in Chapter 2, survivors discussed the feeling of being completely at the mercy of others and subsequent feelings of 'uncontrollability' and 'unpredictability', as expressed in Marcelo Viñar's concept of the destructive power of the 'waiting time'. Lack of control and being at the mercy of others is probably one of the most distressing and damaging elements of psychological torture – more than pain itself, as Liscano, Villani and Larreta emphasised in the texts in Chapter 2.

Learning theory

Fear and the impact of uncontrollability are at the heart of the **learning theory** formulation of psychological torture (Başoğlu and Mineka, 1992), which is based on well-known experiments, conducted by Seligman and others in the 1960s and 1970s, on the effects of inescapable shock on lab animals.[1] According to the learning theory model, torture will have more impact when it includes (1) frequent exposure to multiple, unpredictable, uncontrollable stressors that threaten physical or psychological equilibrium and (2) lack of control over the stressors, leading to a state of total helplessness.

This formulation implies that a particular situation, when considered together with other contextual elements, constitutes torture to the extent that it maximises helplessness and lack of control. It also implies that the traumatic impact of torture depends on the uncontrollability of the stressor (i.e. torture technique) and the extent of the helplessness it induces (Başoğlu et al., 2007).

The effects of the stressor depend on the context. This means that the impact of specific threats to the detainee increases when combined with other factors (such as sleep and food deprivation, or restriction of movement) that *emphasise the victim's lack of control* over the environment. The term 'torture' refers to an entire context that induces helplessness, lack of control and fear. These overwhelming emotions are inscripted in the brain and appear as flashbacks, traumatic memories of torture and conscious or unconscious avoidance of situations and stimuli that recall past trauma (Brewin, Dalgleish, and Joseph, 1996). Moreover, the production of fear begins at the moment of detention – often at night or in the early morning – by creating an atmosphere of uneasiness, extreme anguish and fear. This fear is at the core of techniques that might at first seem to be purely physical. In wet-asphyxia (called the 'submarino' in Argentina, the 'tacho' in Uruguay, and 'waterboarding' in the US), the victim is submerged in a water tank, or water is poured over his or her mouth and nose. This torture method leads to a near-death experience in which victims feel suffocated, a situation that survivors describe as one of the most terrifying experiences that a human being can endure (Pardo, 2014). The acute physical suffering produced during the immediate infliction of 'waterboarding' overlaps with the often unbearable terror of the expected repetition of the experience. In the aftermath, the experience may lead to horrific memories that persist in the form of recurrent flashbacks and nightmares[2] (Reyes, 2008).

As fear increases, it leads to shock, confusion, distrust, lack of sleep, mental exhaustion, isolation and startle responses to true or false alarms. It is well documented that this constant tension damages the body in general and the brain in particular through alterations in the neuroendocrine system and especially the dysregulation of the adrenal-cortisol-axis system, and that this damage can be permanent (Fields, 2008).

Do biological markers of psychological torture exist?

Ideally, one way to clarify the concept of psychological torture would be to find biological indicators sensitive and specific enough to distinguish torture from other traumatic events, or to quantify the impact of torture in an objective way. If we could identify torture's biological marker it would, in theory, open the door to assessing credibility and damage. There are new preliminary lines of research using neuro-image procedures (Nuclear Magnetic Resonance, Computed Tomography Scan and others), analysers of neural activity (electroencephalogram, evoked potentials or others), neuroendocrine markers (especially determinations of cortisol and cell markers), psychophysiological measures (the sweating test, cardiovascular reactivity and others) or neuropsychological tests (measures of attention, cognition, memory and higher-order functions). Some of them are already in use in interrogation processes, but only (as we will see later) to detect lying and deception.

The search for markers has been limited to fear theories, despite the fact that other theories about trauma exist. There is ample research on neural circuits associated with fear and anxiety responses in general and PTSD in particular (Kolassa and Elbert, 2007; Neumeister, Shannan and Krystal, 2007), and research on neuroendocrine correlates of the different clusters of symptoms of PTSD (Ressler et al., 2011; Southwick et al., 2007). The results, however, are mostly discouraging because they are not sufficiently specific.

Kolassa and Elbert (2007), following the fear-based models of torture reviewed above (Başoğlu and Mineka, 1992; Saporta and Kolk, 1992), have argued that there is a neural circuit of fear in the human brain that expands with each accumulative event of trauma. During an event the brain stores neutral or 'cold' memories, which include perceptual and emotional features of the situation and autobiographical context information (dates, external circumstances), and emotionally charged or 'hot' memories, including sensory-perceptual information (fear, helplessness, high pulse). Both hot and cold memories remain linked and form the nucleus of a network associated with the traumatic event. Subsequent traumatic events are associated with similar hot and cold memories, which are integrated into the already existing fear network, enlarging it by increasing the number of neural interconnections. The activation of a single item triggers a response from the entire fear network.

The circuit requires significant neuronal plasticity. This plasticity could be traced through small changes in the size of areas of the pre-frontal cortex, hippocampus and amygdala. A review of available studies (Karl et al., 2006; Neuner et al., 2010) suggest that there could be a significantly smaller hippocampal structure and slight hypertrophy of the pre-frontal cortex and amygdala in people with PTSD, compared to non-traumatised controls and participants traumatised without PTSD. Other reviews, in contrast, find that a majority of studies are inconclusive (Neumeister et al., 2007).

Studies of twins that compare siblings exposed and non-exposed to traumatic events show that the diminished size of the hippocampus appears in both twins and that it might be a trait pre-existing to the exposure to the trauma stressor. It's possible that such slight changes in the brain are a risk factor, and not a consequence of trauma. An alternative hypothesis grounded on a psychoanalytic framework posits that the alterations in the hippocampus may be caused by early childhood traumas shared by twins (Yehuda et al., 2010).

The same German group that conducted the research described above did functional imaging studies with MRIs in groups of torture survivors that show activation of different areas of the amygdala and prefrontal cortex associated with traumatic stimuli linked to their experience (Junghofer et al., 2003). The group also found that among subjects confronted with aversive images, people with PTSD (compared to normal controls and torture survivors without PTSD), produce a specific pattern in the activation of occipital lobe structures (Catani, Adenauer, Keil, Aichinger and Neuner, 2009). Using the same stimuli, but measuring the electric activity of the brain through Visual Evoked Potentials, the team found a pattern of early activation of electric activity in brain areas traditionally associated with fear circuits (Weierstall et al., 2011). There is also preliminary data showing increased peripheral reactivity in torture survivors exposed to disturbing images (Adenauer, Catani, Keil, Aichinger, and Neuner, 2010).

But seeing torture only as a memory-based, fear-conditioned response limits our view of a survivor's experience. Many other predisposing, precipitating and maintaining factors explain why there are different responses among torture victims, from resilience to permanent damage. Fear is a good starting point, but not the only path to a more complete understanding of survivors' experiences.

Self-conscious emotions

Other overwhelming emotions like sadness and anger have been less extensively explored, but there is data showing that they contribute to explaining traumatic reactions independently of fear (Rizvi, Kaysen, Gutner, Griffin and Resick, 2008). Especially important, as seen in Chapter 5, are the emotions of humiliation, embarrassment, shame and guilt (Baer and Vorbrügeen, 2007; Harman and Lee, 2010). These are known as secondary emotions: they are not part of the group of basic emotions that all human beings seem to have at birth, but appear at two to three years of age as a person develops their own identity an independent individual. This means that humiliation, shame and guilt do not appear as priming answers to a menace (as does fear) but require the victim's self-consciousness, as well as an appraisal–evaluative component that connects the relationship with the context (specifically, with the perpetrator and bystanders). These emotions are elicited not by a *physical threat* but by a *threat to self and identity*.

Preliminary data suggests that self-conscious emotions enhance and prolong primary threat feelings (Harman and Lee, 2010). Moreover, different studies have consistently shown that guilt is a better predictor than fear of long-term psychological distress in female survivors of sexual assault (Resick and Miller, 2009). These findings highlight the fact that fear does not play the only role in explaining long-term psychological distress; they point to the necessity of exploring the full range of possible reactions, and the interaction between conditioned responses and higher cortical evaluative processes.

Neuropsychological evidence of torture

The Istanbul Protocol encourages the use of neuropsychological tests as an important adjunctive tool in the diagnosis of torture. Unfortunately, this area of study has been widely neglected. A review on the subject in medical and psychological literature shows very few results regarding best practices, recommended tests, interpretation of profiles, differential diagnoses or research related to the existence of torture.

Neuropsychological tests can provide an accurate picture of the performance of higher brain functions, and clearly distinguish between damage secondary to traumatic brain injury and damage linked to psychological trauma (Mollica et al., 2009; Weinstein, Fucetola and Mollica, 2001). Among many other things, testing can determine the impact of torture on attention and memory, psychomotor functions, learning capacities, symbolic and logical reasoning and other dynamic indicators of the brain at work. It also allows for a differential diagnosis between PTSD and brain contusion (Joseph and Masterson, 1999; Weinstein et al., 2001), or between organic and dissociative amnesia (Sutker, Vasterling, Brailey and Allain, 1995).

Jacobs (2008, see also Jacobs & Iacopino, 2001) has made compelling appeals for neuropsychological testing, unfortunately with little success. Such tests are very time consuming, and a full exploration might require more than a day's work from a dedicated specialist.

Additionally, difficulties are faced when applying tests that need careful calibration and sometimes depend on the education and cultural background of the patient.

In the era of high-tech neuroimaging and detection of the brain's electrical activity, it seems that neuropsychological tests have a limited future. Clinicians prefer tests that can be run in seconds, tests that provide powerful color images of reality. But the truth is that the unexplored possibilities of neuropsychology are enormous. Inexplicably, its use has been limited and scarce research has been conducted.

Conclusions: from nonspecific to specific correlates

Different theories explain trauma and traumatic responses, but in the field of torture research only those linked to the circuits of fear and to self-conscious emotions have been explored. This is no surprise: survivors themselves have acknowledged several key features of the experience of torture, including fear, uncertainty, lack of control, humiliation and shame.

With the development of new neuroimaging procedures, it is now possible to find gross biological correlates of torture in the brain: it appears that a diminished size of the hippocampus, an enlargement of pre-frontal cortex and the amygdala, and changes in electric activity are consistent with torture.

The results of these studies, all of which were conducted by the same research group at the University of Konstanz, Germany, are difficult to interpret. They explain all of their findings as convergent and coincident indicators that signal an increase in, and lower activation threshold for, the neural circuits of fear. But it is not clear whether this is a marker of pre-existing vulnerability, a generalisation of a fear-conditioning situation or – as they propose – a sensitisation process through an increase of fear structures by neural adaptation. It is unclear whether there are other, more plausible explanations than the fear hypothesis. Though existing research does point to a promising new path, there is clearly a need for more research by other groups, using different samples and paradigms.

The true significance of this biological data associated with the experience of torture has yet to be demonstrated. All of these lines of research are promising, and it is possible that in the distant future biological markers of brain alterations may be specific enough to be useful for judicial and forensic purposes: x-rays for seeing broken bones and fMRIs for seeing broken minds. But this is far from what we have at the present. Currently, markers are unreliable, and trying to relate neurobiological alterations to certain events in the past, to symptoms or to diagnoses is, at best, risky. In any case, the cost and feasibility of these kinds of procedures make them completely unrealistic for actual work with torture survivors.

In the meantime, the potential use of neuropsychology as a diagnostic tool for better understanding psychological torture remains largely untested.

Notes

1 Inescapable shock experiments involved giving electric shocks to an animal placed in a box while not allowing it to stop the shocks (e.g. by pressing a lever). Exposure to such stressors causes certain associative, motivational and emotional deficits in animals that closely resemble the effects of traumatic stress in humans. These deficits include a phenomenon characterised by failure of animals initially exposed to uncontrollable shocks to learn to escape or avoid shocks later.
2 Despite the intense suffering they cause, these so-called 'fear-up' methods are considered part of a normal interrogation both in the KUBARK Manual and the list of authorised methods in CIA interrogation manuals.

9

TRAUMA THEORY AND THE CONCEPT OF PSYCHOLOGICAL TORTURE

The concept of 'trauma'

The debate surrounding the definition of psychological torture closely resembles the debate on the concept of trauma. After decades of international consensual classifications, psychiatry still lacks a satisfactory definition of trauma. For some authors, torture is simply a very specific kind of traumatic event (Gerrity, Keane and Tuma, 2001), while others have debated the pros and cons of developing specific diagnostic criteria for torture survivors (including diagnostic criteria for a 'torture syndrome') and the suitability of granting torture specific status as a complex traumatic event (Genefke and Vesti, 1998). We will briefly review the debate on the definition of psychological trauma in clinical psychiatry in order to understand the lessons and insights that psychiatry can offer for a general theory of psychological torture.

Who defines trauma? Etic and emic approaches

The main theoretical difficulty with finding a universal definition of what constitutes a 'traumatic event' is that trauma (i.e. the psychological damage associated with a threatening event) is far from a universal response. People can react to many different *potentially* traumatic events with a wide range of possible responses.

Most psychologists and psychiatrists working with torture survivors apply standard diagnostic criteria (e.g. the International Classification of Diseases (ICD-11), or the Diagnostic and Statistical Manual for Mental Disorders (DSM-V)) in their daily work to fulfil specific clinical or legal requirements, but feel more comfortable working with symptoms and narratives. A narrative is the personal 'story' that a person narrates to him or herself about what happened, as well as the feelings and cognitions around that 'story'.

This purely subjective experience of trauma is exactly what allows mental health professionals to become closer to the patient and to work together in the special kind of dialogue called psychotherapy. A *narrative-constructionist* view of reality approaches reality as a mental phenomenon and not a given fact. Elements associated with context are encoded in the mind: sensory inputs, cognitions, feelings; sometimes they are encoded in a fragmented and chaotic way. They are later recalled and narrated in quite difficult conditions: traumatic experiences are, in themselves, often unspeakable and sometimes unthinkable. Most people do not find the words to express these feelings and experiences or find them lacking and disconnected from the events. The final narrative that emerges is a mix of what happened, what can be told and what has been heard from similar past experiences and from other survivors who were present at the time (Fernández Liria and Rodríguez Vega, 2001; Herlihy and Turner, 2006; Pérez Sales, 2006). The shape the narrative takes depends on the group and audience that provides feedback on the narrative (Laney and Loftus, 2013). It is heavily influenced by the survivors' coping mechanisms – whether they are more active and confrontational or more focused on emotion regulation (Muller, 2010). And, of course, the narrative's form is also linked to the amount of 'truth' that the cognisant mind can deal with and the parts that remain in the unconscious mind as dissociated material. In terms of a definition, in our daily work, something is traumatic in as much as the patient feels that it is traumatic and reacts accordingly to it.

This explains why there are infinite ways of reacting and psychologically processing the same event, and why a certain traumatogenic experience can have a small impact on one survivor while changing another survivor's worldview.

In a recent qualitative study among 30 Argentinians that underwent long-term political imprisonment and torture in the 1980s, most considered themselves to be survivors and rejected the idea that they continued to endure psychological sequelae from torture (Arnoso, 2010). In contrast, Gudjonsson (2003) described treating a patient who was severely traumatised and needed long-term support psychotherapy after one incident in which he was called in for two hours as a witness (but not charged) for a routine investigative interrogation in a police station. The patient associated this routine procedure with an intense feeling of dishonour that he could not overcome. For most people, rape is the worst traumatic experience, and many studies show its long-lasting consequences. But it is also well known that some rape survivors report that in retrospect, they felt that their reaction at the time of the rape made them stronger (Wasco, 2003), and that this prevailed over feelings of damage or trauma. The percentage of resilient survivors of even the most horrifying experiences is larger than is generally thought. This is the reason why concepts such as 'rape syndrome' and 'torture syndrome' were finally abandoned.

Working with a narrative model is an essentialist subjective position, and many psychiatrists and psychotherapists will defend it as the only logical position, especially if they work in complex multicultural contexts (Kleinman, 1999).

The debate over whether to work with objective categories versus subjective narratives is an old one in other disciplines. Anthropology has debated the etic–emic dichotomy (or the tension between Comparatists and Particularists) for decades. An emic position assumes that the informant's version is the nucleus of knowledge. An etic position assumes that the theory and the categories of the anthropologist, as a person external to the culture under examination, are the nucleus of knowledge. In the end, we need an emic position to be close to the population we work with, but we need an etic position if we want science to advance. Infinite studies on subjective experiences can hardly build new knowledge.

On the other hand, this radically subjective position confronts us with a paradox: if trauma is what the patient defines as trauma, then everything is potentially traumatic. This has led to the appearance of dozens of new 'trauma' syndromes associated with various everyday experiences: discovering a lover's affair, the dissolution of a romantic relationship (Chung, Farmer and Grant, 2002), fear or pain associated with normal delivery of a healthy baby (Reynolds, 1997), or teasing by peers in the classroom or workplace (Hershcovis, 2011), for example. Can we equate the experience of a Rwandan genocide survivor to any of these everyday, normal life experiences of crisis or adaptive pain? From a subjective point of view, the answer is yes. One can certainly suffer permanent psychological consequences from any quotidian situation (even the most banal) provided there are specific vulnerability factors and circumstances. Medicalising human life is not a good idea: we do not medicalise grief and mourning, and we shouldn't do so with trauma. Pérez–Sales (2006) has defined trauma as:

1. An experience constituting a threat to a person's physical or psychological integrity that is frequently (a) associated to experiences of chaos or confusion during the event, (b) fragmentation of memory, (c) absurdity, (d) atrocity, (e) ambivalence or (e) bewilderment
2. Having an unspeakable, undiscussable nature incomprehensible to others
3. Breaking one or more basic assumptions serving as points of reference for human beings regarding their safety, specifically (a) beliefs of invulnerability and control over their own life, (b) trust in others, in their kindness and predisposition towards empathy, and (c) trust in the controllable and predictable nature of the world.
4. Causing questioning of views of the self in the world

The traumatic experience is also often associated with:

1. A subjective, conscious or unconscious yet indelible scar
2. Feelings of alienation towards others who have not had the traumatic experience
3. Isolation and estrangement
4. Affective and emotional withdrawal
5. Confrontation with experiences of personal responsibility and guilt
6. Confrontation with feelings of humiliation and shame, or questioning one's personal dignity
7. A process of personal rebuilding and integration of the experience and ability to foster posttraumatic growth

A view combining biology and subjectivity, centred on the person and considering an experience traumatic when it is an extremely threatening situation physically or psychologically that, for whatever reason, cannot be integrated into one's memory and personal narratives and therefore becomes frozen and calls one's self and one's self in the world into question. As we will see later, the idea that trauma changes identity and worldviews is a helpful starting point that combines both positions (Pérez Sales, 2006).

Traumatic events in clinical psychiatry

The concept of trauma in clinical psychiatry can be traced by following the diagnostic criteria of Post-Traumatic Stress Disorder (PTSD), the clinical diagnosis specifically linked to potentially traumatic events. PTSD, as we know it today, first appeared in the third edition of the Diagnostic and Statistical Manual of Mental Disorders (American Psychiatric Association, 1980). It defined trauma as a recognisable stressor 'that would evoke significant symptoms of distress in almost everyone' and that was 'generally outside the range of usual human experience' (Criterion A). The logic behind this definition was to protect victims and prevent blaming them as suffering from weakness or character flaws by appealing to a kind of universal vulnerability to certain experiences. But epidemiological studies (Breslau et al., 1998) showed that the concept of 'usual human experience' was a vague and indefinite expression heavily dependent on cultural milieu, personal experiences and social class, among other factors (Weathers and Keane, 2007). In other words, being detained and interrogated using physical force can be considered among 'normal', 'logical' or 'expected' events in certain countries where human rights abuses include much more lethal forms of violations. It is not strange to find torture survivors from African or Asian countries who see treatment such as being naked, slapped, shouted at, insulted or not being allowed to eat or sleep as simply part of the 'usual' treatment one can expect in a short-term detention centre (Assistance Association for Political Prisioners [Burma], 2005). From an *etic* point of view – which guides international classifications – the stressor criterion (Criterion A) was considered too indeterminate to be the basis for a universal definition of 'trauma'.

The APA Committee reformulated the 'usual human experience' criterion in DSM-III-R and, ten years later, in DSM-IV. A traumatic event became an incident in which a person has 'experienced, witnessed, or been confronted with an event or events that involve actual or threatened death or serious injury, or a threat to the physical integrity to oneself or others' (American Psychiatric Association, 1994, p. 428). The new emphasis was on *perceiving a threat* to the physical integrity of the person. This definition would specifically exclude non-physical torture as a traumatic event (Priebe and Bauer, 1995). The World Health Organization, in its 10th edition of the International Classification of Diseases, disagreed and considered that trauma should include threats to '*physical and psychological integrity*' (World Health Organization, 2010).

The 'perceived threat' criterion was clearly better than the previous one. Different studies have shown that the severity of a traumatic response does not depend on the *actual* menace to the integrity of the person, but to the subjective perception of the event, and that this is linked to the emotions that the person feels (Beck, Palyo, Canna, Blanchard and Gudmundsdottir, 2006; Rizvi et al., 2008). Freezing emotions or extreme fear (among many other factors) were better predictors of long-term distress than the actual threat or the perception of danger associated with the threat. An injured person could recognise that he was next to die in a very severe car accident, but experienced no fear or perception of lack of control during the event and thus has scarce psychological sequelae. On the other hand, his best friend could be involved in a minor crash in which no one was injured, and feel overwhelmed and blocked, causing long-lasting psychological damage. The long-term impact seems to depend less on the objective risk to life than on the existence of an overwhelming emotional reaction at the moment of the accident which becomes imprinted in the mind.

To overcome this difficulty, the trauma criterion of PTSD (Criterion A) was further revised in DSM-IV to require that the person's response to the event (Criterion A2) involve '*intense fear, helplessness, or horror*' (American Psychiatric Association, 1994). The central point for defining trauma was, then, living or witnessing a life-threatening event associated with an intense *emotional response*. The logic behind this is the conceptualisation of trauma as a fear-based response, as presented in Chapter 8.

The line that separates normalcy from trauma is crossed *when the emotions associated with the event are so overwhelming that they leave a permanent mark on the survivor's mind*. Avoidance reactions, hyperactivity, and especially intrusive symptoms (flashbacks, nightmares) do not tend to disappear with time, but endure as a conditioned response to this extreme fear or helplessness.

The preparation of the next edition, DSM-V, took a new turn when a theoretical dispute arose between two opposite positions. On one hand, several authors argued that overwhelming emotions – specifically fear – should constitute the *core* of any definition of trauma. They proposed strengthening the DSM-IV position, and that the concept of trauma should be strictly limited to fear-induced responses (Brewin, Lanius, Novac, Schnyder, and Galea, 2009). On the other, a group of influential authors proposed exactly the opposite: that any mention of emotions (extreme fear, horror or helplessness) (Criterion A) should be abolished from the definition. They wrote that (1) the criteria confused the traumatic event with the person's response to the inciting event, and (2) the initial emotional response actually reflects the expression of an underlying personal resilience or vulnerability to the stressor. It is a consequence, not a cause. Lastly, they argued that (3) the number of emotional responses to traumatic events is far broader than fear and horror, and also includes emotions like shame, betrayal, guilt and rage (McNally, 2010; Resick and Miller, 2009).

The APA's decisions quite often have more to do with internal disputes over control and power than with science. The DSM-V supported the latter position and, contradicting the DSM-IV, decided that a traumatic event is when a person (1) is exposed to death, death threats, actual or threatened serious injury, or actual or threatened sexual violence; (2) because of direct exposure, personally witnessing, indirect repeated exposure through his or her profession, or learning that a close relative or close friend was thus threatened or injured. In earlier drafts of DSM-V there was a list of traumatic events that could qualify for Criterion A. In the end, only rape was explicitly retained. Criterion A2, related to overwhelming emotions, was deleted because 'it had not proven any predictive value' (American Psychiatric Association, 2013).

This position has its critics, myself among them. Fear is not a *consequence* of trauma (in which case they would be right and it would not make sense to include it in the definition) but rather an *etiological* factor. From this perspective, it is the overwhelming emotion that originates traumatic damage by imprinting a mark in the memory. While trauma is much more than emotions, emotions are, as defined above, an indissociable component of trauma, firmly associated and encoded in memory.

On the other hand, DSM-III-R cited specific examples of situations that would be considered 'traumatic events' including combat, rape, natural disasters and torture. It disqualified stressors falling within the ambit of ordinary life, such as bereavement or marital disputes. This disappeared in DSM-IV, likely because the Committee considered that listing traumatic stressors is an empirical matter, not a conceptual one. The consequence was, as explained in the introduction to this chapter, the proliferation of studies exploring 'trauma' in the most banal daily life experiences. This was not corrected in DSM-V, except for rape, which was specifically cited as a traumatic event.

What we can learn from the debate over the concept of trauma

The evolution of the concept of trauma has been a process of trial and error, of refinement. With each new version of the DSM the definition has changed, from an extensional definition ('extraordinary events'), to a subjective consequentialist definition ('overwhelming emotions'), and now to an objective consequentialist definition ('threat'). The field has shown the difficulties in finding a consensus, but there are very important lessons to be learned from this process.

If the definition of torture had followed the debate on trauma, then

1. It would exclude the criteria of 'severe suffering' from the definition of torture (a definition of trauma does not rely on the objective severity of the threat).

2. It would not include examples of specific torture methods (an extensional definition).
3. It would consider exposure to threat as the core feature, associated (DSM-IV) or not (DSM-V) with overwhelming emotions (subjective experiences) that leave permanent marks.

It is important to note that the position reflected in these three points is not new in jurisprudence. As seen in Chapter 3, the European Court of Human Rights embraced that same position in the famous *Selmouni v. France* sentence: severe suffering (physical or psychological) was not a relevant factor in defining torture, or, in their words, 'proof of the actual effect may not be a factor' (ECHR, 1999). The Human Rights Committee has also emitted similar pronouncements (Rodley and Pollard, 2009) and the definition of the Inter-American Convention is clear on this.

Clinical consequences of torture

There are more than one hundred studies on the clinical prevalence of psychiatric disorders in general, and PTSD in particular, in torture survivors. Most of them offer data from mixed samples of refugees fleeing from war who were attended to in different specialised and non-specialised health care settings; data from epidemiological studies in refugee camps; or data from post-conflict settings in which it is difficult to isolate the effect of torture from other stressors. Additionally, most studies use general screening tools for any kind of traumatic events linked to war or violence (like the Harvard Trauma Questionnaire) and do not include a comparison group (Gorst-Unsworth and Goldenberg, 1998; Holtz, 1998; Mollica et al., 1993; Pfeiffer and Elbert, 2011). This helps explain why the results are so divergent.

A review of some of these uncontrolled studies showed a prevalence of PTSD ranging from 15 to 85 per cent, in most cases associated with anxiety or depressive syndromes (Başoğlu, Jaranson, Mollica and Kastrup, 2001). In a recent collaborative study conducted in five centres from the IRCT network (Gaza, Egypt, Mexico, Honduras and South Africa) that provide health, social and legal services to torture survivors, the overall prevalence of PTSD across samples was 40 per cent with important differences among centres (McColl et al., 2010). De Jong et al. (2001) studied post-conflict populations in Algeria, Cambodia, Gaza and Ethiopia, and found rates of PTSD ranging from 16 to 37 per cent. On average, taking into account that the prevalence of PTSD in the general population is less than 2 per cent (Alonso et al., 2004), there is a very high prevalence of PTSD among torture survivors with figures ranging from 10 to 80 per cent.

Controlled studies consistently show that refugees who have suffered torture are at greater risk of mental disorder than non-tortured refugees (de Jong et al., 2001; Jaranson et al., 2004; Shrestha and Sharma, Van Ommeren, 1998). For instance, in a classical case-control study with Turkish political prisoners, 33 per cent of the tortured group had lifelong post-traumatic stress disorders, as compared with 11 per cent of the non-tortured group (Başoğlu et al., 1994). Jaranson et al. (2004) found six times more prevalence of PTSD (25 per cent vs. 4 per cent) in tortured (n=502) versus non-tortured (n=632) Oromo and Somali refugees in the US state of Minnesota. Masmas et al. (2008) found a similar proportion in Denmark (63 per cent vs. 10 per cent) among new asylum seekers from 33 countries (n=142). And Van Ommeren et al. (2001) found 10 times more instances of PTSD (43 per cent vs. 4 per cent) in a sample of 810 (418 tortured and 392 non-tortured) Bhutanese refugees in Nepal.

Two reviews and a meta-analysis of post-conflict studies concur that torture and cumulative trauma are the strongest predictors of PTSD when compared to other pre-migration stressors

(Johnson and Thompson, 2008; Rousseau et al., 2011; Steel et al., 2009) with post-migration stressors contributing independently.

Finally, as we saw in Chapter 7, survivors who suffered psychological torture had a similar or higher prevalence of PTSD than people who had suffered physical torture (Başoğlu et al., 2007; Punamäki et al., 2010), which raises the question of whether or not there can be any meaningful medical or psychological distinction drawn in the legal distinction between torture and CIDT.

In short, the prevalence of PTSD in uncontrolled studies with torture survivors ranges from 15 to 85 per cent with an estimated average of around 40 per cent. In controlled studies there is a threefold prevalence in tortured versus non-tortured refugees. Torture predicts PTSD, and psychological torture predicts more than physical torture.

The torture's impact on identity and worldviews

The applicability of psychiatric categories to torture survivors is vigorously debated (Williams and van der Merwe, 2013). The early works of pioneering therapists in Latin America did not even consider the possibility of applying psychiatric diagnoses to torture survivors. There is no mention of PTSD in any of the writings of Elizabeth Lira or Paz Rojas (in Chile), Diana Kordon, Dario Lagos or Lucila Edelman (Argentina), or Marcelo and Maren Viñar (Uruguay), among many others who worked in the nearly 30 centres for the rehabilitation of torture victims that appeared in the 1980s and 1990s in Latin America. Some of these writings were compiled by Martín-Baró (1990) in his seminal book *Psicología Social de la Guerra: Trauma y Terapia* (*Social Psychology of War: Trauma and Therapy*) and in the collective text *Paisajes de Dolor, Senderos de Esperanza (Landscapes of Pain, Paths of Hope)*[1] (EATIP, 2002). The use of clinical diagnoses in work with torture survivors was seen as a medicalisation of reality that deprived torture survivors of something more central and decisive in therapy: the political nature of what happened to them, and the need to interpret the medical consequences in context to find a meaning in suffering and, ultimately, to cope.

The debate was at the forefront of torture research in the 1980s, and the IRCT decided to convene a special Consensus Group (Genefke and Vesti, 1998). The group conducted an international survey among all torture centres linked to the network in order to cement an official common position. It was the age of DSM-III and DSM-III-R. Allodi (1982), in a description of the symptoms in a Canadian sample, described a 'torture syndrome' that 'closely resembles PTSD as defined in DSM-III', although some years later he said that there was not enough evidence for proposing a 'torture syndrome' as a diagnosis in DSM-IV, and in most cases the PTSD diagnosis would suffice. This position was quite close to the final position adopted by the IRCT Consensus Group. Although they acknowledged the important reservations that came mainly from Latin American professionals, the IRCT considered that the category of PTSD was a suitable tool and recommended its use. Many studies at that time (e.g. Gorst-Unsworth and Goldenberg, 1998; Mollica, Gaspi-Yavin, Bollini and Truong, 1992) debated the 'torture syndrome' but considered the use of the standard category of PTSD the preferable option.

But that was also a time when research on the psychological consequences of torture needed scientific recognition, and the IRCT had a pragmatic position: torture needed to be accepted as a medical issue in the academy, and torture victims deserved recognition and compensation. This could be achieved if there were scientific studies that convinced politicians, academics and the population in general of the severe psychological and psychiatric consequences of torture (Genefke and Vesti, 1998). At the same time, the group also acknowledged that without medical findings, the core symptoms of patients (low self-esteem and guilt, changes in personality that affected the wholeness of the self, physical sequelae without organic substrate, and physical complaints – and especially pain) were of marginal value in the diagnostic criteria of PTSD. So they proposed using PTSD, even though the concept of PTSD did not capture all of the essential elements of the psychological suffering of torture survivors.

It became increasingly evident that the diagnosis of PTSD failed to capture the full range of psychophysiological symptoms linked to the brain's immediate defense response in the face of an aggression (as seen in Chapter 8). A PTSD diagnosis did not capture the impact torture had on patients who were struggling to make meaningful sense of what happened to them and process their experiences, or survivors whose identity and worldviews had been transformed (Herman, 1992; Janoff-Bulman, 1992; Pelcovitz et al., 1997).

Over time, the IRCT soon began to reconsider its early, mostly clinical position and accept alternative perspectives that complemented mainstream diagnostic categories. Academic trauma theorists from the US developed concepts like Complex PTSD and Adult Cumulative Trauma, which attempted to define new ideas that were quite close to what Latin American psychologists proposed in the 1980s, albeit from a more humanitarian, non-political point of view.

However, as these concepts gained renewed recognition, many of the key questions posed by Latin American psychologists were lost. But their key elements are valid and remain fully valid today. First, trauma is not an individual phenomenon, but a psychosocial problem (Martín-Baró, 1990) that must be understood within the dialectical relationship between society and the individual. Torture (as perpetrated by the state) can only be understood as part of the local – and global – fight against political oppression. To deprive the survivor of this perspective is to be complicit with the perpetrators, and doing so furthers the physical, psychological and social death of a political activist or human rights defender. Second, although the symptoms of PTSD do exist, there are strong objections to the idea that they can be gathered into one coherent syndrome that excludes all consideration of the deep psychological meaning of trauma. Third, the psychological consequences of torture cannot be understood without tracing a history of trauma that includes early trauma experiences and attachment, family history and transgenerational trauma. Furthermore, the impact cannot be understood without an understanding of the current circumstances of the survivor's social and economic deprivation or exile. Lastly, in a clinical context, it is the torture survivor's interpretation that matters, especially in multicultural contexts. Being able to listen is more important than the ability to diagnose. The concept of PTSD leads to models of cognitive behavioural therapy and narrative exposure that reduce trauma symptoms, but quite often do not go deep into the survivor's experiences. It might consider the painful lessons of a traumatic experience of struggle and oppression to be 'cognitive errors' amendable to correction by middle-class, well-off therapists who hardly understand what the survivor has endured.

We need PTSD and other DSM-V/ICD-11 diagnoses as a reflection of part of what happens to a torture survivor, and as a consensual tool for forensic and academic purposes. However, we must be aware that it skims the surface of reality, and if used as the sole conceptual reference, it definitely blinds us in our daily work.

Complex Post-Traumatic Stress Disorder, EPCACE, DESNOS, mental death and beyond

Part of this alternative view that Latin American authors put forward and IRCT has lately collected has been included in official classifications, under the ICD-10 category of Enduring

Personality Change After Catastrophic Experience (EPCACE) (F62.0). The World Health Organization defines EPCACE as a disorder 'present for at least two years, following exposure to catastrophic stress. The stress must be so extreme that it is not necessary to consider personal vulnerability in order to explain its profound effect on the personality. The disorder is characterised by a hostile or distrustful attitude toward the world, social withdrawal, feelings of emptiness or hopelessness, a chronic feeling of "being on edge" as if constantly threatened, and estrangement.' Post-traumatic stress disorder (F43.1) may precede this type of personality change, but the two diagnoses are considered by ICD to be mutually exclusive.

The WHO specifically states that EPCACE appears after 'concentration camp experiences, prolonged captivity with an imminent possibility of being killed, exposure to life-threatening situations such as being a victim of terrorism and torture'. The Istanbul Protocol recommended using the EPCACE diagnosis, but unfortunately there are very few studies that include it as a relevant category, probably because the ICD-10 definition is not operational and relies on the clinicians' expert criteria to decide whether or not a patient has EPCACE. In 1999, an expert survey (Beltran and Silove, 1999) explored the pros and cons of this newly created diagnosis. Many respondents acknowledged interest and 91 per cent (n=65) agreed that it could be a good diagnosis to describe the clinical consequences of torture, but only 16 per cent of experts had in fact ever used it. The survey showed that many experts recognise that PTSD may be too limited in its coverage of the possible adaptational consequences of human-engendered trauma and that EPCACE filled the gap in many ways, but the lack of operational criteria precluded its use. The same research group, 10 years later, reassessed their results in a new sample of 28 experts (Beltran, Llewellyn and Silove, 2008) and proposed additional criteria for a better definition of EPCACE (Table 9.1).

TABLE 9.1 Enduring Personality Change after Catastrophic Experience (EPCACE): proposed criteria after an expert survey

---

Criteria A. Hostile or mistrustful attitude towards the world
A hostile attitude is manifested through aggression, rage, anger and/or hatred. A distrustful attitude is shown by fear, sense of withholding and/or paranoia. The hostile or distrustful attitude is directed toward society and its structures, toward individuals, toward perpetrators, toward other groups and toward the self.

Criteria B. Social withdrawal
Tendency to isolate or social isolation. Impact on survivor's ability to communicate and to develop and maintain relationships. Apathy. Does not communicate with anyone and holds the view that there's nothing to talk about.

Criteria C. Feelings of emptiness or hopelessness
Lack of self-worth, a sense of nothingness, and anhedonia. Hopelessness is characterised by a sense of powerlessness and passivity, of futility and despair, and of foreshortened future. May be associated with prolonged depression.

Criteria D. Chronic feeling of being 'on edge' as if constantly threatened. Increased vigilance. Restlessness, hypersensitivity and permanent fear underlie this behavior. Anxious mood. Cognitive problems (difficulty concentrating, remembering and thinking clearly) and sleep disturbance (insomnia, nightmares and tiredness).

Criteria E. Estrangement. Alienation from someone that they were before, who they no longer are. Additional criteria: (a) somatisation, (b) self-injurious/self-damaging behaviors, (c) sexual dysfunction, (d) enduring guilt.

Adapted from Beltran, R. O., Silove, D. and Llewellyn, G. M. (2009).

The task group on Anxiety Disorders of the DSM system have also been debating the necessity of introducing the category of 'complex traumatic stress disorder', now referred to in the literature by several names such as complex PTSD (Herman, 1992), Disorder of Extreme Stress (DES) (Pelcovitz et al., 1997; van der Kolk et al., 2005), Disorder of Extreme Stress Not Otherwise Specified (DESNOS), Developmental Trauma Disorder (DTD) or Mental Death/ Adult Onset Complex Post Traumatic Stress Disorder (AO-CPTSD).

The Disorder of Extreme Stress Not Otherwise Specified (DESNOS) includes a broad range of symptoms reflecting disturbances in affective and interpersonal self-regulatory capacities (e.g. difficulty with anxious arousal, anger management, dissociative symptoms, somatic complaints and socially avoidant behaviours) thought to develop after exposure to ongoing interpersonal trauma. Although it has been proposed as a new category for the DSM on different occasions, it has been criticised (and excluded) for lack of specificity in its criteria and its overlap with dissociative disorders, borderline personality disorders, and PTSD (Jongedijk et al., 1996; Roth et al., 1997), and weak cross-cultural validity (de Jong et al., 2005). Currently, DESNOS is not in the DSM as a stand-alone syndrome but the symptoms are listed as associated features of PTSD that are likely to occur when an individual is exposed to chronic interpersonal trauma.

The Developmental Trauma Disorder (DTD) describes the symptoms that may occur in children exposed to interpersonal trauma (e.g. abandonment, betrayal, physical and/or sexual assault). It includes symptoms of emotion dysregulation in response to traumatic events in affective, somatic, behavioural, cognitive, relational and self-attribution domains. The proponents of DTD sought to add a children's version of Complex PTSD to the DSM-V. It was included in field trials for the DSM-V, but ultimately discarded (Sar, 2011).

The ideas behind DES and DESNOS are connected to the dissociative experience linked to extreme trauma and the theories of structural dissociation (Van der Hart, Nijenhuis and Steele, 2005), while the idea of EPCACE is more closely related to enduring changes in identity and worldviews. They depart from different paradigms and cover different areas of the response to torture.

Adult Onset Complex Post-Traumatic Stress Disorder (AO-CPTSD) or 'mental death' defines the long-term consequences of exposure to coercive control in adulthood, focusing primarily on examples of torture and experiences in concentration camps (Ebert and Dyck, 2004). Mental death or 'mental defeat' (Ehlers, Maercker and Boos, 2000) is defined by the loss of the victim's pretrauma identity, loss of core beliefs and values, distrust and alienation from others, shame and guilt, and a sense of being permanently damaged (Table 9.2). Mental defeat represents a more severe form of damage to the self (Ehlers et al., 1998, 2000), and possibly an intermediate step towards mental death or complete loss of identity. It has been defined in survivors of rape as the opposite of 'mental planning' (i.e. coping). Mental planning is defined as thinking about or planning in one's mind what one might be able to do to minimise physical or psychological harm, to make the experience more tolerable or to influence the response of the assailant, whether or not the plan is successful. Mental defeat refers to the victim's perception that he or she gave up in his or her own mind and was defeated and left completely at the assailant's will; it includes losing the sense of being a person with autonomy and will, or no longer feeling human (Ehlers et al., 1998).

Evans (2012), in an unpublished doctoral dissertation, compared criteria for DESNOS, EPCACE and AO-CPTSD in a small sample (n=27) of refugees, most of them torture survivors. The results showed that DESNOS and AO-CPTSD failed to properly address the clinical changes that appeared in torture survivors. DESNOS was uncommon (3.7 per cent of sample) and there was wide variability in how often individual DESNOS symptoms occurred;

TABLE 9.2 Mental death: core domains/AO-CPTSD

1. Acting and living in ways that are inconsistent with the person's core beliefs, assumptions and values, which leads to a discontinuity of identity and can cause the person to feel shame and guilt during and after traumatic events.
2. Perceiving others differently from how they were previously perceived, especially in terms of diminishing a person's capacity to trust and become attached to other people.
3. Major changes to a person's view of the world, including beliefs related to social order, justice and safety.
4. Change in a person's behavior such that continuity is lost between pretrauma and posttrauma patterns of behavior and consequently perceptions of self.

Adapted from Ehlers, A., Maercker, A. and Boos, A. (2000).

it lacked consistency and coherence. AO-CPTSD was difficult to define and included items that did not contribute to the definition of the syndrome. In contrast, EPCACE exhibited satisfactory internal consistency and all items made an important contribution to defining the construct.

The results reflect the fact that the concept of mental death, although well described and reviewed (Ebert and Dyck, 2004) has not been operationalised or applied in any systematic research. In theory, it is probably the most promising construct to understand and work with the experiences of torture survivors. The name might be too dramatic and nonspecific, and attempts by the creators of the concept to link it to the controversial idea of 'complex PTSD' in order to make it more similar to mainstream psychiatry and research may not have worked in its favor. Nevertheless, it has not had the success in trauma literature that it likely deserves.

On a related note, the ICD criteria state that the diagnosis of EPCACE specifically excludes PTSD. In contrast, Evans finds that most people showing signs of EPCACE also have chronic PTSD and that both syndromes can be clearly distinguishable. She proposes that in future revisions, the ICD classification should allow for both diagnoses to be applied simultaneously – a practice that coincides with clinical experience.

The future

A World Health Organization working group proposed the inclusion of Complex PTSD in ICD-11, as reflecting 'A disorder which arises after exposure to a stressor typically of an extreme or prolonged nature and from which escape is difficult or impossible. The disorder is characterised by the core symptoms of PTSD as well as the development of persistent and pervasive impairments in affective, self and relational functioning, including difficulties in emotion regulation, beliefs about oneself as diminished, defeated or worthless, and difficulties in sustaining relationships' (Maercker et al., 2013). The working group found that the concept should replace the overlapping ICD-10 category of EPCACE which 'has failed to attract scientific interest and did not include disorders arising from prolonged stress in early childhood'.

The proposal considers three core features (Table 9.3).

Assessment of the impact of torture on worldviews

In the 1990s, the academic world began to develop tools for measuring the ontological and human side of trauma experiences, though none of these measurements were specifically

TABLE 9.3 Complex PTSD (F62.0): proposal of WHO-Working Group for ICD-11

1. **Cluster A. Difficulties in emotion regulation**. Manifested either as heightened emotional reactivity, or as a lack of emotions and lapses into dissociative states. Behavioural disturbances can include violent outbursts and reckless or self-destructive behavior.
2. **Cluster B. Problems in the self-concept**. Persistent negative beliefs about oneself as diminished, defeated or worthless. They can be accompanied by deep and pervasive feelings of shame, guilt or failure related to, for example, not having overcome adverse circumstances, or not having been able to prevent the suffering of others.
3. **Cluster C. Disturbances in relational functioning**. Exemplified primarily by difficulties in feeling close to others. The person may consistently avoid, deride or have little interest in relationships and social engagement more generally. Alternatively, the person may occasionally experience close or intense relationships but have difficulties sustaining them.

Adapted from Maercker, A., Brewin, C. R. et al. (2013).

tailored for survivors of torture. Among these tools are the World Assumptions Scale (WAS) (Janoff-Bulman, 1992; Kaler et al., 2008; Magwaza, 1999; Matthews and Marwit, 2004), the Post Traumatic Cognitions Inventory (PTCI) (Beck et al., 2004; Foa et al., 1999; Startup, Makgekgenene, and Webster, 2007), and more recently the Vital Impact Assessment Questionnaire (VIVO) (Pérez-Sales et al., 2012), among others.

World Assumption Scale (WAS)

Only one study, to our knowledge, used the WAS[2] in this context; none used the PTCI. Magwaza (1999) compared the long-term consequences of detention and torture in 29 survivors from the South African Apartheid government as compared to 36 people who had witnessed the violent death of a close relative (sibling, mother or father) using the WAS and an ad-hoc scale to cover specific cultural aspects linked to violence. In both groups (Torture and Bereavement) there was a significant impact on participants' basic assumptions about the meaningfulness and benevolence of the world. The tortured and detained group had lower feelings of self-worth as compared to the bereaved group. About 77 per cent of torture survivors expressed inner feelings of apathy and hopelessness. They lacked a coherent value system. For some participants, things no longer mattered, and they felt that they themselves did not matter to anybody. About 83 per cent of the participants viewed the world as malevolent and as a source of sadness. They were more bitter and cynical about life than they had been before the trauma and perceived the world as more treacherous than they would have thought. Most survivors (91 per cent) disagreed with the Just World assumption; 89 per cent of the participants experienced fear that if bad things had happened to them once, they could happen again. Regarding personal consequences, there was a marked sense of threat perception and hypersensitivity to danger; 73 per cent of the participants believed that events in life were uncontrollable and unpredictable. They had an inclination to view themselves not as victims but as heroes, martyrs of society, and resilient people. However, they appeared to have a strong need for the acknowledgment of their integrity by other people. About 35 per cent of the participants experienced survivor guilt.

Vital Impact Assessment (VIVO) questionnaire

The **VIVO questionnaire** (Pérez-Sales et al., 2012) is a 116-item measure of the dimensions of the trauma experience linked to identity and worldviews of survivors. It provides scores for 10 conceptual blocks and 35 subscales: View of the World, Attitude Towards the World, View of Human Beings, Coping Strategies, Cognitions and Emotions During and After Trauma, Communicability, Ability to Share the Experience, Daily Consequences, Perceived Social Support, and Identity. It provides a comprehensive framework for the analysis of extreme traumatic experiences. It aims to provide an overall view of the deep experience of surviving trauma.

Its potential is exemplified in the study of a female survivor of prolonged torture and rape during the military dictatorship in Uruguay. The woman did not fulfill criteria either for PTSD or depression, but 30 years after torture subtle sequelae were evident to her family, colleagues, partners and friends. Though she was proud of her resilience during and after torture, she had radically changed her view of the world and human beings, had deep feelings of shame and survivor guilt related to other women who were disappeared after torture, and prominent feelings of rage against society in general because it looked away while all this happened. All this led her to self-criticism and periodic non-depressive suicidal thoughts. None of this was captured in a clinical diagnosis, but it was collected in the profile of the VIVO questionnaire.

In a study conducted in Spain, 45 torture victims who had suffered incommunicado detention (from 5 to a maximum of 13 days) under the Anti-Terrorist Law in the Basque Country were assessed using the Istanbul Protocol and measures of PTSD, depression, and the VIVO questionnaire (Navarro et al., 2014). Over half of the examinees (57.7 per cent) fulfilled ICD-10 criteria for PTSD at some point, 13.4 per cent had a diagnosis of depressive disorder (from mild to very severe), 6 per cent suffered from anxiety disorder, and a similar per centage had somatoform disorder. The VIVO questionnaire showed that despite the presence of identifiable psychological impacts of detention, about two thirds of the survivors showed, overall, mild changes in their identity and worldviews, or were resilient.[3] Some had flashbacks and avoidance behaviour, but the experience had not substantially changed them. However, approximately one third of survivors showed severe psychological impacts *which were uncorrelated to PTSD* responses. Table 9.4 shows the mean value of each subscale for resilient and non-resilient categories (and the differences, as measured by a t-test), providing a picture of the impact of torture as measured by the VIVO.

In general, torture survivors tend to express that (1) they were blocked during their detention; (2) they now have a greater tendency to think about what happened and to try to seek a logical explanation; (3) they have new and unspecific fears; and (4) they have feelings of guilt. They tend to see themselves as victims and lack hope that this might change in the future. This is partly because other people do not want to know about what they went through and because they feel that part of society blames them, as activists, for what happened to them. The statistical analysis shows that the people most severely affected by torture were those who got blocked or (in retrospect) failed to respond during the days of the arrest, who consider that the suffering they endured was personally and politically useless, and who perceived less social or community support after what happened. For them, communicating what happened was not only relevant, but also part of fulfilling their need to be heard. Making the truth known, guarantees of non-repetition, and the abolition of incommunicado detention were all part of justice and reparations for the victim.

One unpublished study compared the results of the VIVO questionnaire of the Basque detainees with samples of survivors of torture from Argentina and Uruguay using the same statistical analysis of the VIVO questionnaire. In Argentina (n=12), also, about one-third of survivors were severely affected and two thirds mildly affected or resilient. The subscales that best predicted mental health problems were, in this order: rumination (e.g. 'I spend a lot of time thinking about things that have happened to me'), alienation from society (e.g. 'I don't care enough about things that happen around me'), shame (e.g. 'Looking back, I'm embarrassed to think about how I reacted'), and the way they coped with torture (e.g. 'When something serious happens to me, I tend to freeze up'). In Uruguay (n=20), no one was severely affected, probably because members of the social and revolutionary movement that was prosecuted, detained and tortured in the past had just won the elections by a large majority. Social support was a problem in the past, but not at present. Of those who suffered mild to moderate impacts, these were linked to skepticism, loss of confidence in human beings and rejection of their own negative feelings.

The results show the complexities of human responses to torture and how PTSD and other clinical disorders, though relevant categories for research and forensic purposes, are far from capturing the broader psychological world of a survivor, especially regarding changes in their worldviews, identity and self.

TABLE 9.4 Dimensions of human experience in torture survivors: key subscales of the VIVO questionnaire in resilient vs. non-resilient subgroups of Basque Torture Survivors (Navarro et al., 2014)

Selection of relevant subscales	Means / T Test	Selected quotations from interviews
Worldviews Negative worldview Life lacks meaning	63 vs. 51★★★ 52 vs. 47★	'I feel a little strange in society. (. . .) I feel people are distant, they don't understand the context I have suffered (. . .) maybe I am the strange one . . . I don't know.' (MNEG01) 'I didn't know if it was good or bad for me [to develop political activities with other torture victims], but the truth is that I had no strength, because I've noticed that I needed to heal, without knowing how and from what, and for a while I was just going to pursue that. I am lost.' (OBAM04)
Attitudes towards the world Need to find a logic behind what happened Suffering is useless Loss of confidence in people	45 vs. 51★ 52 vs. 47★ 53 vs. 46★	'I think about them, they were psychopaths. You wonder about who he is, how many others he has done the same thing to, if he has a family and if he goes home quietly feeling like a hero for doing what he does . . . I'd like to know who they are and I would like to know their stories.' (OBIM07)
Coping Rumination	64 vs. 51★★★	'The physical aspect, it hurts, there are some days that you cannot walk, but the psychological aspect is one thing that to this day I can't cope with. It's very hard, very hard.' (JGGL03)

Selection of relevant subscales	Means / T Test	Selected quotations from interviews
Impact of the past Guilt Unable to learn from the events Non-specific fears	55 vs. 49★★★ 54 vs. 46★★★ 57 vs. 49★★	'[Memories of the torturers] come in and I can't get them out of my head … what I did, everything. … ' (MTRGL10) 'Honestly if I feel affected, I'm not denying it, yeah I'm emotionally affected … there has been a change in me and I sincerely believe that I'm paying for what has happened.' (BOB12) 'I was afraid of what they could do to me. I was also very nervous, I was blocked, scared, and physically hurt, and my body ached.' (ILMW01)
Emotions Rejection of negative feelings Communicating what happened is unimportant	52 vs. 46★★ 39 vs. 51★★★	'I used to be more affectionate, now it is hard for me to have physical contact, to show my feelings through physical contact; I used to give hugs and kisses to my friends … Now I can't bring myself to do that.' (BOB12) 'All around me I see people continuing with their lives as if nothing had happened, it brings me a sense of despair. To see that people are like this, that they are so insensitive to certain things that exist.' (MIIA02)
Identity Lack of social support Negative future: no hope Changes in identity since the event Identity: victim's outlook on the event	51 vs. 42★★★ 57 vs. 49★★ 56 vs. 49★ 57 vs. 46★★	'You feel, above all, that society judges you. The arrest being broadcast on TV and the information [the media] gave didn't help. In the end, people will always think that you did do something or that you deserve it, and that's hard.' (NLMAP02) 'Now I live life one day at a time, I don't have many goals, right now I am not getting fired from my job and that's it. My goal this year is to not lose my job, and that's how it goes.' (MNEG04) 'So far my life has been normal, I consider myself a person who wants to overcome these things, and the last few years different things in my life have gone relatively well. Over time things go on healing, I'd even say they are sort of forgotten. You give more importance to, or you focus on other things that continue happening to you, then you leave the rest behind.' (JZLV05) 'There is a before and an after experiencing [torture], something changes inside us, we don't relate in the same way, life values change, things that didn't matter before do now, or vice versa, something within changes.' (AMRGL09)

★ $p < 0.05$,
★★ $p < 0.01$,
★★★ $p < 0.001$

Functional measurements

An additional approach to assessing the impact of torture is to measure disability and functioning. The IRCT undertook a project to adapt the International Classification of Functioning, Disability and Health (ICF) to describe the overall health condition of traumatised refugees (Jørgensen et al., 2010). The study showed that such a measure was feasible and could include physical, mental and social indicators. The publication (which is available online) includes the detailed core symptoms, codes and preliminary testing, and is being used for assessing the impact of rehabilitation programs in IRCT centres (Arenas, 2009; Jaranson and Quiroga, 2011), although it has been considered too lengthy and complex (Jørgensen et al., 2010).

In a community study in Bangladesh (Wang et al., 2009) 236 torture survivors were assessed using an abridged 14-item version of the ICF scale[4] and the WHO-5 well-being questionnaire. Both tools proved easy to administer, fast and feasible.

Mental harm as a sign of psychological torture

The existence of psychiatric sequelae is a powerful indicator of psychological torture. Depression, anxiety and posttraumatic symptoms coherent with the alleged treatment support the reliability of the statements.

The data in this chapter reveal that a lack of sequelae does not rule out torture. If an average of approximately 40 per cent of torture survivors have endured PTSD, this means that around 60 per cent are *resilient*. In other words, the absence of a clinical diagnosis does not mean that a person did not suffer torture. The person may have been able to cope or the sequelae may not be related to the standard diagnostic syndromes but to more existential aspects of their lives, i.e. the irrevocably changed way in which they view the world after what happened to them (Elsass et al., 2009) measured, for instance, by the VIVO questionnaire.

This is important to keep in mind because sometimes there has been a tendency to equate suffering and harm, and use harm as an indicator of suffering. When the Bush administration tried to find legal support for the Enhanced Interrogation program, two of its legal advisors, John Yoo[5] and Jay S. Bybee, issued three legal memoranda (called the Torture Memos,[6] the Bybee Memos or the 8/1/02 Interrogation Opinion) that, among other things, discussed the language of the torture statute (18 U.S.C. sections 2340-2340A) to conclude that torture was defined by 'extreme acts' that involved 'severe' pain. This was defined in the Memo as '*serious physical injury, such as organ failure, impairment of bodily function, or even death*'. The Memo asserted that mental suffering should be of a similar intensity as '*severe pain*', and this involved '*prolonged mental harm*', which is harm that must last for '*months or even years*' (p. 7). Falling below these levels, the Enhanced Interrogation Techniques would be considered 'only' CIDT, which was not subject to prosecution under their particular interpretation of the Convention.

The memo has been widely criticised from all sectors inside the US, and the authors have even been indicted for what has been considered cooperation with torture by purposely providing legal advice that was flagrantly wrong.

In summary:

- A review of the debate over time on the concept of trauma shows that a definition of torture would not include severity of suffering criteria but instead threat with or without overwhelming emotions as core features. The ICD-10 EPCACE diagnosis seems to reflect this.[7]

- Torture is one of the most devastating human experiences. The per centage of survivors with long-term sequelae surpasses that of any other traumatic experience.
- On average, and across studies, around 40 per cent of survivors develop enduring PTSD and one in five suffer profound impacts on their identity, belief system and worldview.
- These elements must be added to conventional clinical elements when assessing torture survivors. The VIVO questionnaire appears to be a complex and appropriate measurement of them.
- While acute, chronic consequences are a consistent indicator in torture allegations, mental harm is not a pre-requisite for concluding that a person was tortured. Most survivors are resilient (when measuring resilience based on the absence of PTSD). A lack of a diagnosis does not indicate a lack of torture.
- The on-site detection of mental harm cannot guide an interrogation assisted by a psychologist. Even if mental harm was present in all cases of torture – which isn't the case – it would not manifest itself immediately. The most severe forms of mental damage can (and usually do) appear months or years after torture.

Notes

1 Full text available for free at www.psicosocial.net/.
2 The WAS has three main subscales: Benevolence of the World (whether or not the world is a good place, and the person believes that people are basically good, kind, helpful and caring); Meaningfulness of the World (whether the world is a fair place where justice is fairly distributed and a person can maintain control over his or her life, providing an overall sense of meaning); and Self-Worth (individuals' beliefs that they themselves are good, worthy and highly moral people).
3 K-Means Cluster Analysis (SPSS 19.0). The best analysis involved two groups, which we labelled the resilient and the damaged group. The program calculated the group each participant belonged to and compared mean scores subscale by subscale (see Table 9.4).
4 The items chosen were body function: b130, b280 and b760; activity: a340, a450 and a740; participation: p930, p940, p950 and p798; environmental factors: e299, e320, e330 and e470.
5 Yoo was Deputy Assistant Attorney General of the United States; Jay S. Bybee was head of the Office of Legal Counsel of the United States Department of Justice.
6 John Yoo to William J. Haynes, 14 March 2003, 'Memo Regarding the Torture and Military Interrogation of Alien Unlawful Combatants Held Outside the United States', ACLU.
7 Although it seems doomed to disappear in future editions of the WHO-ICD classification and substituted with the idea of Complex Trauma, which is not equivalent.

SECTION 5

Psychological torture techniques

10

THE HISTORICAL ROOTS OF PSYCHOLOGICAL TORTURE IN MODERN HISTORY: THE SLOW ROAD TO CONVERGENCE

To understand where we are now and how we came to be here, a quick overview of the contemporary history of torture is useful. There are excellent reviews of the topic (Rejali, 2007); in this chapter we will focus on the historical origins of psychological torture. Contemporary torture is the result of the combined work of torturers around the world who share experiences and techniques: they learn from one another, in some cases through competition and copying, in others through direct cooperation.

We will review four initial styles of creative improvisation from different countries that began sharing information about torture methods and, over the years, converged into a quite similar corpus: the French school, the British, the American and the Russian. Of course, each country has developed its own variations and local peculiarities. The Khmer Rouge in Cambodia, the South African Apartheid regime, the Argentinian military Junta and different Turkish governments have all developed their own styles of torture.

An historical road map of torture is summarised in Tables 10.2 and 10.3 at the end of the chapter. Anecdotally, we have included in the tables key data on the organisation of academic and humanitarian research on the consequences and treatment of torture, which helps visualise how mental health and human rights workers are, on average, one to two decades behind military psychologists and interrogators in their understanding of torture.

The French school: the rule of pain

Marnia Lazreg (2008) is the author of *Torture and the Twilight of Empire: From Algiers to Baghdad*, a crucial text which traces how torture and colonial domination were intimately intertwined in Algiers and how this is reproduced in present-day Iraq and Afghanistan. She shows how torture was officially sanctioned as a legitimate tool in war, part of a well-established national policy of the occupying forces that served psychological, sociological, political and cultural objectives. Torture was the organising axis of the French colony and targeted both individuals and society (Figure 10.1).

She paints a picture of a French nation that had just lost its colonies in Indochina, and commissioned the army to avoid a second failure and control the incipient Algerian revolution at any price. During the eight years preceding its liberation (1954–1962),

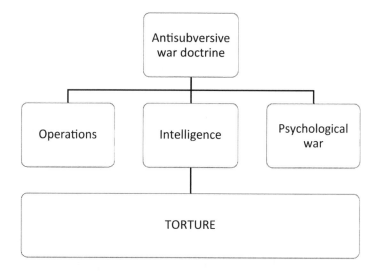

FIGURE 10.1 Torture and social control. The French model in Algeria.

Adapted from Marnia Lazreg (2008). *Torture and the Twilight of Empire: From Algiers to Baghdad.*

Algeria lived under a reign of terror. According to historians, around 300,000 people were tortured (Vidal-Naquet, 1975). In July 1968, the French government approved an amnesty law that exonerated their military from any responsibility regarding the 'counterinsurgency' work. Covered by the amnesty, some of the leading French torturers have had no problem in calling their past actions torture and publishing popular books on how torture was organised, both justifying their actions and arguing for torture's merits (Aussaresses, 2010) – though not without creating polemic.

The Algerian Revolution began in 1954 and soon became a widespread national movement. The French decided to resort to torture in December 1956, completely removed the primary officials in charge at the time, and appointed new generals from Paris who arrived with clear orders from de Gaulle:[1] torture as state policy in France was a fait accompli. French officers not only applied torture, but also systematised it and theorised about it. The person responsible for counterinsurgency in the town of Algiers was Roger Trinquier, a parachutist who wrote an influential book, *La Guerre Moderne (Modern Warfare: A French View of Counterinsurgency)*, in which he claimed the situation in Algiers was that of an 'asymmetric war': a regular army would lose confronted with an enemy that appeared and disappeared, that merged into in the population of a town. In his mind, torture was a legitimate resource (Trinquier, 1961). David Galula (1964) published *Counterinsurgency Warfare* soon afterwards defending the need to target an entire population to defeat revolutionary groups.

According to this policy, in 1957 around 40 per cent of the male population of the old quarter of Algiers were tortured and an estimated of 5,000 killed, some of them left dead in the streets with clear signs of torture, while the rest were abandoned in hospitals or disappeared.[2] Torture was the foundation on which policies of social control were built (Lazreg 2008).

In his book, Trinquier was among the first to propose the ticking time bomb scenario and the legitimacy of torture if used 'to save lives'. Aussaresses, director of the French secret service in Algiers, wrote in his memoir, *The Battle of the Casbah*: 'We were given a free hand to do what we considered necessary. And we did.' He went on to describe the techniques:

> First, a beating, which in most cases was enough; then other means, such as electric shocks, known as the famous 'gegene'; and finally water. Torture by electric shock was made possible by generators used to power field radio transmitters, which were extremely common in Algeria. Electrodes were attached to the prisoner's ears or testicles, then electric charges of varying intensity were turned on. (p. 16)

Torture was, in Algiers, simply about producing pain. The French torturers used electricity devices (the 'magneto'), different methods of simulated drowning (buckets, wet clothes on the face with water), hard beatings – sometimes to death, sexual torture and rape. 'Water torture . . . was the most dangerous technique for the prisoner. He never lasted for more than one hour and the suspects would speak in the hope of saving their own lives. They would therefore either talk quickly or never' (p. 128). As Aussaresses and Trinquier have described, there was no formal interrogation. The purpose was confessing, obtaining names and killing (see addendum at the end of the chapter): 'Fearing these methods or because of their use, the prisoners began providing very detailed explanations and even other names, allowing me to make further arrests.' Showing no remorse for having resorted to torture, Aussaresses stated: 'This is Algeria, our mission demands results, requiring torture and summary executions.'

In the 1950s, numerous accounts already testified to the systematic use of torture in Algeria. In 1958, a French-Algerian journalist, Henri Alleg, published the most influential book *La Question (The Question)*, in which he exposed his own torture at the hands of the French Army with a prologue by Sartre. The film *The Battle of Algiers* reflects the pattern of French torture in a brutal and detailed manner. Frantz Fanon, a French-Algerian psychiatrist wrote *Les damnes de la Terre* (*The Wretched of the Earth*) in 1961 (Fanon, 1963); it was the first book to describe the impact of torture from the testimonies of the people (tortured and torturers) that he treated in his practice.

The French school of torture's expansion and influence around the world

The investigative documentary and subsequent book *Escadrons de la mort: l'école française* (*Death Squads: The French School*) interviews former French torturers and documents how their network expanded (Robin, 2004).

Roger Trinquier's *La Guerre Moderne* (*Modern Warfare*) was published in French in 1961 (Editions de la Table Ronde), translated into Spanish in 1962, then published in Argentina (Editorial Rioplatense) and Barcelona (Editorial Herder); it was published in English in 1964 in London (Pall Mall Press) and New York (Praeger), and distributed in India through Praeger-India. The Italian version appeared in 1965 (Brossura Editorial) and subsequent editions appeared in other countries. The book was soon put to use by Spanish police under Franco's dictatorship; they adopted most of Trinquier's lessons for torturing political opponents. It also expanded throughout Francophone Africa and his book and theories on torture became influential in Central Africa. Trinquier was hired by the Katanga secessionist movement in the Democratic Republic of Congo in 1964 to train its officers (Trinquier, Duchemin and Bailley, 1963).

The Latin America branch. The main area of expansion of French methods was Latin America. As early as 1958, Trinquier supported the creation of a paramilitary group based in Buenos Aires formed by French mercenaries of the OAS.[3] Based on their extensive experience in torture, they offered training and strategic support in the area. In 1959 the government of Paris and Buenos Aires signed an agreement that created a 'permanent French military mission', comprised of French army personnel who had fought in the Algerian War (1954–1962) that would train the Argentinian Army (Robin, 2004). The agreement was publicised in the press and on television in both countries. The mission was located in the offices of the chief of staff of the Argentine Army. Soon military officers from Chile, Uruguay, Paraguay and Brazil travelled to receive training from French officials in Buenos Aires. Most torturers from the Argentine Escuela Superior de Mecánica de la Armada (ESMA) and the Chilean Dirección de Inteligencia Nacional (DINA) attended these courses.

The US adopts French theories and takes the lead

Trinquier's defense of torture as a necessary tool in asymmetric war and his justification of counterintelligence methods that target civilian populations were very influential in the United States. The 1964 edition of his book included a foreword by Bernard B. Fall, an American expert on Indochina who described Trinquier as a 'centurion', a 'hard-bitten French regular who had survived the Indochina war, had learned his Mao Tse-tung the hard way, and later had sought to apply his lessons in Algeria or even in mainland France' (p. 5). He suggested that *Modern Warfare* should serve 'as a timely warning in the United States, of the incredible difficulties a regular army must face when committed to a long series of revolutionary wars' (p. 6) and encouraged the US Army to adopt the methods Trinquier used in Algiers. It was incorporated into lessons on how to torture: Pall Mall Press printed a special edition for the School of the Americas in 1985, converting it into the textbook for officers across Latin America.

Galula was personally invited to the US, where he lived periodically between 1960 and 1963. He had a military appointment at Harvard's Center for International Affairs, where he wrote one of his two books, and participated in the early stages of American counterterrorism. Field Manual FM 3–24, *Insurgencies and Countering Insurgencies*, made constant references to the 'French lessons' and cited Trinquier and Galula's books nearly 40 times.[4] A US Army officer recently wrote that 'Galula's perspective on the war in Algeria dominates [the] intellectual space' at the United States Army Combined Arms Center in Fort Leavenworth, Kansas, and that dozens of copies of Trinquier and Galula's book were available in the Combined Army Research Library (Demarest, 2010).

Paul Aussaresses was appointed in 1961 as a military attaché to the French diplomatic mission in the US, alongside ten veterans of the Algerian War who were formerly under his charge. In the documentary *Esquadrons de le Mort* he explained that he served in Fort Bragg, North Carolina, and trained people at the 10th Special Forces Group, a military unit for unconventional warfare. He suggests that his lessons included interrogation tactics. Copies of Trinquier's books were part of the training material used by CIA interrogators in Vietnam, some of whom had received training courses from Aussaresses (as part of the 'Phoenix Program'[5]).

Aussaresses relocated to Brazil in 1973 during the military dictatorship, where he trained officers from Chile and other countries, according to former head of the Chilean DINA General Manuel Contreras.

The French model in Guatemala. France's influence was also decisive in Central America. Trinquier's ideas on how to control civilian populations to isolate insurgent forces were the theoretical basis upon which Guatemalan Dictator Efraín Ríos Montt built his scorched-earth policy ('tierra arrasada'). Rios Montt referred to this practice as 'taking away the fish's water' ('quitar el agua al pez'); it led to the killing of approximately 200,000 people in more than

2,000 massacres documented in reports by both the Truth Commission and the Guatemalan Archbishop's report, *Guatemala Never Again*. In 1982 the Guatemalan Army implemented the 'Sofia Plan'[6] that literally followed the French doctrine by ordering systematic torture, forced disappearances, rape of Mayan women and massacres of entire villages.

David Mitrione and the role of the United States. Beginning in 1960 the US began to do its own on-site training in torture techniques. FBI officer David Mitrione was assigned to the State Department's International Cooperation Administration. Over the course of seven years, he traveled to various South American countries to teach 'advanced counterinsurgency techniques'. He was based in Brazil, where he worked inside Brazilian Army facilities, first in Belo Horizonte then in Rio de Janeiro. Mitrione also had a house in Montevideo, Uruguay, where he built a soundproofed room in the cellar in which he trained police and members of the military in different torture techniques using political prisoners borrowed from the Uruguayan Army. Several descriptions of his seminars based on the recollections of Uruguayan torturers have been published (for example, see the description by Hugo Rivas, a former torturer, in Chapter 3). With logistical support from the CIA, he traveled to Chile, the Dominican Republic, Panama and Honduras. He returned to the US in 1967 to share his experiences and expertise on 'counter-guerilla warfare' at the US Agency for International Development (USAID), in Washington, and in 1969 returned to Uruguay as part of a USAID cooperation mission. He was kidnapped and killed in Montevideo by Tupamaros guerrillas in 1970.

Mitrione strictly adhered to the French school. He has been repeatedly quoted by people trained by him and his team as saying: 'The precise pain, in the precise place, in the precise amount, for the desired effect.' According to Gordon Thomas, an intelligence researcher, Mitrione also trained US interrogators involved in Cold War operations, using homeless people who were later disappeared (Thomas, 2001). Those involved were mostly Army officers to be deployed in foreign missions.

Today's influence. General David Petraeus, chief officer in command of the American troops in Afghanistan, was quoted as saying that Galula's book has been the most influential source of knowledge for writing FM 3-24 (Marlowe, 2010). Two high-ranking US officials have recently published a review of Trinquier's theories on counterinsurgency, defending his views as a landmark and a point of reference for the current work of the US Army in Iraq and Afghanistan, noting that the chapter 'Counter-guerrilla Operations' was 'especially enlightening'. Despite specifically rejecting the use of torture, which they call 'unacceptable', they argue that

> Our employment of Trinquier's legitimate principles during our 14 months of counterinsurgency operations has brought significant improvements to the Mada'in Qada. (. . .) By selectively applying the moral lessons of *Modern Warfare* and heeding the wisdom gained by other American units over the last five years, we have made good progress. (Fivecoat, 2008)

The British school: implementing and training in psychological torture

The British Army has always practiced torture. When the ECHR sanctioned the interrogation practices of the British Army in Ireland as CIDT (see Chapter 4), the Parliament made an official inquiry and commissioned it to Lord Parker.

The Parker Inquiry, an official investigative report, more or less reconstructed the history of British torture in the 20th century, despite the fact that most of the documentation had been lost. The Parliament banned the use of the so-called 'five techniques' (standing against a wall for hours, hooding, subjection to noise, sleep deprivation and restriction of food and drink) in 1971.

These 'five techniques' were developed by officials in the Joint Services Interrogation Wing (Britain's only official interrogation training school), drawing from the experience of British campaigns in the colonies. They were restricted to what in intelligence language were called 'emergencies', a euphemism for popular uprisings or anti-colonialist movements. The first reports on the use of some of the five techniques are from the Kenya Emergency (1953–1954). There are also reports from the Malayan Emergency (1955–1960), which was 'successfully' controlled, and the Cameroon Emergency, in territory mostly belonging to present-day Nigeria (1960–1961). They were considered 'very successful' according to internal reports collected by the Parker inquiry. In Cameroon, according to official reports, 15 of every 20 suspects 'confessed'. There are additional reports of its use in Swaziland (1963), Aden – now part of Yemen[7] (1964), and, very likely, in Palestine (Newbery, 2009).

In 1963 the British Army developed a large-scale interrogation operation in Brunei involving more than 2,000 suspects, with three interrogation centers working simultaneously. Hooding and white noise were used with all the detainees, and the five techniques were used with 'high value' suspects. It was the first time that reports distinguished between two basic components of psychological torture: 'environment manipulation' and 'handling of prisoners'. The detainees were deprived of food and sanitary facilities, and subjected to high temperatures. Detainees were also brutally beaten. The process was coordinated by the Special Branch Headquarters, the organisation directing the interrogations.

The Parker inquiry showed that once the five techniques had been established as a successful method, *they were always used in combination*, never individually. By the time the techniques were finally implemented in Northern Ireland, British intelligence officers were proud that they had developed such an invaluable method: 'Hoods, wall-standing and noise . . . were used on each occasion to ensure complete isolation and consequent security, and to impose a degree of discipline which helped to create a proper working environment [during interrogation].' For British intelligence officers, the method was in fact based on three techniques: hooding, wall-standing and noise; the other two were just additional features to increase efficacy.

The British model in Latin America

The British model cannot be called no-pain torture. Wall-standing inaugurated what were later called *stress positions*, which were included as a key element in US Interrogation Manuals of the 1970s and 1980s. The five techniques were most influential in Anglophone Africa and countries of the Commonwealth, although their relatively 'high sophistication' precluded wider use.

The influence of the 'British model' was particularly strong in Brazil. The model's true impact can be traced in the documents of the Brazilian truth commission and the testimonies of survivors of the Brazilian dictatorship. *Tirando o Capuz (Taking Off the Hood)* is the testimonial book of Alvaro Caldas (1981), a journalist who was arrested in 1970 and detained for more than two years in Rio, where he was repeatedly tortured based on Mitrione's teachings. He was subjected to severe beatings, electric shocks, and the 'parrot's perch' (being tied to a horizontal pole and hung upside down for hours). He was released in 1972, only to be arrested again the following year.

When Caldas was brought back to the same building in Rio upon his arrest, he found that it had been completely transformed. Now Brazil followed the British model.

> This time the cell was clean and sterile with a nauseating, sickly smell. The air conditioning was very cold. The light was on permanently so I had no idea whether it was day or night. There were alternating very loud and then very soft sounds . . . I couldn't sleep at all.[8]

Caldas describes being hooded permanently and in constant fear and terror during repeated and exhausting interrogations. He wrote in his memoirs that this 'new method' was much worse than the physical torture he had endured three years previously under to the pain model, and that 'the aim was to destabilize the personality'. During the interrogations he confessed to something he had not done. 'Luckily I was only there a week, if I had been there for two weeks or a month I would have gone mad,' he declared to the Brazilian Truth Commission.

Paulho Malhaes, a former torturer killed shortly after giving his testimony to the Truth Commission, explained that he learned the new model in a course in England, where Brazilian and other Latin American officers went for training. He had also received training in Germany, France, Panama and the US, but in his words 'the British methods are by far the best'. He stated that 'Those prisons with closed doors, where you can modify the heat, the light, everything inside the prison, that idea came from England,' and 'The British recommended interrogating a prisoner when he was naked as it left him anguished and depressed, a state favorable to the interrogator.' The British school successfully competed with the French 'old style'.

But that was only the tip of the iceberg. The British government provided military assistance and training to most military regimes in Central and Latin America. While the US has had a prominent and visible role, the UK has maintained a low profile while training interrogators as part of a broader program of selling arms and military technology (Phythian, 2000). There is documentation regarding training courses by British mercenaries in Argentina, Chile and Colombia, among other countries (Almond, 2013).

The British Army still trains officers in the UK and abroad using manuals that encourage the widespread use of these seemingly unauthorised techniques, as an investigation by *The Guardian* discovered after an Iraqi prisoner died during a torture session in British headquarters in Baghdad (Cobain, 2012; Redress, 2007).

The American school of psychological torture

Since the 1940s there has been a constant exchange between British, American and Canadian researchers, including visits and discussions among experts in human investigation and torture. The history of US torture is well known. Prominent scholars have done extensive research and there are over a dozen books on the subject (e.g. McCoy, 2012; Otterman, 2007; Thomas, 2001).

1945: Interrogation in other countries through the eyes of US intelligence officers

From the beginning of the 20th century, US military personnel compiled and documented interrogation procedures in enemy countries. Information came from handbooks obtained during operations or interrogations of liberated prisoners of war (POWs) after liberation.

- **Japan**. An official report by an intelligence officer (Mueller, 1946) describes how Japanese intelligence officers were encouraged to scale up procedures. Three stages are noted: (1) isolation, immediate interrogation, undermining the morale of detainee (e.g. reminding him or her of the days before the war, casting doubts on religion, family); (2) threats of increasing severity; (3) beatings and good cop/bad cop. The report also includes stress positions (kneeling for hours); 'cases' of force-feeding with water, sometimes until death; obligating the prisoner to run while tied to a car; forcing the prisoner to beat another prisoner with a stick; and other atrocities, including decapitation of extremely non-cooperative POWs in front of others. Most of the space in the report is devoted to detailing the cruelties of Japanese interrogators and lacks analysis.

- **Gestapo**. Different reports by intelligence officers reveal that the Gestapo used 'psychological interrogation' more than physical interrogation (NDS, 1940). They describe, for instance, that a person was detained along with all of his or her relatives and acquaintances. They were interrogated one by one, and later confronted over any inconsistencies until some piece of information emerged, then the people named by victims were detained and interrogated as well. They used 'a constant bombardment of questions' ultimately 'exhausting the person by shifting interrogators'. The detainees were held in isolation for days without knowing when they would be interrogated. According to a directive by Gestapo Chief Commander included in the Nuremberg Trials, the procedure was called 'sharpened interrogation' and included the 'simplest rations (bread and water), hard bed, dark cell, deprivation of sleep, exhaustion exercises, blows with a stick (in case of more than 20 blows, it specifies that a doctor must be present)'. After World War II a group of Nazi researchers, doctors involved in human experimentation, and hard interrogators were recruited by the US Army (called 'Operation Paperclip') under the pretext of 'avoid[ing] the risk of rearmament of Germany' (Hunt, 1991).

- **China** attracted a great deal of interest from US Army officers with both academic papers (Hunter, 1951; Schein, 1960) and the still-influential book by Jay Lifton (1961) on indoctrination processes in China. The term 'brainwashing' was coined to name the process of changing a person's worldviews (see Chapter 15), and described the use of isolation, fear and pressure from small groups (neighborhood, relatives) and big groups (community, workplace, society) to foster ideological change, using strong social control, incentives and positive rewards for adjusting ideas and behavior in the approved direction.[9] There have been repeated reports of the use of physical and psychological torture from the last 50 years from inside China, where the debate on the illegitimacy of torture is just beginning (Beken and Wu, 2010).

- **The Soviet Union** drew the most attention from US scholars with its very detailed reports and monographic research projects funded by public and private institutions (Beck and Godin, 1951). The reports describe how Russia's secret police began isolating prisoners in the 19th century, then at the beginning of the 20th century abandoned the use of brutal force and began to develop sophisticated psychological techniques based on persuasion and the exploitation of the intimate interrogator-prisoner relationship. The description of a 'standard procedure' includes: absolute isolation except during interrogation; harsh conditions of detention (small cell, no blankets, constant electric light, shortage of food, salty and distasteful meals, no sanitary facilities, very cold or very hot temperatures); strict schedules (early awakening); and stress positions (sitting most of the day in a rigid chair without being able to move). One of the reports states: 'Pain may result from fixed positions during sleep and when awake'

(Hinkle and Wolff, 1957). This combination of 'isolation, fear and harsh conditions' leads to breaking down the individual in one to three days, or in some exceptions, up to ten days. Longer periods, the report claims, have devastating consequences: 'there is a complete disorganization of the prisoner in a period of three to six weeks . . . the reaction may go on to frank delirium' (p. 23). Interrogations would begin 'when the interrogator feels that the prisoner is ready to talk, but before he has become completely disorganized'. These interrogations lasted for weeks, to the point of exhaustion. They involved reviewing the prisoner's entire life, rejecting answers that did not lead in the 'proper' direction (and rewarding those that did), incriminating questions and deceitful strategies. Then a confession was finally written, signed and filmed for broadcasting if necessary.[10]

Albert Biderman's early model

As a psychologist and official in the US Air Force, Albert Biderman interviewed subjects who had been prisoners of war in Korea and Russia. He synthetised his findings in a paper (Biderman, 1957) which he began by affirming: 'the most new and spectacular is the finding that essentially there was nothing new or spectacular about the events we studied' (p. 617). He stated that the interrogation process 'can be understood as essentially a teaching procedure without making the lessons explicit – a lesson teaching the prisoner how to comply' (p. 618), and he outlined eight methods (see Table 10.1).

Biderman introduced concepts that have since been adopted as some of the classic tenets of torture: 'Where physical violence was inflicted during the course of such an attempt, the attempt was particularly likely to fail completely' (p. 621). The ever-present fear of violence

TABLE 10.1 Communist interrogation techniques according to Biderman

	Effects (purposes?)	*Variants*
1. Isolation	• Deprives victim of all social support of his ability to resist • Develops an intense concern with self • Makes victim dependent on interrogator	• Complete solitary confinement • Complete isolation • Semi-isolation • Group isolation
2. Monopolisation of perception	• Fixes attention upon immediate predicament; fosters introspection • Eliminates stimuli competing with those controlled by captor • Frustrates all actions not consistent with compliance	• Physical isolation • Darkness or bright light • Barren environment • Restricted movement • Monotonous food
3. Induced debility and exhaustion	• Weakens mental and physical ability to resist	• Semi-starvation • Exploitation of wounds • Induced illness • Sleep deprivation • Prolonged constraint • Prolonged interrogation • Forced writing • Over-exertion

	Effects (purposes?)	Variants
4. Threats	• Cultivates anxiety and despair	• Threats of death • Threats of non–repatriation • Threats of endless isolation • Vague threats • Threats against family • Mysterious changes in treatment
5. Occasional indulgences	• Provides positive motivation for compliance	• Occasional favors • Fluctuations of interrogators' attitudes • Promises • Rewards for partial compliance • Tantalising
6. Demonstrating omnipotence	• Hinders adjustment to deprivation; suggests futility of resistance	• Confrontations • Pretending cooperation taken for granted • Demonstrating complete control over victim's fate
7. Degradation	• Makes cost of resistance more damaging to self-esteem than capitulation; reduces victim to 'animal level' concerns.	• Personal hygiene prevented • Filthy, infested surroundings • Demeaning punishments, insults and taunts • Denial of privacy
8. Enforcing trivial demands	• Develops habits of compliance	• Forced writing • Enforcement of minute rules

Source: Biderman, A. (1957) Communist Attempts to Elicit False Confessions from Air Force Prisoners of War, *Bulletin of the New York Academy of Medicine*, 33, p. 619.

in the mind of the prisoner appears to have played an important role in inducing compliance. The Communists generally 'fostered such fears through vague threats and the implication that they were prepared to do drastic things' (p. 621). According to him, 'Physical punishment was very limited. Generally, it appears to have been limited to cuffs, slaps and kicks, and sometimes merely to threats and insults' (p. 622). 'The prisoners were required to stand, or sit, at attention for exceedingly long periods of time – in one extreme case, day and night for a week at a time with only brief respites. In a few cases, the standing was aggravated by extreme cold. This form of torture had several distinct advantages for extorting confessions. Where the individual is told to stand at attention for long periods, an intervening factor is introduced. The immediate source of pain is not the interrogator but the victim himself. The contest becomes, in a way, one of the individual against himself. The motivational strength of the individual is likely to exhaust itself in this internal encounter' (p. 620). This interrogation method 'is consistent with formal adherence to principles of legality and humaneness (. . .) [the Communists] can gain a considerable propaganda advantage when victims who are released truthfully state that no one ever laid a hand on them' (p. 621).

Biderman's model was an instant success, and was repeatedly quoted in experimental research and served as the basis for CIA torture manuals in the 1960s, 1970s and 1980s. The KUBARK Manual constantly references his work.[11]

Biderman was commissioned by the US Army in 1961 to edit *The Manipulation of Human Behavior*, a collection of essays. The book remains a crucial text on the subject. Though Biderman himself did not contribute to the volume, he invited prominent psychologists to review various topics related to the manipulation of the physiological state of detainees, including sensory deprivation, use of drugs and hypnosis in interrogation, analysis of deception, interpersonal manipulation and counter-manipulation tactics. In the book's introduction Biderman pretended that he had no access to classified information and that the reviews are based only on information published in public scientific sources.[12] He stated that most people – especially people with clear convictions – are resilient. When this was not so, he argued that in most cases sequelae were either part of a transitory state linked to confusion, or an adaptive response called 'opportunistic conformity', not to be confused with a 'true sincere conversion' (p. 16). This was, in his view, very difficult – if not impossible – to achieve, and always required long periods of time.

1950–1960: CIA research and related work

The Central Intelligence Agency created the Office of Scientific Intelligence, which coordinated research projects with more than 100 universities from the US, the UK and Canada. Some of the most well-known projects include:

1. **Project Artichoke (1951–1953).**[13] The project aimed to 'gain absolute control of a person's mind' and involved researchers from divisions of the Army, Navy, Air Force and FBI. It focused on the study of hypnosis, forced morphine addiction (and subsequent forced withdrawal), LSD, mescaline and other chemicals. It explored ways to induce amnesia and other vulnerable 'brainwashed' states in subjects. After hundreds of people were subjected to these chemical experiments, the project was closed due to lack of results.

2. **Project MK-Ultra (1953–1963), later renamed MK-Search (1964–1973)**. Most of the work was done during Project MK-Ultra. The project, with an investment of 25 million dollars,[14] had many branches and sub-branches of research involving 80 private and public institutions, including 44 colleges, universities, hospitals, prisons and pharmaceutical companies, and 185 private and public researchers – most of them unaware of where the funds came from or how their research would be applied. Most of the research was done using unwilling subjects. The project was coordinated by Sidney Gottlieb; its archives were destroyed in 1973 by special order of CIA director Richard Helms. Parallel to external commissioned research, the Central Intelligence Agency developed its own internal program that involved several prominent psychologists from the time, including collaboration with British and Canadian researchers.

MK-Ultra maintained an interest in LSD and other mind-altering drugs, but its main focus was on **behaviour manipulation** through the control and alteration of sensory environments. Some of the most well-known researchers involved include:

1. Donald Hebb at McGill University conducted a series of CIA-funded investigations into the effects of **complete sensory deprivation**. He worked initially with student volunteers. The results were devastating. Psychotic states were induced in less than 48 hours in most of the participants and sequelae were sometimes long-lasting. As Hebb wrote, absolute sensory deprivation (including soundproof spaces, goggles, gloves, and earmuffs) makes 'the subject's very identity disintegrate' (Mausfeld, 2009).

2. Donald Ewen Cameron, also at McGill University, experimented with 'brainwashing' using multiple techniques, ostensibly in the search of a cure for schizophrenia. The experiments involved two branches: erasing memory and introducing new content. Erasure was done with different techniques: insulin-induced comas, paralytic drugs or electroconvulsive therapy (ECT, commonly known as shock treatment). In some of his experiments, he administered up to 120 sessions of ECT at different levels (using up to thirty or forty times higher power than was standard for the treatment of schizophrenia). He created 'psychic driving', a room in which one subject was put in a coma and kept for weeks (up to three months in one documented case) while forcing him or her into listening to simple, repetitive statements. Patients were unaware of the final purpose of the treatment – they thought they were being treated for depression or anxiety (Thomas, 2001). Cameron worked jointly with William Sargant, a British psychiatrist at St. Thomas' Hospital in London. Some of the people who were subjected to 'brainwashing' treatments developed permanent amnesia and severe mental sequelae. Years later they organised and sued for millions of dollars. This, in conjunction with the scandal in newspapers and the lack of any useful results, led to the secret closing of this branch, and in 1973, to the destruction of the project's archives (Collins, 1988).

MK-Ultra had a branch for experiments abroad (MK-Delta),[15] which have been documented in Japan, France and the UK – some of them as covert research using unknowing civilian populations (Albarelli, 2009).

The MK-Ultra project might at first appear to be an historical failure: huge amounts of money invested in unethical research that damaged many people for very few results. But its legacy lives on. In a review of various studies, Lawrence Hinkle (1956, 1961) described absolute sensory deprivation as

> the ideal way of breaking down a prisoner, because . . . it seems to create precisely the state that the interrogator desires: malleability and the desire to talk, with the added advantage that one can delude himself that he is using no force or coercion. (Quoted in McCoy, 2008)

The images of Guantanamo detainees wearing gloves, earmuffs and blindfolds shows that the behavioral psychologists at the Behavioral Science Consultation Team (BSCT) unit shared Hinkle's opinion and decided to produce experiments of their own.

3. In 1955, the US Air Force began to develop **SERE (Survival, Evasion, Resistance, Escape)**, a program to train pilots to resist psychological torture. The program focused on how to defend oneself from 'brainwashing' and how to resist under harsh conditions. It is part of present-day US Army training and is presumably one of the theoretical bases behind the design of the conditions of detention in Guantanamo (Morris, 2009).

The review reveals that at the time, there was a great deal of academic information related to the process of *destroying a detainee's mental resistance and will,* and researchers had learned both how fragile and how resilient the human mind can be. But much less was known about how to produce the changes in the identity and thoughts of the detainees that brain manipulators desired. A scientist could quite easily reduce a person to a pre-psychotic or regressive state. But the key questions were: *What for?* And, *What next?* Sometimes, it was possible for the interrogator to achieve 'opportunistic conformity' (i.e. when detainees say 'yes' in order to try to save themselves) and the cooperation of an enemy; the famous Milgram experiments are one example. But forcing the desired response is not about changing the *ideology* of a person. In the exceptional cases in which detainees *do* change (as is the case when religious conversions occur), other relevant variables come into play, factors related to individual characteristics of the person (patterns of attachment in infancy, cognitive vulnerabilities, sensibility to group pressure and personality traits).

The CIA produced a manual that synthesised state-of-the-art practices in the interrogation of suspects, the **KUBARK Counterintelligence Manual (1963)**—KUBARK means CIA in the language of the agency. It quotes Biderman's book as the most authoritative source, and based on the scientific evidence found in his work, the manual establishes a group of techniques that they found to be the most successful in 'breaking the resistance' of uncooperative sources. The KUBARK Manual collects lessons from American psychologists and experienced interrogators to produce a comprehensive structure for psychological interrogations.

1970–1980s: The implementation of US-supported torture on a massive scale

The KUBARK Manual places strong emphasis on the manipulation of the environment to attack the mind (temperature, light, noise and hunger), the use of stress positions, and a pattern of highly coercive interrogation. Ojeda (2008) has summarised the practices recommended by the manual (see Appendix 2). In brief, the manual gives instructions for arresting suspects early in the morning by surprise, blindfolding them and stripping them naked. Suspects should be held incommunicado in small spaces and deprived of any kind of normal sleeping or eating routines. Interrogation rooms should be windowless, soundproof, dark and without toilets. It cites scientific research to describe the use of stress positions and exhausting exercises, and recommends the use of threats of pain instead of pain itself.

The authors know perfectly well what these techniques are for. Their aim is

> to induce psychological regression in the subject by bringing a superior outside force to bear on his will to resist. Regression is basically a loss of autonomy, a reversion to an earlier behavioral level. As the subject regresses, his learned personality traits fall away in reverse chronological order. He begins to lose the capacity to carry out the highest creative activities, to deal with complex situations, or to cope with stressful interpersonal relationships or repeated frustrations. (CIA, 1963; Kleinman, 2006 p. 64)

The purpose of interrogation (as explained in Chapter 3) is to find the precise equilibrium between the disorganisation of the person's mind and extraction of information. If the person's mind is still structured and keeps some control, he or she will not voluntarily provide information. If the person's mind has been seriously affected and loses too much of its structure, the information will be unreliable. The interrogator maintains the fantasy that he or she will intuitively find this point and will thus find the imaginary 'security zone' between the breaking of the will and the breaking of mind (see Chapter 3).

This was not, in fact, the way interrogations were usually conducted. The KUBARK Manual represented the scientific, 'educated' way of doing things. Surprisingly enough, *this is not what US advisers taught military interrogators.* If the KUBARK Manual had been used, one would expect to find it translated into other languages (at the very least into Spanish) or to find copies, notes or adaptations in the headquarters of most Latin American armies that send their commanders to be trained in Panama or the School of the Americas. But this is not the case. The KUBARK Manual was of limited use to American interrogators. African, Asian and Latin American militaries demanded more direct approaches and most likely preferred Mitrione's pain-producing methods, linked to the old French school: the 'picana', the 'tacho', the 'caballete', and the 'pau de arara'. These were the techniques taught and used by North American advisers at the time. In 1971, Brazilian torturers were admired for having learned the impact of isolation and manipulation of environment from the British, though these methods had already been described in the KUBARK Manual eight years earlier. It was not until 1975 that US Army created Mobile Training Teams (with support from USAID) to provide on-site training using these 'new techniques'; historical reports of systematic training of Nicaraguan Contras and Guatemalan and Honduran officers in 'the new' methods of interrogation detailed in the KUBARK Manual did not emerge until the early 1980s.

In 1979 and 1980, US trainers began to systematically introduce psychological torture into their workshops. In 1983 the information was updated and the CIA issued a new interrogation manual, the *Human Resource Exploitation Manual*, which included stronger warnings about improper use of the techniques. The roughest physical methods were abolished in the text, although testimonies show that in practice they were never truly abandoned. Parts of the manual were translated into Spanish and found in the hands of US-supported Contras.

The CIA exchanged information with Israel and allied governments in the Middle East, trained torturers in North Africa and developed a large-scale program for outsourcing torture. People were delivered to secret detention centers in Libya, Yemen, Pakistan and later Poland, where (under USAID funding) teams of both local and US interrogators implemented measures that would be difficult to hide or tolerate on North American soil.

Israel's role in training torturers in Latin America

We have seen how French, British and US torturers competed to exert their expertise and influence in Latin America. But the country that has deployed more personnel to train interrogators and torturers in Latin America is Israel. Different teams of Israeli trainers were based in Guatemala, where a large permanent mission operated since General Ríos Montt's coup d'état in 1982 (Hunter, 1987). Ríos Montt's 'scorched earth' policies were part of the legacy of Trinquier's theories (not to mention US experience in the Vietnam War), and were also largely influenced by Israeli assistance. The idea of relocating populations in army-controlled 'aldeas modelo' (model villages) after mass killings came from the experience of the Kibbutz. In a review on Israel's involvement in torture in Latin America, Almond (2013) wrote that more than 50,000 Mayan men, women and children were killed with Galil assault rifles and Uzi submachine guns bought from Israeli military enterprises (Bahbah, 1986; Nederveen, 1984). In 1982, Ríos Montt told ABC News that his success was due to the fact that 'our soldiers were trained by Israelis' (Jamail, 1986). Israel supplied napalm to El Salvador's government, and Israeli trainers conducted torture workshops in Honduras, Nicaragua and Guatemala with the Contras, mostly working as subcontractors for the US government with funding from USAID. Approximately 150 top high-ranking officers from Brazil, Guatemala, Peru and Bolivia were trained in interrogation techniques in Tel Aviv, also with USAID funds (Thomas, 2001). Israel provided military assistance to almost every country in the Southern Cone. This support continues to this day. Carlos Castaño, founder of the paramilitary group Autodefensas Unidas de Colombia (AUC) – responsible for more than 50 massacres and thousands of killings – was trained in Israel, as he explained in his memoirs (Castaño, 2001), and received Israeli arms and assistance for his fight 'against communism'. Israeli interrogators were 'extremely technical and cruel', according to the testimonies of the soldiers they trained (Almond, 2013). Though Israel acted independently, most of its work was done indirectly by serving as agents of outsourced US torture training, in exchange for funding and huge commercial and military contracts in the Latin America (Cockburn and Cockburn, 1991).

The 2000s: Guantanamo and beyond – enhanced interrogation methods

The peculiarities of US laws

In 1994, the US finally ratified the UN Convention against Torture, but included four 'reservations' (just for the United States) that narrowed the definition to only four kinds of acts: the infliction of physical pain, the use of drugs, death threats and threats to harm another person (see Chapter 1). Thus, the United States excluded most of the psychological techniques developed in the KUBARK Manual, especially sensory deprivation and stress positions, from *their* definition of torture. These 'reservations' were the Bush Administration's legal basis for authorising waterboarding – an old technique taught by Mitrione in Uruguay and Argentina – because it 'did not produce physical pain' (Bradbury, 2004).

2002 – Enhanced interrogation methods

When the US began to transfer detainees to Guantanamo in 2001, the legal point of reference for the Army was the *FM 34–52 Manual*. It allowed the use of 18 interrogation techniques. However, the interrogators were apparently unsuccessful and asked to use methods not contemplated in the manual.

The Bush administration built a justification through a series of memos issued in 2002 in which legal advisors Yoo and Bybee produced ad-hoc definitions of torture, defining 'serious physical pain' as the 'significant loss or impairment of the function of a bodily member, organ, or mental faculty'. Based on this idea, and the intentional confusion of terminology between torture and CIDT, the Bush administration approved an initial group of ten 'Enhanced Interrogation Techniques' (EIT) that went far beyond FM 34–52, supposedly under the scientific scrutiny and oversight of psychologists working for the army and CIA. These methods were considered insufficient due to the lack of evident results, and in April 2003 Secretary of State Donald Rumsfeld convened a working group that proposed the use of 35 EIT, though not all of them were ultimately approved.[16]

The people in charge of the EIT program had absolutely no experience (Miles, 2009), and Guantanamo soon became a place for experimentation, informed in part by reversing the military's SERE program, as well as ideas taken from reference texts from the 1970s and the KUBARK Manual, but mainly through crude trial and error. For instance, testimonies from Guantanamo show that detainees were subjected to sensory deprivation following the extremely dangerous Hebbs model (complete isolation and deprivation of sight and sound through the use of blindfolds, earmuffs and hoods). The detainees were also forced to undergo nudity, public exposure and shame, sleep deprivation, dietary manipulation and harsh interrogations. The objective was – as the KUBARK Manual explained – to induce a state of regression, to induce a parent-child relationship in which the interrogation could be 'successfully' conducted.

The Guantanamo Base was officially established as a laboratory with the creation of the Behavioral Science Consultation Teams (BSCTs) in which military psychologists had ample authorisation to try new techniques, in addition to classical ones such as isolation, environment manipulation and fear, and painful stress positions. According to a booklet about the 'Arab character' intended for briefing American personnel, the members of the BSCTs learned that Arab people feared dogs, and the importance of religion and avoiding nakedness. In addition to the basic KUBARK program (that already included nakedness and humiliation), they added specific forms of sexual humiliation (like the use of female interrogators to violate detainees' personal space, debasement, beatings and inappropriate touching), and exploited phobias of darkness, insects and dogs.

Guantanamo detainees were subjected to different levels of torture that included (1) beatings and ill treatment; (2) stress positions; (3) attacks on the senses, including periods of extreme sensory deprivation; (4) threats; (5) sexual humiliation; (6) debasement and feral treatment; (7) attacks on religion and culture; and (8) use of phobias and fear of animals. This was combined with hours of lengthy interrogations (analysed in detail in Chapter 14) (Center for Human Rights and Humanitarian Law, 2006, 2009; Dehn, 2008; FBI Review Division, 2008; Fletcher and Stover, 2008; Iacopino and Xenakis, 2011).

Guantanamo was a space of unrestricted experimentation in which psychologists imposed their fantasies on 'uncooperative sources'.[17] Some inmates, for instance, were subjected to a 'new' method: they were forced to sit down while staring at a wall at close range (from 50 centimeters to 2 meters away) for hours, and they were forbidden to look away until they began to shout and have hallucinatory episodes.[18] Today, these practices continue at Guantanamo, albeit under stricter control; experimentation is more common in other detention centres abroad.

The full program from Bagram and Guantanamo was brought to Abu Ghraib prison in Iraq, where the process became completely uncontrolled, all professionalism was abandoned, and the most bizarre parts of the Guantanamo model were imported and implemented for use against more than 1500 detainees.

Abu Ghraib, Guantanamo and other detention centres where Enhanced Interrogation Techniques were applied have not solved the central conflict facing interrogators: they know how to break detainees, how to induce regressive states and dependence. *But then what?* How to direct behavior in a desired direction? Experimentation at Guantanamo did not bring significant advances towards this goal. Interrogators wanted to fine-tune and slow the process of demolishing the mind to increase the 'safety zone' (see Chapter 3), obtain 'actionable' information, and try out new methods of destruction that keep the subject defeated and submissive yet 'useful'. No one could answer the question: *What happens if the source does not cooperate simply because he or she does not know anything?* Many interrogators finally began to recognise that their victims were simply not involved in any relevant activities or able to offer any information (Pardo, 2014).

The Obama Administration tried to close the debate by issuing *Army Field Manual 2 22.3*, which substituted all previous texts. It authorised 18 techniques, devoted ample space to warn against abuses, and emphasised the need to respect international law regarding prisoners (see Appendix 2). A full analysis of *Army Field Manual FM 34–52* and *FM 2-22.3* (and their derivations), and the lessons they offer in the search to better understand the concept of psychological torture, is included in Chapter 14.

Conclusions: lessons from history

Several conclusions arise from the brief and schematic history of psychological torture outlined in this chapter. Table 10.2 summarises these historical lessons.

Networks

Distinct histories of torture can be traced chronologically for individual countries, but in the end most of these histories intertwine, revealing constant exchanges between nations at all levels – from government headquarters to operations on the ground. The worst French and Gestapo torturers were contracted by the US Army. Most of the MK-Ultra program was based on Canadian and US soil, funded by the CIA and other US agencies, and involved permanent exchanges among researchers from the UK, Germany, France and other countries.

Training for interrogators (i.e. torturers) has been regularly included in aid programs. The French and Argentine governments signed a public agreement. USAID, the official US agency for humanitarian aid, funded most of Mitrione's work in the Southern Cone. Mobile teams of Israeli and US torturers trained Nicaraguan Contras and Honduran torturers, and served as advisers to Ríos Montt in Guatemala. A 1979 review identified 26 countries in five continents where US advisers had offered interrogation training in the preceding decade using funds allocated for 'humanitarian aid' (Amnesty International, 2002; Herman and Chomsky, 1979). The motivation behind such extensive international cooperation is easy to understand: training the military of a foreign country is an undeniably powerful source of political influence. Moreover, it paves the way for the future outsourcing of torture while avoiding scandal at home.

Methods

We have briefly shown that there are different *styles* of torture. But when they are analysed together (Table 10.3), it becomes clear that there are no significant differences between methods. What differences exist lie in the *severity* of methods, the emphasis on certain *kinds* of methods and, of course, the legal guarantees of the people detained.

Over the decades, knowledge of torture has converged to form a shared corpus of techniques and methods. Over half a century has passed since the wars in Algeria, Malaysia and Vietnam, and today the practice and methods of psychological torture have been firmly established – although there are variations, the basic building blocks are on the table. Going through the columns in Table 10.3, on one side we find isolation; sleep deprivation; brutal conditions of detention; manipulation of environment (light, heat, time); pain (harsh beatings and stress positions); nakedness and other forms of humiliation; threats; and fear. On the other side we see long, exhausting, manipulative and deceptive interrogations. We will review this techniques and methods in more detail in Chapters 11 to 15.

This is what the landscape of psychological torture looks like after 50 years of international exchange and experimentation.

Similar does not mean the same

The full history of the evolution and exchange of torture techniques worldwide has yet to be written. This chapter offered a basic outline, revealing the convergence over time and similar aspects of psychological torture across countries. But similar does not mean the same.

The Organization of Intelligence and National Security of Iran (SAVAK) was a secret police, domestic security and intelligence service established by Iran's Mohammad Reza Shah Pahlevi, who controlled the country with a firm hand from 1957 to 1979 with help from the CIA. The ties between SAVAK and the CIA were extremely close, and US trainers led a permanent mission in Tehran. In 1972 the Shah inaugurated Evin Prison. Its intended purpose was to serve as a detention centre for those awaiting trial, but many people were held there for years (and even died inside) without ever going to trial. Soon Evin Prison became known for its harsh torture methods, and there is ample documentation of the brutality of the methods used in the search for information from communist dissidents. As part of the collaboration between the US and Iran, a special pavilion was built in Evin where the CIA experimented with white torture. According to testimonies,[19] the experiments were conducted in a small, three-floor building, separated from the rest of the prison. There were special cells painted entirely in white or uniform yellow tones, without any furniture. Detainees were dressed in white clothes and held under constant electric light; food was served at random hours, and interrogations took place at irregular intervals.[20] This treatment was reserved for 'high value' prisoners.

After the Ayatollah's revolution, CIA advisers were forced to leave and SAVAK was refunded and renamed SAVAMA, but Evin Prison remained. Testimonies reveal that the cells for sensory deprivation were maintained and continue to be used to this day (Amnesty International, 2004), though they now receive technical assistance from Russian advisers, and methods have changed. Currently the detainee, after detention, is kept alone for two to four weeks with only sporadic contact with the person who brings them food or allows access to the toilet. The detainee is then interrogated, but interrogations are 'soft', and ask for the cooperation of an inmate who is increasingly broken. As a patient explained:

> They ask you for information. If the answer does not satisfy them, you are brought to the isolation cell for two or three days, and then back again. Once I told my torturer, who was always the same: 'C'mon, hit me.' He laughed: 'We do not do these things in Iran.' They get what they want without having to hit you. Once you give them a small piece of information they have informants inside every organization and cross-check the information, and over and over again they confront you and ask for details, showing you that they know everything beforehand. They can make you believe whatever they want. It takes two to three months, but sooner or later you break and then you begin to provide information. (K.S., Personal interview, September, 21, 2014)

Despite occurring in the same place, using the same basic principles and similar methods, SAVAK and SAVAMA torture play out in very different ways. One has less information about the victim prior to detention, and asks open questions without knowing exactly what they are searching for, with the understanding that time is important and a confession must be obtained as soon as possible. The other draws from a dense network of infiltrated informants who gather 'evidence' about the detainee. Interrogators then slowly proceed to destroy the detainee in a process that can take weeks, combining total and partial isolation with interrogations in an indefinite time frame. Victims of these practices will show different scars in the future – though sequelae from current practices are likely much longer lasting.

One constant between these two groups is that interrogators during both the SAVAK and SAVAMA years raped many of the female detainees (Iran Human Rights Documentation Center, 2011). Rape is a universal torture technique that does not change with political regimes or the nationality of advisers.

Actions

We have added a column in Table 10.2 with data on the work of mental health networks who work with torture survivors. There is a delay of approximately 20 years between *innovations* in torture methods developed by intelligence services and the psychology departments working

TABLE 10.2 Psychological torture: historical evolution, and scientific and mental health work

	France	US	UK	Scientific and mental health work
1940–1950		Reports by US researchers on torture in Germany (1940), Japan (1946), USSR (1950), China (1950).	Reports by UK researchers on German and Soviet interrogation techniques.	
1950–1955	1954. Algerian revolution	1951–1953. Project Artichoke 1954–1957. Reviews of communist 'brainwashing' – Biderman, Lifton.	1953–1954. Kenya 'emergency'	
1956–1960	1956. New French policy 1958. Henry Alleg – *The Question* 1959. Permanent French mission in Buenos Aires – Training of Southern Cone Military	1955. SERE Program begins 1955–1960. Project MK-Ultra Canada/US Donald Hebb –Sensory deprivation Donald Cameron – 'Psychic Driving'	1955–1960. Project MK-Ultra William Sargant works 1955–1960. Malaya 'emergency' 1960–1961. Cameroon 'emergency'	1961. Frantz Fanon – *The Wretched of the Earth* 1965. Film – *The Battle of Algiers*
1961–1965	1961.Trinquier – *La Guerre Moderne*. Worldwide influence. 1961.Aussaresses – military attaché in United States. Involved in training US interrogators. 1964. Galula invited to US *Counterinsurgency Warfare*	1961. Biderman – *Manipulation of Human Behavior* 1963. Milgram experiments 1963. CIA – KUBARK Manual 1959–1969. David Mitrione (US officer) trains torturers in the French model. Based in Brazil and Montevideo	1963–1964. Swaziland, Yemen and Brunei 'emergencies' – 'five techniques' defined	
1966–1970	French officers involved in training in Africa and Latin America.	1959–1969. David Mitrione (US officer) on-site seminars 1970. (approx.) Israeli training assistance	Use of "five techniques" in Ireland. Expansion in Africa.	

	France	US	UK	Scientific and mental health work
1971–1980	1973. Aussaresses involved in on-site training of Southern Cone interrogators (Brazil, Chile).	1974. USAID Army Mobile Teams provide on-site training to Southern and Central American interrogators (Panama, Honduras). Training provided in more than 20 countries including Israel, Iran and Egypt. Israeli assistance, based in Guatemala, a major source of on-site training all over Latin America.	1971. British interrogators involved in on-site training of Southern Cone interrogators (Brazil).	1979. Early works of Amnesty International – Denmark
1981–1990		1982–1984. Plan Sofia – Scorched earth policy 1983. CIA – Human Resource Exploitation Manual – translated and key source for training		1981. RCT founded in Copenhagen 1982. Early works by Chilean therapists 1984. Early works by EATIP – Argentina 1986. Early introduction of the idea of 'Psychological Torture'. 1989. Martin Baró killed.
1991–1995		1987. Army FM 34-52. Intelligence Interrogation Manuals		1990s. Theoretical discussions mainly focus on the epidemiology of physical torture, the appropriateness of using PTSD as a category, and therapy strategies in centers for torture victims. 1991. *Torture* journal launched.
1996–2000				1997. IRCT established as an independent network.
2001–2005		2000. First detainees in Guantanamo 2002. Enhanced Interrogation Techniques; creation of Behavioral Science Consultation Teams 2006. Army FM 2.22-3 Human Intelligence Collector Operations reviews US policies	British Army involved in allegations of torture in Iraq.	2004 – *Torture* journal re-launched.

TABLE 10.3 Torture techniques: sharing knowledge among countries

France: 1950s	Early accounts: 1940s	United Kingdom: 1950s	United States: 1960s–2000s	Guantanamo and Abu Ghraib
Algeria • Beating to death • Electric torture (Magneto) – ears, testicles • Water torture/simulated drowning (using buckets, wet clothes on face, water, etc.) • Sexual torture/rape **Latin America** • Pain torture: 'picana', 'tacho', 'caballete', 'pau de arara' **West Africa** • Beatings • Electric torture • Sexual torture • Hunger	**USSR** • Isolation • Fear • Cells/interrogation rooms (small, no blankets, light, temperature, starving, no toilet facilities) • Interrogation lasting weeks. Harsh and deceptive interrogation techniques • Stress positions (rigid chair) **Gestapo** • Isolation • Fear • Cells/onterrogation rooms • Beatings • Strenuous exercises • Exhausting interrogations with deceptive techniques **China** • Isolation • Fear • Group pressure for change • Strong social control/incentives **Japan** • Isolation • Immediate interrogation • Undermine morale of detainee • Threats • Beatings and good cop/bad cop • Stress positions (kneeling for hours) • Pain torture	**'Five Techniques'** • Stress positions – standing against a wall for hours • Hooding • Subjection to noise • Sleep deprivation • Restriction of food and drink And also: • Isolation • Manipulation of environment (heat, light, etc.) • Fear • Nakedness • Exhausting interrogations	**Mitrione** *'The precise pain, in the precise place, in the precise amount, for the desired effect.'* • Harsh cell conditions • Beating to death • Pain (electric, water, and other) • Prolonged stress positions • Manipulation of environment • Nakedness **KUBARK** *Induce psychological regression by:* • Shock of capture • Isolation/solitary confinement • Fear • Cells/interrogation rooms are windowless, soundproof, dark, and without toilets • Blindfolding, manipulation of environment to attack the mind (temperature, light, noise and hunger) • Nakedness • Deprivation of any kind of normal eating and sleeping routine • Stress positions and exhausting exercises • Pain and threats of pain • High pressure, coercive interrogations	• Beatings and ill treatment • Stress positions • Attacks on the senses, including periods of extreme sensory deprivation • Threats • Sexual humiliation • Debasement and feral treatment • Attacks on religion and culture • Use of phobias and fear of animals • Lengthy and deceptive interrogations

for them, on the one hand, and the *reaction* by civil society and organisations working with survivors, on the other. Organisations were still discussing the epidemiology of physical torture when torturers had already shifted to using primarily psychological methods.

Today, with better access to information thanks to the Internet, there is hope that this gap will diminish. The work of organisations like Physicians for Human Rights (PHR) to produce scientific documentation and new theories on the use of psychological torture in Guantanamo and the Middle East detention centres is a wonderful example of this shift towards a faster understanding of, and reaction against, torture.

The CIA is highly invested in promoting the idea that torture led to the capture of Osama Bin Laden; it even commissioned a commercial film (*Zero Dark Thirty*, released in 2012), echoing the old-fashioned propaganda of the film *I Am Not Alone*. This has become one of the primary concerns of the torture debate: utilitarians argue that the ends justify the means, and ethicists find torture wrong regardless of its eventual 'results'. It becomes more clear that torture is ineffective and there are strong scientific grounds to discard it as useless (O'Mara, 2015). Not only does it does not help in providing information, the information is unreliable and can be better obtained through other more efficient and successful ways. But what if the intentional destruction of human beings is ultimately a useless exercise? If torture does not meet its ostensible goal, then further investment, research, and resources are even more clearly unjustifiable. This is why the majority of current research is devoted to new technologies that aim to detect deception, in the hopes that imaging, thermal and neurophysiological devices might be able to distinguish between 'high' and 'low' value detainees, helping to screen sources prior to interrogations. Some cling to the fantasy that in the future, technical implements will direct interrogations based on subtle in vivo measurements of the detainee's bodily functions. These technologies will be reviewed in detail in Chapter 16.

Addendum: excerpts from *Modern Warfare: A French View of Counterinsurgency* by Roger Trinquier (1961)

Counterinsurgency warfare, interrogation and torture. '*Each man [in the revolutionary war] has a superior whom he knows; he will first have to give the name of this person, along with his address, so that it will be possible to proceed with the arrest and interrogation without delay. No lawyer is present for such an interrogation. If the prisoner gives the information requested, the examination is quickly terminated; if not, specialists must force his secret from him. Then, as a soldier, he must face the suffering, and perhaps the death, he has heretofore managed to avoid. The terrorist must accept this as a condition inherent in his trade and in the methods of warfare that, with full knowledge, his superiors and he himself have chosen*' (p. 23).

Interrogation in modern warfare '. . . *should be conducted by specialists perfectly versed in the techniques to be employed. (. . .) Science can easily place at the army's disposition the means for obtaining what is sought (. . .). It is deceitful to permit artillery or aviation to bomb villages and slaughter women and children, while the real enemy usually escapes, and to refuse interrogation specialists the right to seize the truly guilty terrorist and spare the innocent*' (p. 24).

Use of state terrorism. '*Terrorism in the hands of our adversaries has become a formidable weapon of war that we can no longer permit ourselves to ignore*' (p. 36).

Controlling the population. *[When we arrive at a location]'we cannot wait, however, until an intelligence network has been set up before obtaining from the population the information we need. Operations must begin as soon as the army has taken up its position. (. . .). The inhabitants are first mustered entirely by city district. They are quickly interrogated, individually and in secret, in a series of previously arranged small rooms. Any non-commissioned officer of the unit can ask them simple questions (. . .). As time goes on, we increase the number of interrogation teams. Certain inhabitants, assured that their identities will not be disclosed, will readily give the information requested. After verifying this data, we proceed to the arrest of the individuals who have been singled out and to force information from them. In this manner, we can capture the first-echelon elements of the enemy organization (. . .). Except for rare cases of emergency, the arrests should take place at night, facilitated by a curfew. (. . .) Anyone found away from his home at night is suspect, and will be arrested and interrogated. (. . .) Numerous small patrols will move about rapidly and securely apprehend most of the individuals sought in their homes. These are interrogated on the spot by specialized teams. They must give quickly the names and addresses of their superiors, so that the latter may be arrested before the lifting of the curfew. During the day, they would surely be forewarned* (pp. 45–46).

Collective torture. *'When we arrest important leaders, we carefully disguise them and line up before them all persons picked up in the course of police raids. The leaders will be able to point out members of their organization they recognize, whom we can arrest on the spot. At other times, we may place the leaders in concealed "observation posts" set up at heavily trafficked points in a city, from which they will indicate (by radio or other means) recognized individuals to surveillance teams who will quickly apprehend them'* (p. 77).

In villages *'the entire population, men and women, is called together and prohibited from leaving for the duration of the operation. Every inhabitant is individually and privately interrogated (. . .). If this first interrogation is well handled, several people will readily make the desired replies. Quite often, since guilty individuals hope to escape detection, the ones we seek will be among those assembled. We will therefore have no difficulty in arresting them. Those who have succeeded in leaving the village will not have gotten very far. Deprived of any contact with the population, they may very likely fall into our night ambushes when they attempt to find out what is going on or try to escape. The first echelon of the enemy politico-military organization will also fall into our hands (. . .)'* (pp. 77–78).

'At least a week is needed for the specialized teams to destroy a village politico-military organization (. . .). Parallel to the work of destruction, we lay the foundation of our own system by selecting intelligence agents and organizing the populace' (. . .) (p. 91).

Training. *'The intervention units are elite troops who will seek out the bands in their refuge areas and destroy them'* (p. 91).

'Cadres of the highest quality are needed to conduct an effective police operation, to interrogate interesting prisoners quickly at the very point of their capture, and to exploit the situation without losing any time. This difficult and costly training will be available to only a small number of units. They should be utilized judiciously so that they do not suffer unnecessary wear and tear. (. . .). The commanding general of an important theatre of operations ought to have at least four divisions at his disposal. Consolidated under the command of a dynamic leader, well up on the combat procedures of modern warfare, they will be capable of successfully handling within a few months the most threatened and vulnerable areas' (pp. 91–92).

Notes

1 'Regarding the use of torture, it was tolerated if not actually recommended. Francois Mitterrand, as minister of justice, had a de facto representative with General Massu in Judge Jean Berard, who covered our actions and knew exactly what was going on during the night. I had an excellent relationship with him, with nothing to hide' (Aussaresses, The Battle of the Casbah, pp. 128–30).

2 Soon the Front de Libération Nationale also began to torture French collaborators, though not with the same systematic methods or on the same scale.

3 The so-called Secret Army Organization, or Organisation de l'Armée Secrète (OAS) in French, was a right-wing terrorist organisation led by General Raoul Salan that led counterinsurgency par-amilitary operations in Algeria. It had more than 1,000 active members, perpetrating both selective killings and terrorist attacks against civilian targets. After the independence of Algeria, the OAS was dismantled. The main leaders moved to fascist Spain, Argentina and Chile, while some of them continued to work for more than two decades for the French Government that protected them.

4 It was not until the last review of the FM 3–24 in May 2014, after strong campaigning both from inside and outside the US Army, that all references to the French school have been completely erased (Department of Army, 2014, FM 3–24. Insurgencies and Countering Insurgencies. Washington DC).

5 The Phoenix Program followed the Algerian model and was designed, coordinated and executed by the CIA during the Vietnam War. The two major components of the program were Provincial Reconnaissance Units (PRUs) and regional interrogation centers. PRUs would kill or capture sus-pected Vietcong members, as well as civilians who were thought to have useful information. Many of these suspects were then taken to interrogation centres where they were tortured. The program was in operation between 1965 and 1972. According to official data, 81,740 suspected Vietcong operatives, informants and supporters were 'interrogated', of whom between 26,000 and 41,000 were killed during or after 'interrogation'.

6 The original 358-page text of the Sofia Plan was found in 2010 as part of the Guatemalan Documentation project. Full text available at www2.gwu.edu/~nsarchiv/NSAEBB/NSAEBB297/.

7 Amnesty International denounced a broad campaign in Yemen in 1964–1965 (Newbery, 2009).

8 www.twcenter.net/citingBBCnews (www.bbc.com/news/magazine-27625540).

9 There is a strong discussion within present-day China regarding the use of torture in police interro-gations, with at least five open access academic journals debating the issue. Most of the information is available on the Internet in Chinese. In a recent review of studies (Beken, Vander, and Wu, 2010), the authors (who do not live in China) find that torture is a serious matter of concern for two reasons: lack of clear regulations at all levels, and 'cultural reasons', both among the population and police officers, revealing that pressure and ill-treatment during detention is seen as customary, and is therefore not questioned.

10 Communist interrogations and brainwashing became part of the folk knowledge of American society in the 1950s. The 1956 film *I Am Not Alone* (directed by Arnold Laven) was inspired by these reports and was created specifically for an American audience; it is a fictional representation of the Soviet Union's interrogation and torture of a Polish Catholic nationalist until he embraces communism.

11 His influence has continued to this day. Some contemporary manuals on domestic violence and abuse still use Biderman's categories as a point of reference.

12 Biderman was a CIA contractor and received generous funding, but apparently did not have access to the results of other CIA contactors like Hebb or Cameron.

13 www2.gwu.edu/~nsarchiv/NSAEBB/NSAEBB54/.

14 25 million dollars in 1953 would be 179 million in 2014 according to the mathematical formula described in www.measuringworth.com/uscompare/relativevalue.php.

15 One of the most well-known experiments in MK-Delta is Project SPAN, which involved the con-tamination of food supplies and the spraying of a potent aerosolized LSD mixture in the village of Pont-Saint-Esprit, France in August, 1951. The Pont-Saint-Esprit incident resulted in mass psychosis,

32 committals to mental institutions, and at least seven deaths. It was officially attributed to some poisoning by a local bakery. The head of the project, a chemist working for the military (Frank Olson), died soon after. It was officially considered a suicide, although the family disputes this version (Albarelli, 2009, pp. 686–92).

16 The process and techniques approved at each stage and memorandum can be found at www.hrw .org/legacy/backgrounder/U.S./0819interrogation.htm.

17 Several 'low value' Guantanamo survivors who were assessed six months after release were literally destroyed. They had been reduced to a kind of childish regressive state, unable to hold basic meaningful conversation, recall an emotion or express feelings, and most of the time they remained in an absent, confused state. It took more than two years after their release for them to begin reassuming a semblance of a normal life (author's own assessment and follow-up).

18 Nothing is really new in the field, and psychologists already understood the effects of these kinds of procedures. When the patient submits voluntarily to this exercise, it can induce a pre-hypnotic state, useful for certain memory-processing techniques linked to past traumatic experiences. When it is not a voluntary process, it leads to confusion, destructuration, and psychosis (as seen in Henry Engler's testimony in Chapter 2).

19 Personal account of patients.

20 The method closely resembles the F-1 Type prisons operated in the past in Turkey.

11

PRIMARY NEEDS AND RELATIONSHIP TO THE ENVIRONMENT

We will briefly review key points on how detention conditions can be leveraged as part of interrogation and torture, and the potential impacts of these conditions. In Chapter 4 we examined the detention conditions found to amount to CIDT or torture by tribunals. Each country has domestic legislation that establishes rules regarding the treatment of prisoners and codes of practice. Although they are not uniform and some offer more protection than others, they usually adhere to international standards, which are sometimes deliberately vague – as the Special Rapporteur against Torture (Mendez, 2010) denounced. It is impossible, for instance, to find agreement regarding minimum cell size, or the minimum quantity of food to be provided. Reference texts mostly deal with *recommendations* (American Bar Association, 2011; Association of Chief Police Officers, 2012; Council of Europe, 2006; Coyle, 2002, 2008; Mendez, 2013; Rodriguez, 2007; UNHCR, 2005). Thus, it is difficult to define psychological torture in detention centres as those aspects which fall outside the authorised legal framework. In spite of this, it is worth reviewing some of the more essential aspects of these international standards and their guidelines regarding the limits of ill-treatment and torture in detention centres.

Detention conditions

The *UN Standard Minimum Rules for the Treatment of Prisoners*,[1] updated in December 2015 (the *Nelson Mandela Rules*[2]) and the *European Prison Rules* are the main points of reference when judging conditions of detention. They are applied to both long-term and short-term detention centres (like police stations), as well as during the transportation of persons in custody. Both systems of rules are effectively applicable to all people held under any form of detention or imprisonment, including detention for criminal or civil reasons; if the person is detained prior to trial, while on remand or after conviction; or if the individual is subject to so-called special security measures (see Table 11.1). Both the Inter-American and the European Court have recognised the presence of CIDT and torture in contexts were the person was retained in locations that did not comply with these minimum standards (Coyle, 2008). We reviewed this legal corpus in Chapter 3.

TABLE 11.1 UN Prison Standard Minimum Rules and Conditions (2015) – Mandela Rules: excerpts relevant to the definition of torture

Basic principles

Rule 1. All prisoners shall be treated with the respect due to their inherent dignity and value as human beings. No prisoner shall be subjected to, and all prisoners shall be protected from, torture and other cruel, inhuman or degrading treatment or punishment, for which no circumstances whatsoever may be invoked as a justification. The safety and security of prisoners, staff, service providers and visitors shall be ensured at all times (. . .)

Rule 7. No person shall be received in a prison without a valid commitment order. The following information shall be entered in the prisoner file management system upon admission of every prisoner: (a) Precise information enabling determination of his or her unique identity, respecting his or her self-perceived gender; (b) The reasons for his or her commitment and the responsible authority, in addition to the date, time and place of arrest; (. . .) (d) Any visible injuries and complaints about prior ill-treatment;

Rule 8. The following information shall be entered in the prisoner file management system in the course of imprisonment, where applicable: (a) Information related to the judicial process, including dates of court hearings and legal representation (. . .) (d) Requests and complaints, including allegations of torture or other cruel, inhuman or degrading treatment or punishment, unless they are of a confidential nature; (e) Information on the imposition of disciplinary sanctions; (f) Information on the circumstances and causes of any injuries or death and, in the case of the latter, the destination of the remains.

Rule 9. All records referred to in rules 7 and 8 shall be kept confidential and made available only to those whose professional responsibilities require access to such records. Every prisoner shall be granted access to the records pertaining to him or her, subject to redactions authorised under domestic legislation, and shall be entitled to receive an official copy of such records upon his or her release.

Conditions of imprisonment

Rule 12. Accommodation. 1. Where sleeping accommodation is in individual cells or rooms, each prisoner shall occupy by night a cell or room by himself or herself. If for special reasons, such as temporary overcrowding, it becomes necessary for the central prison administration to make an exception to this rule, it is not desirable to have two prisoners in a cell or room. 2. Where dormitories are used, they shall be occupied by prisoners carefully selected as being suitable to associate with one another in those conditions. There shall be regular supervision by night, in keeping with the nature of the prison.

Rule 13. All accommodation provided for the use of prisoners and in particular all sleeping accommodation shall meet all requirements of health, due regard being paid to climatic conditions and particularly to cubic content of air, minimum floor space, lighting, heating and ventilation.

Rule 14. In all places where prisoners are required to live or work: (a) The windows shall be large enough to enable the prisoners to read or work by natural light and shall be so constructed that they can allow the entrance of fresh air whether or not there is artificial ventilation; (b) Artificial light shall be provided sufficient for the prisoners to read or work without injury to eyesight.

Health services

Rule 24. 1. The provision of health care for prisoners is a State responsibility. Prisoners should enjoy the same standards of health care that are available in the community, and should have access to necessary health-care services free of charge without discrimination on the grounds of their legal status.

Rule 25. (. . .) 2. The health-care service shall consist of an interdisciplinary team with sufficient qualified personnel acting in full clinical independence and shall encompass sufficient expertise in psychology and psychiatry. The services of a qualified dentist shall be available to every prisoner.

Health services

Rule 26. 1. The health-care service shall prepare and maintain accurate, up-to-date and confidential individual medical files on all prisoners, and all prisoners should be granted access to their files upon request. A prisoner may appoint a third party to access his or her medical file. (...)
Rule 27. (...) 2. Clinical decisions may only be taken by the responsible health-care professionals and may not be overruled or ignored by non-medical prison staff.
Rule 30. A physician or other qualified health-care professionals, whether or not they are required to report to the physician, shall see, talk with and examine every prisoner as soon as possible following his or her admission and thereafter as necessary. Particular attention shall be paid to (...) (b) Identifying any ill-treatment that arriving prisoners may have been subjected to prior to admission; (c) Identifying any signs of psychological or other stress brought on by the fact of imprisonment, including, but not limited to, the risk of suicide or self-harm and withdrawal symptoms resulting from the use of drugs, medication or alcohol; and undertaking all appropriate individualised measures or treatment.
Rule 32. 1. The relationship between the physician or other health-care professionals and the prisoners shall be governed by the same ethical and professional standards as those applicable to patients in the community, in particular: (a) The duty of protecting prisoners' physical and mental health and the prevention and treatment of disease on the basis of clinical grounds only; (b) Adherence to prisoners' autonomy with regard to their own health and informed consent in the doctor-patient relationship; (c) The confidentiality of medical information, unless maintaining such confidentiality would result in a real and imminent threat to the patient or to others; (d) An absolute prohibition on engaging, actively or passively, in acts that may constitute torture or other cruel, inhuman or degrading treatment or punishment, including medical or scientific experimentation that may be detrimental to a prisoner's health, such as the removal of a prisoner's cells, body tissues or organs. (...)
Rule 33. The physician shall report to the prison director whenever he or she considers that a prisoner's physical or mental health has been or will be injuriously affected by continued imprisonment or by any condition of imprisonment.
Rule 34. If, in the course of examining a prisoner upon admission or providing medical care to the prisoner thereafter, health-care professionals become aware of any signs of torture or other cruel, inhuman or degrading treatment or punishment, they shall document and report such cases to the competent medical, administrative or judicial authority. Proper procedural safeguards shall be followed in order not to expose the prisoner or associated persons to foreseeable risk of harm. (...)

Restrictions, discipline and sanctions

Rule 41. 4. Prisoners shall have an opportunity to seek judicial review of disciplinary sanctions imposed against them.
Rule 42. General living conditions addressed in these rules, including those related to light, ventilation, temperature, sanitation, nutrition, drinking water, access to open air and physical exercise, personal hygiene, health care and adequate personal space, shall apply to all prisoners without exception.
Rule 43. 1. In no circumstances may restrictions or disciplinary sanctions amount to torture or other cruel, inhuman or degrading treatment or punishment. The following practices, in particular, shall be prohibited: (a) Indefinite solitary confinement; (b) Prolonged solitary confinement; (c) Placement of a prisoner in a dark or constantly lit cell; (d) Corporal punishment or the reduction of a prisoner's diet or drinking water; (e) Collective punishment. (...)
Rule 44. For the purpose of these rules, solitary confinement shall refer to the confinement of prisoners for 22 hours or more a day without meaningful human contact. Prolonged solitary confinement shall refer to solitary confinement for a time period in excess of 15 consecutive days.

(continued)

TABLE 11.1 UN Prison Standard Minimum Rules and Conditions (2015) – Mandela Rules: excerpts relevant to the definition of torture (*continued*)

Restrictions, discipline and sanctions

Rule 45. 1. Solitary confinement shall be used only in exceptional cases as a last resort, for as short a time as possible and subject to independent review, and only pursuant to the authorisation by a competent authority. It shall not be imposed by virtue of a prisoner's sentence. 2. The imposition of solitary confinement should be prohibited in the case of prisoners with mental or physical disabilities when their conditions would be exacerbated by such measures. The prohibition of the use of solitary confinement and similar measures in cases involving women and children, as referred to in other United Nations standards and norms in crime prevention and criminal justice, continues to apply.
Rule 46. 1. Health-care personnel shall not have any role in the imposition of disciplinary sanctions or other restrictive measures. They shall, however, pay particular attention to the health of prisoners held under any form of involuntary separation, including by visiting such prisoners on a daily basis and providing prompt medical assistance and treatment at the request of such prisoners or prison staff. (...)

Instruments of restraint

Rule 47. 1. The use of chains, irons or other instruments of restraint which are inherently degrading or painful shall be prohibited. (...)

Searches of prisoners and cells

Rule 52. 1. Intrusive searches, including strip and body cavity searches, should be undertaken only if absolutely necessary. (...) 2. Body cavity searches shall be conducted only by qualified health-care professionals other than those primarily responsible for the care of the prisoner (...).

Other relevant elements

Rule 57. 3. Allegations of torture or other cruel, inhuman or degrading treatment or punishment of prisoners shall be dealt with immediately and shall result in a prompt and impartial investigation conducted by an independent national authority in accordance with paragraphs1 and 2 of rule 71. (...)
Rule 68. Every prisoner shall have the right, and shall be given the ability and means, to inform immediately his or her family, or any other person designated as a contact person, about his or her imprisonment, about his or her transfer to another institution and about any serious illness or injury. The sharing of prisoners' personal information shall be subject to domestic legislation.
Rule 71. 1. Notwithstanding the initiation of an internal investigation, the prison director shall report, without delay, any custodial death, disappearance or serious injury to a judicial or other competent authority that is independent of the prison administration and mandated to conduct prompt, impartial and effective investigations into the circumstances and causes of such cases. The prison administration shall fully cooperate with that authority and ensure that all evidence is preserved. 2. The obligation in paragraph 1 of this rule shall equally apply whenever there are reasonable grounds to believe that an act of torture or other cruel, inhuman or degrading treatment or punishment has been committed in prison, irrespective of whether a formal complaint has been received. 3. Whenever there are reasonable grounds to believe that an act referred to in paragraph 2 of this rule has been committed, steps shall be taken immediately to ensure that all potentially implicated persons have no involvement in the investigation and no contact with the witnesses, the victim or the victim's family (...).
Rule 82. 1. Prison staff shall not, in their relations with the prisoners, use force except in self-defence or in cases of attempted escape, or active or passive physical resistance to an order based on law or regulations. Prison staff who have recourse to force must use no more than is strictly necessary and must report the incident immediately to the prison director. (...)

Other relevant elements

Rule 83. 1. There shall be a twofold system for regular inspections of prisons and penal services: (a) Internal or administrative inspections conducted by the central prison administration; (b) External inspections conducted by a body independent of the prison administration, which may include competent international or regional bodies (. . .).

Rule 89. 3. It is desirable that the number of prisoners in closed prisons should not be so large that the individualisation of treatment is hindered. In some countries it is considered that the population of such prisons should not exceed 500. In open prisons the population should be as small as possible.

Rule 109. 1. Persons who are found to be not criminally responsible, or who are later diagnosed with severe mental disabilities and/or health conditions, for whom staying in prison would mean an exacerbation of their condition, shall not be detained in prisons, and arrangements shall be made to transfer them to mental health facilities as soon as possible.

Rule 111. 2. Unconvicted prisoners are presumed to be innocent and shall be treated as such.

Adapted from *UN Standard Minimum Rules for the Treatment of Prisoners*. A/RES/70/175.

The UN (Nelson Mandela) Rules provide a detailed framework (see Table 11.1) but they have a 'non-binding nature'[3] suggesting that Member States may adapt the application of the Rules in accordance with their domestic legal frameworks, as appropriate, bearing in mind the spirit and purposes of the Rules. The European Prison Rules are defined in broader terms (Council of Europe, 1973, 2006; Coyle, 2002; Mendez, 2013; Economic and Social Council, 1957). They are only *recommendations* (Council of Europe, 2006), and limit their scope to enouncing global principles. Their concretion (their nature, specifications, duration, the grounds on which they may be applied or any other aspect) are determined by domestic laws, and depend on national security and domestic policy concerns. Additional specifications can be deduced from the European Court's sentences, though the judges' rulings are usually vague. These guidelines can be important tools when implemented together with domestic enforcement mechanisms, but unfortunately most countries lack such mechanisms.

The European Committee for the Prevention of Torture (CPT) has developed specific norms for pre-trial detention and police custody through its annual reports and country visits (Morgan and Evans, 1999, 2001). The Committee is of the view that, in places of detention intended for short-term custody,[4] the '*physical conditions. . . cannot be expected to be as good. . . as in other places where persons may be held for lengthy periods*' and accepts some limitations to the general European Prison Rules.

The US lacks any kind of universal law or general rule that protects prisoners in their legal system. The American Bar Association (2011) has provided a set of independent rules for US prisons based primarily on domestic jurisprudence that discusses local minimums of protection for prisoners; these rules are a useful guideline for best practices.

These standards are of great help in monitoring visits, although it must be kept in mind that it is the interaction among all of the elements what will ultimately be relevant.

Social isolation, solitary confinement and sensory deprivation

The first element that most torturing systems share is the use of isolation. In almost all torturing systems not based on the simple and direct production of pain, total or partial isolation can be considered the foundation on which psychological torture is built. It was the cornerstone of Biderman's classical model of human manipulation and thought control (1957; see also Biderman and Zimmer, 1961), and a central focus of the MK–Ultra research project. From incommunicado detention to the F and maximum security prisons, isolation has always been at the centre of the debate on torture.

There are three different situations which are all commonly referred to as 'isolation' that are best understood separately: **social isolation**, defined by preventing detainee contact with any person except the interrogator; **sensory deprivation**, defined by creating an environment in which all of the senses are obliterated, and the person has some or all of his or her sensory afferences blockaded; and a **controlled environment**, in which every minute detail of a person's life is fully controlled. Of course, these three categories sometimes overlap.

Social isolation is distinct from **solitary confinement**. Social isolation is a strategic process during detention and interrogation of a suspect, aimed at avoiding contact with the outside world. Solitary confinement is a category of legal penalty applied to certain inmates, ordered by a court or by prison authorities, in which the person has no contact with any other *prisoner*. In incommunicado detention this restriction is extended to any *person*, including lawyers or trusted doctors. It is a form of legal punishment. Because it is authorised by law, it cannot technically be categorised as a form of torture, although there are many interesting studies (which we will review below) that help shed light on the effects of social isolation.

Social isolation

Social isolation is a strategic process during detention that, officially, seeks to prevent the detainee from sharing information or preparing an alibi with other detainees. In the context of a coercive interrogation, social isolation serves to:

1. Exploit the strong, basic human need for belonging. The person is abandoned to his or her own fears, with no possibility to share his or her thoughts. He or she may feel scared and alone.
2. When social isolation is prolonged, it increases the need for contact and creates a predisposition towards the captor, who is always the only source of human contact. The detainee will then be compelled to establish bonds and talk.
3. The need to talk will eventually make him or her more likely to speak with interrogators.
4. Any small sign of attention, positive reward or sign of recognition from the captor can be interpreted in positive terms and have an impact on cooperation. Sometimes it can even lead to emotional dependence on the captor through an ambivalent tie.
5. During the time between interrogations, the person is again left alone with his or her thoughts for an indefinite period of time. The detainee likely goes over the interrogation in his or her mind, remembering what was said and what wasn't. Over time, this makes it more difficult to remember the interrogations accurately, and it is easier to become confused, contradict oneself or provide new information.
6. The lack of stimulation induces a rapid, progressive state of weakness and lethargy in which the person does not have the mental strength needed to resist suggestion.

Social isolation is, then, a pre-condition for a successful interrogation.

In a review of classical studies Kubzansk (1961) showed that short periods of social isolation (from one to a maximum of four days) did not deteriorate the quality of the information recalled by the subject, but did affect his or her ability to reason through the complexities of the interrogator-prisoner relationship, and thus decreased the ability to cope rationally and effectively with being interrogated. The studies regarding social isolation and suggestibility (the success of social isolation in modifying beliefs and convictions) showed inconclusive results, probably because the periods of isolation were too short to provide evidence of significant changes.

The Enhanced Interrogation procedures in Guantanamo avoid the word isolation and use 'segregation' to refer to the idea of *social isolation*. 'Segregation' was officially authorised for up to 30 days, but the duration could be extended indefinitely with special permission. According to independent reports, some detainees were kept in isolation from periods ranging from three to eighteen months (Physicians for Human Rights, 2005). The practice was widespread, and, according to the International Committee of the Red Cross (ICRC) there were around 500 detainees in complete isolation in the Camp Five facilities.

Honigsberg (2013) coined the term *linguistic isolation* (Koenig calls this cultural isolation) to describe the situation of a 16-year-old Uzbek adolescent held in Guantanamo for eight years with inmates who only spoke Arab or English, even though there were other Uzbek people who were also detained.

Solitary confinement and incommunicado detention

Solitary confinement (SC) is a lawful regime in prison that involves the deprivation of social contact. The *Istanbul Statement on the Use and Effects of Solitary Confinement* defines it as 'physical isolation in a cell for 22 to 24 hours a day' (Task Group, 2008). In SC, meaningful contact with other people is minimised, and any contact is often monotonous and not empathetic[5] (Smith, 2008b). The Special Rapporteur proposed that 15 days marks the limit between 'solitary confinement' and 'prolonged solitary confinement' (Mendez, 2011) that could be considered by itself as ill-treatment or even torture.

There is ample anthropological, historical and medical documentation of solitary confinement since the early 19th century which provides strong evidence of its severe mental health effects on the vast majority of subjects. We reviewed the testimony of Henry Engler (2012), a member of the Tupamaro movement in Uruguay, in Chapter 2, and his descent into psychosis during isolation.

Studies show that between 33 and 90 per cent of prisoners in solitary confinement experience mild to severe adverse symptoms (Grassian, 2006; Haney, 2003; Shalev, 2008; Smith, 2008a). Psychiatric symptoms can appear after only a few days in solitary confinement; although the literature suggests some risk factors, it is impossible to predict which people will experience symptoms (Shalev, 2008).

Kubzansk's (1961) review shows that there are two broad patterns of detainee responses to SC: those who, in general, adapt well to isolation, who may even reach equilibrium over time, and prefer not to be held together with other prisoners; and those who soon become distraught, and experience steadily increasing anguish over time, leading to despair and self-aggression.

To date, there are no reliable epidemiological data on the mental health consequences of SC. There are few studies and they cannot be compared. Some provide data from people in absolute social and sensory deprivation (which commonly occurs in specially-designed maximum security jails in some countries). Other studies offer data from people who are deprived of human contact but still allowed to keep a minimum of intellectual activity (access to books, radio, TV, one hour of exercise). There are even studies that suggest that SC does not have a negative impact – these are based on violent prisons, where social isolation without losing other rights is seen as a privilege. Currently, a meta-analysis summarising all available data remains impossible.

Patterns of psychological response: from aggression to learned helplessness. There are at least 50 different studies which document the impact of isolation on adult animals (Mortensen, 2012). Negative impacts affect all areas of a living being, from brain functioning to bodily diseases. In human beings there are two different broad patterns of reaction when all stimulation and control is removed. Some prisoners have increased anxiety and unease and resort to aggression (leading to self-mutilation) as a way of obtaining sensory input and feeling alive, while others fall into a state of learned helplessness and become submissive, passive and apathetic. They become so reliant on the external world of the prison to organise and control their lives that they ultimately lose the capacity for self-determination and autonomy; their capacity to exert will, to plan and to act is permanently damaged (Rodriguez, 2011).

Grassian (2006) conducted a classical review of studies, which remains the primary point of reference on the subject. Table 11.2 summarises the key clusters of symptoms, with per centages derived from a qualitative review of available studies.[6] Some of these symptoms carry over as permanent damage – especially irritability, impulsiveness, pervasive sleep disorders, dependency and lack of autonomy, and severe difficulties in establishing trusting bonds and social relationships (Shalev, 2008).

Although the vast majority of literature is convergent with their descriptions and it can be said beyond a reasonable doubt that confinement practices in prison have detrimental health effects in a significant per centage of inmates (Smith, 2008a), the difficulties in separating solitary confinement (social isolation) from sensory deprivation make the data difficult to interpret.

The impact of solitary confinement depends on the following factors, among others (Grassian, 2006):

1. Medical surveillance. A doctor should certify that there is no contraindication for SC and should perform regular visits. This undoubtedly poses ethical problems for the doctors involved (Elahi, 2004; Metzner and Fellner, 2010).
2. Conditions in the cell. Space according to standard minimum rules for prisoners, access to books, TV, newspapers, radio, etc. (American Civil Liberties Union, 2012; Haney and Lynch, 1997).

TABLE 11.2 Cluster of symptoms in detainees in SC (SC by Solitary Confinement)

1. Inability to distinguish the internal and external word. Merging of reality, fantasy and illusions (60%) (Shalev, 2008).
2. Hyper-responsivity to external stimuli. Progressive inability to tolerate ordinary stimuli (50%).
3. Perceptual distortions, illusions and hallucinations: voices, often whispering frightening things (30%) leading to acute psychotic, confused states (Grassian, 2006; Shalev, 2008).
4. Anxiety and nervousness. Panic attacks (50%) (Haney and Lynch, 1997; Haney, 2003; Toch, 1992).
5. Helplessness and despair. Anomia (Toch, 1992), leading to full clinical depression (Shalev, 2008).
6. Severe difficulties with thinking, concentration, and memory.
7. Intrusive thoughts (Grassian, 2006).
8. Obsessional thoughts. Primitive aggressive ruminations (50%) (Grassian, 2006).
9. Overt paranoia (50%).
10. Problems with impulse control. Self-mutilation, aggressions (40%) (Grassian, 2006; H. Miller and Young, 1997).

Adapted from Shalev, S. (2008).

3. Restricting contact with other inmates (and also with lawyers, doctors, educators or relatives in incommunicado detention).

4. Total or partial sensory isolation (access to natural light/windows, sounds from outside (locked metal door designed to cause sensory isolation), plain walls and floor with uniform color).

5. Adequate justification of SC based on security measures. Grassian (2006) suggests that inmates present more psychiatric symptoms when they perceived that this is an arbitrary decision whose only purpose is punishment.

6. Periodic review by judicial authorities who supervise internment (Rodley and Pollard, 2009).

7. Length of stay. Some authors (Haney, 2003; Shalev, 2008) suggest seven to ten days as the maximum limit for most subjects before clear and evident damage appears, although symptoms can appear after only one day. In extreme sensory deprivation, experimental subjects present psychotic symptoms in the first 48 hours. The consequences are much worse when the person is confined without any information about the length of SC (Shalev, 2011; Toch, 1992).

Sensory deprivation

Sensory deprivation (SD) is the confinement in spaces where there is a deprivation of sensory stimulation, leading to a state of anomia and lack of stimulation. It may include noise elimination, 24-hour monotonous light and an environment without visual stimulation (rounded objects; no furniture; uniform color for walls, ceiling and floor; plain or similar colors for clothes and implements; etc.).

We briefly reviewed studies in the 1950s and 1960s that dealt with sensory deprivation as part of the MK–Ultra Project in Chapter 10.

Citing Biderman, the KUBARK Manual recommends sensory deprivation as a central tenet of coercive interrogations. For especially rapid results, the manual endorses the use of a 'cell which has no light (or weak artificial light which never varies), which is sound-proofed, in which odors are eliminated, etc., (. . .) the subject has a growing need for physical and social stimuli; and some subjects progressively lose touch with reality, focus inwardly, and produce delusions, hallucinations, and other pathological effects' (p. 87). The manual warns that 'everyone has read of prisoners who were reluctant to leave their cells after prolonged incarceration. Little is known about the duration of confinement calculated to make a subject shift from anxiety, coupled with a desire for sensory stimuli and human companionship, to a passive, apathetic acceptance of isolation and an ultimate pleasure in this negative state. Undoubtedly the rate of change is determined almost entirely by the psychological characteristics of the individual. In any event, it is advisable to keep the subject upset by constant disruptions of patterns.'

The Human Resource Exploitation Manual (Central Intelligence Agency, 1983) warns against the use of SD, saying that it 'acts on most persons as a powerful stress. A person cut off from external sensory stimuli turns his awareness inward and projects his unconscious outward. The symptoms most commonly produced by solitary confinement are superstition, intense love of any other living thing, perceiving inanimate objects as alive, hallucinations, and delusions.'

Records of prolonged sensory isolation with terrorist suspects

The first record of the modern use of prolonged sensory isolation is that of the members of the Bader-Meinhoff group in Germany. Astrid Poll, one of the members, declared: '*I was taken to an empty wing, a dead wing, where I was the only prisoner. (. . .) I could not hear any noises apart from the ones that I generated myself. Nothing. Absolute silence. I went through states of excitement, I was haunted by visual and acoustic hallucinations. There were extreme disturbances of concentration and attacks of weakness. I had no idea how long this would go on for. I was terrified that I would go mad.'*

She was sent to a psychiatric hospital, and she escaped two years later. Recaptured in England after three years, she wrote: '*During the two and a half years of remand I was completely isolated [for more than four months] in the Dead Wing of Cologne-Ossendorf. Not even today, six years later, have I completely recovered from that. I can't stand rooms which are painted white because they remind me of my cell. Silence in a wood can terrify me, it reminds me of the silence in the isolated cell. Darkness makes me [depressed], as if my life were taken away. Solitude causes me as much fear as crowds. Even today I occasionally [feel] as if I can't move'* (Croissant, 1975).

Sensory isolation has always been used. It was well documented in Uruguay against the leaders of the Tupamaros Guerrillas (who were held in solitary confinement which lasted up to ten years, with long periods of almost complete sensory isolation) and Peru (where most MRTA and Shining Path members were held in sensory isolation in high-security prisons for years). We saw the consequences of this in Henry Engler's testimony in Chapter 2.

The Turkish government designed special cells that included sensory deprivation in the F-Type prisons (Erol, 2010), but international pressure and recommendations from the CPT and the ECHR lead to their closing. In Iran, the use of sensory deprivation in Evin Prison has been documented for over thirty years (Medical Foundation for the Care of Victims of Torture, 2013).

Sensory deprivation was also one of the Enhanced Interrogation techniques authorised in Guantanamo Bay, although there were legal warnings that it would violate the Geneva Convention. Sensory deprivation was considered 'relative' and to be used for a 'short time'. The term could refer to anything from being left alone in a room to being subjected to complex outfits combining goggles, earmuffs, mittens and darkened cells that quickly drive subjects into psychotic states. According to Physicians for Human Rights (PHR) people were immobilised individually in small, soundproof rooms and dressed in blacked-out goggles and earmuffs. There are documented cases in which this induced permanent psychotic states (Physicians for Human Rights, 2005).

The question was whether or not sensory isolation might be used for short periods of time without mental health risks, and how long those periods could be. Mason and Brady (2009) conducted an experimental research study in London. They classified normal students in low versus high susceptibility to hallucinations using a psychometric measure, and placed them in a full isolation device for 15 minutes. The test showed significant increases on three subscales of the Psychotomimetic States Inventory: perceptual distortions, anhedonia and paranoia in both groups – though clearly the effect was greater in hallucination-prone individuals. Participants saw 'faces even though no one was in fact there' (two strongly); six participants saw 'shapes and forms even though they weren't there' (four strongly); four participants felt that their 'sense of smell was unusually strong or different' (one strongly) and two participants 'sensed an evil presence even though they couldn't see it'. The authors raise the question of what effect would result when a person is subjected to conditions of extreme fear without knowing the length of time he or she would remain in sensory isolation.

Solitary isolation and solitary confinement in international human rights law

From a legal point of view, solitary confinement is part of the lawful sanctions in the penitentiary system of most countries. Between 5 and 20 per cent of inmates across countries are held in solitary confinement, depending on the strictness of domestic laws. It is a legal, widespread practice.

Justifications for solitary confinement include pre-trial confinement to avoid informing others of aspects related to the alleged offense, isolation of dangerous and conflictive inmates to prevent conflict and control misbehaviour, or confinement as a disciplinary measure. In any case, the decision must always be taken by a competent body, in accordance with the law and in adherence with the requirements of due process. The authority making the decision should justify its decision in writing, and be held accountable for the decision. In the case of pre-trial detention, only a court should authorise solitary confinement. If these rules of due process are not respected, solitary confinement may amount to ill-treatment or torture.

Prisoners are protected by the International Covenant on Civil and Political Rights (ICCPR) monitored by the Human Rights Committee (HRC). Under Article 10, the ICCPR states that a person in detention shall be treated with humanity and with respect for the inherent dignity of the human person, and that the essential aim of the penitentiary system shall be social rehabilitation.[7]

Case law

The effects of SD have been found to be so devastating that almost all international human rights bodies have stated that its use produces 'severe or serious mental pain and suffering' that can amount to torture.

The UN Human Rights Committee found a specific isolation regime to violate both Article 7 and Article 10 of the ICCPR (*Campos v. Peru*, 9 January 1998).

The Inter-American Court of Human Rights has repeatedly and consistently found that solitary confinement amounts to cruel, inhuman and degrading treatment. For instance, in *Castillo Petruzzi et al. v. Peru* (1998),[8] there is a lengthy discussion on the subject, with references to previous sentences. In *Suárez Rosero v. Ecuador* the Court establishes that '*isolation from the outside world produces moral and psychological suffering in any person, places him in a particularly vulnerable position, and increases the risk of aggression and arbitrary acts in prison*'.

Judge Myjer (2004), member of the ECHR, reviewed cases of solitary confinement from 1980 to 2003. He concludes that the Court case law suggests that complete sensory isolation coupled with total social isolation can destroy the personality, and constitutes a form of inhuman treatment which cannot be justified based on the security requirements or for any other reason. He states that SC can even amount to torture by itself, but that the deprivation of social contact for security, disciplinary or protective reasons *while providing contact* with lawyers and relatives and basic facilities for leisure does *not* amount to inhuman treatment or degrading punishment – especially when dealing with detainees suspected of participating in terrorism, the mafia or international criminal organisations. The Council of Europe stated that a system of isolation called FIES[9] (established in Spain to control supposedly dangerous inmates for periods of up to a year[10] in very austere material conditions of detention with little or no activities) constituted 'inhuman treatment'.[11] In all case law the European Court has demanded the claimant document that prolonged segregation caused marked psychological effects amounting to cruel, inhuman or degrading treatment. In circumstances of prolonged solitary confinement, the Court has held that the justification for solitary confinement must be explained to the individual and the justification must be 'increasingly detailed and compelling' as time goes on.[12]

Additionally, European Prison Rule 38(1) requires that *'punishment by disciplinary confinement . . . shall only be imposed if the medical officer after examination certifies in writing that the prisoner is fit to sustain it'* and Rule 38(3) requires the medical officer *'to observe prisoners in such confinement daily, monitoring any change in their psychological state, which prompts immediate termination or alteration of punishment'*. Medical organisations have objected to this on ethical grounds, and the World Health Organization discourages doctors from accepting involvement in these kinds of procedures, or even working for prison systems (WHO-EU, 2007). In 2002, the International Center for Prison Studies, ICPS, distributed a handbook for prison staff, reiterating that solitary confinement is inappropriate punishment save for the most exceptional circumstances, and emphasising that careful monitoring of prisoners' mental states is integral to maintaining the welfare of inmates (Vasiliades, 2004).

The American Psychiatric Association has proposed to ban solitary confinement for inmates previously diagnosed with a severe mental disorder and especially those diagnosed with a psychotic disease (American Psychiatric Association, 2005).

In 2011 the Special Rapporteur presented a thematic report discussing whether solitary confinement would be considered cruel, inhuman or degrading treatment *in itself* (Mendez, 2011). He proposed that, based on medical evidence showing that prolonged solitary confinement produced long-term damage to the mental health of most inmates subjected to it, *any imposition of solitary confinement beyond 15 days constitutes torture or cruel, inhuman or degrading treatment or punishment, depending on the circumstances.* He called on the international community to agree to this standard and impose an absolute prohibition on solitary confinement exceeding 15 consecutive days.

Short-term solitary confinement amounts to CIDT or torture in the following circumstances:

1. When used for the purpose of punishment, including as a result of a breach of prison discipline, *'as long as the pain and suffering experienced by the victim reaches the necessary severity'.* (Mendez, 2011)
2. If the purpose of the solitary confinement is to coerce the person or to extract information or a confession from him or her. *'The practice of solitary confinement during pretrial detention creates a de facto situation of psychological pressure which can influence detainees to make confessions or statements against others and undermines the integrity of the investigation (. . .)* and *'it amounts to torture (. . .) or to cruel, inhuman, or degrading treatment or punishment'* (Mendez, 2011; Reyes, 2008; Smith, 2008b).
3. When the conditions are disproportionately harsh (limited space, no social contact at all/ incommunicado detention, sensory deprivation, prolonged confinement, etc.); short-term solitary confinement also amounts to CIDT or torture, according to the European Court and the SRT, in all cases where there is *sensory deprivation*.

Incommunicado detention requires unique analysis. Sentences from the Human Rights Commission, the Inter-American Commission and the European Court of Human Rights (e.g. *Onoufriou v. Cyprus* (2010)) find that *complete* social isolation, which includes preventing access to a lawyer or to medical or psychological assistance, amounts to Inhuman Treatment and must be ceased regardless of the circumstances (Open Society, 2012; Rodley and Pollard, 2009).

Sleep regulation

Sleep regulation, also referred to as sleep adjustment, sleep manipulation or sleep deprivation, is a coercive method used mainly in contexts in which interrogations and confessions are important. It requires the captors to be present constantly to keep the detainee awake. It is not an effective strategy if used solely for punishment.

Sleep regulation can be defined as not allowing a person to obtain complete rest. An adult human being needs between 6 and 10 hours of continuous sleep (8 hours on average[13]). Sleep deprivation is the use of maneuvers aimed to prevent normal rest, including:

- Shackling
- Spraying with water
- Forced walking or exercise
- Stress positions (like wall-standing with hands held above the head, or standing on a small surface with the risk of falling)
- Loud music
- Allowing the person to fall asleep and then waking them immediately with shouts, slaps, beatings, etc.

A variant is *sleep dysregulation*, in which the detainee's ordinary sleep schedule is disturbed by, for example, reversing the sleep cycles from night to day without depriving the detainee of sleep. The hours he or she is awake, provided with food, or allowed to go to the toilet differ from his or her normal routine. Consequently, the person is constantly disoriented (similar to continuous jetlag). The person remains awake and is interrogated in the hours when studies show that it is easier to induce a confession, from 3:00 to 6:00 AM.

The purpose of sleep deprivation can, of course, be simply to punish the victim. Not being able to sleep is an unpleasant experience, one that provokes an internal battle. The person would like to stay awake, but the need to sleep is sometimes insurmountable. In normal conditions, this can often be solved by a brief 15-minute nap, which allows for a slight recovery. If even such brief respite is prevented, the person becomes painfully trapped and may suffer intense headaches and desperation, cognitive exhaustion and brief periods of disconnection. In those periods, the detainee may fall asleep for as few as one to three minutes, in which his or her brain will attempt to reach REM phase. He or she may experience dreams that merge fantasy and reality, with hypnagogic and hypnopompic perceptual alterations and confusion of the inner and the outer world. It becomes difficult for him or her to know what is real and what is a dream. The will is suppressed, and the person feels deeply irritable and exhausted.

But keeping a person awake requires effort. Though it can be used as punishment, the main function of sleep deprivation is to facilitate the interrogation of suspects. It is among the short-term measures that prolong the *shock of capture* and prevent the detainee from recovering, regaining control or making decisions.

Sleep deprivation affects almost every function of the human body (Table 11.3). It has cognitive effects and makes the person more vulnerable to cognitive manipulation; it has negative effects on mood and produces irritability and anger that can be directed inwards; it increases the perception of pain; and it diminishes the capacity to react in complex adverse situations.

For this reason, the KUBARK Manual (Central Intelligence Agency, 1963) notes that sleep deprivation should not be prolonged over time, and recommends imposing shorter periods of *absolute* sleep or patterns of repeated *interruptions* of sleep: '*Another objection to the deliberate inducing of debility is that prolonged exertion, loss of sleep, etc., themselves become patterns to which the subject adjusts through apathy. The interrogator should use his power over the resistant subject's physical environment to disrupt patterns of response, not to create them. Meals and sleep granted irregularly, in more than abundance or less than adequacy, the shifts occurring on no discernible time pattern, will normally disorient an interrogate and sap his will to resist more effectively than a sustained deprivation leading to debility*' (p. 98).

TABLE 11.3 The psychological impact of sleep deprivation

Cognitive: General cognitive slowing; impaired attention span; diminished concentration; impaired decision-making involving dealing with the unexpected, innovation, revising plans, processing competing distractions and communicating effectively; reduced capacity for logical and sequential thought; decreased accuracy when estimating time; increased suggestibility.
Emotional: Negative effects on mood.
Physical: Alteration of the body's immune system, increased perception of physical pain (hyperalgesia).
Drive: Decreased motivation.

Mckenna, Dickinson and Orff (2007) offer an experimental example of how this works. Different tasks related to a risk game were completed by 26 young volunteers. Half were then subjected to 23 hours of complete sleep deprivation while the others maintained a normal sleep pattern. Then both groups repeated the assignment. The persons subjected to sleep deprivation incorrectly evaluated risks and benefits: they assumed excessive risks if they thought they would win, and were overly conservative if they thought they would lose. The authors explore different explanations for this behaviour; the most plausible is that the exhaustion of the brain reduces the many subtle cognitive tasks involved in making risky decisions to a minimum and the person shifts from being able to modulate answers to being limited to a *yes/no* mindset that requires less concentration and effort, but causes more errors.

In the context of interrogation, the detainee may be more easily convinced by minimisation arguments, deceptive reasoning or lose–lose questioning, and more likely to make a false confession. Just 24 hours of sleep deprivation produces significant results.

The results confirm previous empirical evidence that people deprived of sleep are significantly more suggestible, as measured by the Gudjonsson Suggestibility Scale, than normal controls. The degree of suggestibility increases with the amount of sleep deprivation (Blagrove and Akehurst, 2000). Hunger, thirst and other techniques targeting the body to reach the conscious mind all work in the same way: they cause painful punishment while altering the capacity for emotional and cognitive self-regulation.

Sleep deprivation has been considered torture in the United States since the 1944 *Ashcraft v. Tennessee* case, in which a detainee confessed after 36 hours of sleep deprivation and the court considered this to amount to 'torture'. This contrasts with the legal 40-hour continuous interrogations that the Enhanced Interrogation Techniques allow when two 20-hour periods are conducted consecutively (Reyes, 2008).

An integrated model of environmental manipulation and coercive interrogation

Davis and Leo (2012) have developed a model that links food and sleep deprivation to confessions called the IBRD (Interrogation-Related Regulatory Decline) which proposes that a person's self-regulation capacities must remain intact in order to confront stressful situations. There are three situations in particular (emotional overload, sleep deprivation and glucose deficiency) that undermine the capacity to self-regulate, making the person more vulnerable to pressure during interrogation.

Based on this idea, Figure 11.1 offers an overall view of the interaction between attacks on the body, brain debilitation and vulnerability of the conscious self to emotional and cognitive manipulative tactics during coercive interrogation and torture.

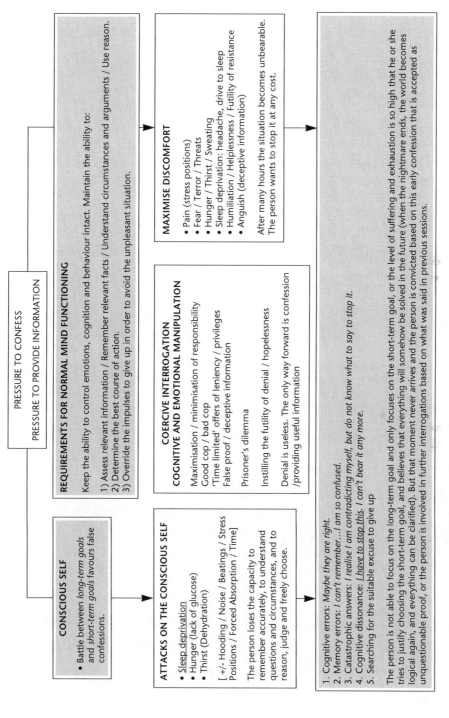

FIGURE 11.1 Interaction between attacks on the body, brain debilitation and vulnerability of the conscious self to emotional and cognitive manipulative tactics, during coercive interrogation and torture.

Adapted from Davis, D., and Leo, R. (2012). Acute suggestibility in police interrogation: self-regulation failure as a primary mechanism of vulnerability. In A. M. Ridley, F. Gabert, and D. La Rooy (Eds), *Suggestibility in legal contexts* (pp. 171–95). John Wiley and Sons.

At the centre there is a balance between long-term goals (the will to overcome interrogation without giving information which incriminates oneself or others) and short-term goals (escaping physical and psychological suffering). The interrogator exerts as much pressure as possible so that the detainee's short-term goal of relief overrides his or her long-term goal of not betraying his or her convictions. There are two paths available to the interrogator: increasing suffering to a maximum, and debilitating the conscious self so that the detainee loses the capacity to understand, judge and make choices.

Once the structure of pressure and debilitation has been created[14] the person is subjected to hours of exhaustive questioning with interrogators shifting roles, taking turns and using emotional and cognitive manipulation tactics (see Chapter 12) until the person either reveals pieces of information (which may be true but are most likely fabricated) in an attempt to stop the situation, or confesses to whatever is demanded of him or her. Even if some of the information is true, the weakness causes the detainee's memory to be partial and unreliable, merging what might be true with what has been suggested, causing inaccurate information.

Notes

1 Approved by the Economic and Social Council by its resolutions 663 C (XXIV) of 31 July 1957 and 2076 (LXII) of 13 May 1977.
2 Resolution A/RES/70/175 adopted by the General Assembly on 17 December 2015.
3 A/RES/70/175 para 8, p. 6/36.
4 A standard paragraph of the European CPT states: '*Police cells should be clean, of a reasonable size for the number of persons they are used to accommodate, and have adequate lighting (i.e., sufficient to read by, sleeping periods excluded) and ventilation; preferably, cells should enjoy natural light. Further, cells should be equipped with a means of rest (e.g. a chair or bench) and persons obliged to stay overnight in custody should be provided with a clean mattress and blankets. Persons in custody should be allowed to comply with the needs of nature when necessary, in clean and decent conditions, and be offered adequate washing facilities. They should have ready access to drinking water and be given food at appropriate times, including at least one full meal (i.e., something more substantial than a sandwich) every day. Those detained for extended periods (twenty-four hours or more) should be provided with appropriate personal hygiene items and, as far as possible, be allowed to take outdoor exercise every day.*'
5 The Special Rapporteur proposed that 15 days marks the limit between 'solitary confinement' and 'prolonged solitary confinement' (Mendez, 2011).
6 Figures are probably overestimates, as authors cannot conduct separate analyses for solitary confinement and sensory deprivation.
7 The Standard Minimum Rules for the Treatment of Prisoners (SMR) adopted by the UN in 1957, although not legally binding, also protect prisoners. They affirm in Rules 64 and 65 that prisoners should be imprisoned as punishment, not for punishment; in Rule 27 that prisons should operate with '*no more restriction than is necessary for safe custody and well-ordered community life.*' Rule 31 prohibits placement in a dark cell and all cruel, inhuman, or degrading punishments for disciplinary offences.
8 www.corteidh.or.cr/docs/casos/articulos/seriec_52_ing.pdf.
9 FIES: Fichero de Internos de Especial Seguimiento (File on Inmates Requiring Special Follow-up).
10 Under a special classificatory status caller FIES.
11 Council of Europe doc. CPT/Inf. (96)9, Part I, para 113. Downloadable at www.cpt.coe.int/documents/esp/1996-09-inf-eng-1.pdf.
12 *A.B. v. Russia,* Application No. 1439/06, European Court of Human Rights, para. 108 (2010)

13 In Enhanced Interrogation Techniques it was considered 'enough' to guarantee 4 hours of sleep per 24 hour period. This is clearly insufficient. Under such measures, it is possible that the detainee is kept awake during the first and last four hours of a two-day period, effectively permitting 40 hours of continuous interrogation in-between and resulting in 4 hours of sleep per 48 hour period.

14 Some manuals call this 'softening up' the prisoner, an expression that trivialises torture and should be avoided.

12

TARGETING THE BODY TO REACH THE MIND: PAIN WITHOUT MARKS

Pain-producing positions and exercises

Pain-producing exercises and positions are among the oldest and most common torture methods. They have been reported in every geographical area, across the historical record. Classic examples are found in the imagery of torture, such as a hooded person tied to a device, hanging for hours in a painful position.

Rejali (2007) proposed four different categories of pain without marks:

1. **Positional torture**, such as forced standing, squatting or kneeling for hours, sometimes holding heavy objects.
2. **Exercising ceaselessly until prisoners are exhausted**. These include push-ups, knee bends and forced crawling.
3. **Restraint torture**, including handcuffing prisoners in standing positions or with the hands positioned above the head ('high cuffing'), or suspending prisoners in uncomfortable ways. This category also includes positional devices, such as forcing individuals into constrained spaces.
4. **Beatings**, including slapping, mild but constant striking of the head with objects that leave no marks, cuffs to the ears, or blows to the abdomen.

These techniques are painful, but may not mark the body permanently. Rejali built a detailed catalogue of horrors, and described the history and variations of techniques in every category in different countries. He classified the methods in Greater Stress and Less Stress traditions based on whether the objective was to produce more or less pain in more or less time. When examining the vast quantity of methods, it becomes clear that the only thing limiting the number of torturing techniques is the sadistic imagination of the torturer.

Positional torture

The psychological effects of positional torture are well known and perfectly described in this early account by the KGB (Hinkle and Wolff, 1956):

> Any fixed position which is maintained over a long period of time ultimately produces excruciating pain. Certain positions, of which the standing position is one, also produce impairment of the circulation. Many men can withstand the pain of long standing, but sooner or later all men succumb to the circulatory failure it produces.[1] Men have been known to remain standing for periods as long as several days. Ultimately they usually develop a delirious state, characterised by disorientation, fear, delusions, and visual hallucinations. This psychosis is produced by a combination of circulatory impairment, lack of sleep, and uremia.
>
> In addition to the physiological effects, this type of torture creates a psychological conflict. When the prisoner is required to stand in one position, there is often engendered within him an initial determination to 'stick it out'. This internal act of resistance provides a feeling of moral superiority, at first. As time passes and pain mounts, the individual becomes aware that, to some degree, it is his own original determination to resist that is causing the continuance of pain. There develops a conflict within the individual between his moral determination and his desire to collapse and discontinue the pain. It is this extra internal conflict, in addition to the conflict over whether or not to give in to the demands made of him that tends to make this method of torture effective in the breakdown of the individual.
>
> The KGB hardly ever uses manacles or chains, and rarely resorts to physical beatings. The actual physical beating is contrary to KGB regulations.

Restraint and positional torture produce permanent damage to the musculoskeletal systems and often cause chronic pain (Skylv, 1992) that does not correspond to any detectable physical damage and is resistant to rehabilitation (Carinci, Mehta and Christo, 2010). Survivors say that this is *embodied pain*: the indelible mark of the pain in the unconscious memory of the body (Theidon, 2010):

> Some days, my whole body hurts. Sometimes it's just my legs that hurt. They hurt at the thighs most intensely, but also along the arches of my feet. I've described the sensation to my doctors as a burning sensation, the kind of pain you feel from muscular exhaustion. There is no medical explanation for my pain. And yet there is.[2]

The main difference between restraint and positional torture is that the latter has always been considered 'torture lite' because the body is not forced into abnormal positions, but rather requires prisoners to assume normal positions for abnormal periods of time. Wall-standing was one of the five techniques reviewed in the *Ireland v. UK* case, and it was not found to constitute torture. It was also one of the techniques authorised in Israel for the interrogation of Palestinian prisoners (later banned in its more crude forms). In Guantanamo these were called 'stress positions' and considered acceptable because they were supposed to produce only 'mild physical discomfort' rather than pain associated with contortions. The BSCTs proposed a variety of methods, among them leaning against the wall with only the forehead touching it (called 'prolonged standing') and not recommended for more than four hours in a 24-hour period (General Counsel of the Department of Defense, 2003). 'Stress positions' were later found to violate the Geneva Conventions (Elsea, 2004) and not recommended as a standard procedure in FM 34–52.

Exhaustion exercises

Exhaustion exercises are also considered to be 'lite' torture and are a routine part of contemporary 'soft' techniques. The detainee is forced to undergo actions and movements that resemble military training. In Spain, the Policia Nacional (*National Police*) and the Guardia Civil have been documented to force suspects of terrorism under incommunicado detention to do endless push-ups until they are exhausted before and during interrogation (Navarro et al., 2014).

Exhaustion exercises induce unbearable muscle cramps and physically weaken detainees. When used during interrogation they cause acute confusion from anoxia, sweating and dehydration, humiliation and fear of painful reprisals – making the detainee vulnerable to deception, suggestion and false confessions. Additionally, these exercises require absolute obedience, fostering submission to orders.

Internal battles: externally-imposed self-inflicted pain, forced absorption, stress positions and emotional exhaustion

Constant beatings and wall-standing that lasted for days were the most frequent torture methods at the hands of Antonio González Pacheco, Jesús Muñecas and other torturers during the 1970s and 1980s under the Franco dictatorship in Spain. Many survivors describe the mixture of pain, terror, disorientation and mental confusion that these methods produced.[3] Although they are not included in the IBRD model (Davis and Leo, 2012) described in Chapter 11, they probably should be.

Externally-imposed self-inflicted pain

The testimonies of survivors in Chapter 2, especially those of Carlos Liscano and Marcelo Viñar, perfectly described the pain generated by stress positions. They explained the internal battles that take place within the victim. As Liscano (2004) said: '*This body, dirty, smelling bad, in pain from beatings and from lack of rest, sleepy, that can't so much as move a foot without asking permission, provokes disgust. It's one thing to think, "This is disgusting." It's different to feel, "Now I am disgusting." (. . .). But one can't ask the body to bear pain and at the same time tell [the body that] it is disgusting. You feel for this animal. It's disgusting but one wants to love it, because it is all one has*' (p. 69).

This internal battle is one of the key elements in the three mindsets we derived from the testimonies of torture victims in Chapter 2.

The KUBARK Manual included prolonged standing in its discussion of 'coercive interrogation' methods, noting that a subject's 'resistance is likelier to be sapped by pain *which he seems to inflict upon himself*', than by direct torture. Borum (2005), a psychologist working for the army, considers this an unproven fact.

Rejali (2007) writes, 'positional tortures are labor-saving devices (the prisoner does the work), but they take time to have their effects'. He notes that 'torturers use them when they have plenty of time, mainly to intimidate prisoners or force a false confession. When they are short of time, torturers normally reach for devices like magnetos that cause immediate pain' (p. 329).

Forced absorption

Confronted with pain, normal human behaviour in such circumstances is evasion, to distract oneself from the noxious stimulus. But torture is designed in a way that makes this impossible, leading to cognitive and emotional exhaustion. The pain is constant. The torturer's work is to shift the circumstances, induce fear and prevent the detainee from escaping into mental disconnection or dissociation. Forced absorption are those measures taken to prevent the detainee to mentally evade and to keep him or her to the here and now of the torture process and thus, in constant cognitive tension maximizing the efficacy of psychological torture. Forced absorption is the necessary link between pain and one's mental state (Jacobs, 2008; Scarry, 1985). It produces an endless cognitive and emotional battle that cannot be maintained for long.

Crampton (2013) considers forced absorption to be one of the indicators of psychological torture. His argument focuses not on the harmful stimuli, but rather on the practice of preventing the detainee's mind from appropriately processing and reacting to stressors, some of which may even be legal.

Notes

1 This is explained because '*After 18 to 24 hours of continuous standing, there is an accumulation of fluid in the tissues of the legs. This dependent "edema" is produced by fluid from the blood vessels. The ankles and feet of the prisoner swell to twice their normal circumference. The edema may rise up the legs as high as the middle of the thighs. The skin becomes tense and intensely painful. Large blisters develop which break and exude watery serum. The accumulation of the body fluid in the legs produces an impairment of the circulation. The heart rate increases and fainting may occur. Eventually there is a renal shutdown, and urine production ceases. The prisoner becomes thirsty, and may drink a good deal of water, which is not excreted, but adds to the edema of his legs.*'

2 Ashana M. *Stress Positions are Torture: Autobiographical Account.* In http://ashanam.wordpress .com/2013/02/03/stress-positions-are-torture/.

3 www.lacomunapresxsdelfranquismo.org/.

13

THE LIMITATIONS OF NORMAL INTERROGATION IN LAW ENFORCEMENT PROCEDURES

If one of the purposes of torture – as stated by the UN Convention – is eliciting information from a detainee, then interrogation is necessarily an essential component of a comprehensive view of torture and deserves reflection.

In interrogational torture, physical and psychological techniques serve the purpose of 'softening' the detainee and setting the stage for 'successful' questioning. The opposite also holds true: interrogation is often conducted in a way that takes advantage (and deepens the effect) of torturing environments, contributing to confusion, distortion and psychological suffering. Therefore, interrogation and torture are often complementary sides of the same process, and interrogation should be studied as one of many elements within the torture process, a practice deeply ingrained in the mechanisms of torture. The interrogation should be understood within the broader framework of torture; it follows predetermined procedures and has strictly defined methods, just like other elements of the torturing process.

Coercive interrogation is paradigmatic of the idea that if there is no physical pain, then torture has not occurred. Although certain interrogation methods within an environment of pressure *constitute psychological torture in themselves*, they rarely appear in the list of torture methods. The Istanbul Protocol does not include interrogation as part of torture and it does not list interrogation (or certain techniques within it) as a defined category in their catalogue of torture methods.

The interrogation of witnesses and suspects in law enforcement procedures, and the process of interrogation in military intelligence collection (HUMINT), correspond to two different worlds with distinct purposes, techniques and systems of legal protection. This chapter offers an overview of general concepts and then focuses on interrogations within the civil legal process building on an analysis of police interrogation manuals. In Chapter 14 we will analyse intelligence collection in military procedures.

Legal precedents

Many sentences have found self-incriminating statements to be invalid because the jury believed that the person was subjected to questioning under 'pressure', or 'coercive interrogation'. There is ample anecdotal, historical and experimental documentation (reviewed below) of the high number of false confessions that coercive interrogation can elicit. Military and police interrogation manuals include codes of conduct that outline, in theory, a definition of the limits of what is *permissible* – and therefore the theoretical limits of psychological mal-treatment or torture. But in practice, there is ample debate among varying national traditions and domestic laws about the different ways of conceptualising what is ethical and admissible in educing information from a detainee.

There are two schools of thought on the subject, which are difficult to reconcile. The first includes those who think that during an interrogation, anything that does not involve overt physical violence is permissible (including interview strategies employing manipulative dialogue, deception, trickery, maximisation, false evidence or other *verbal* tactics). These are seen not only as acceptable, but as complex and valued skills to be acquired as part of elicit-ing a suspect's confession. Most countries adhere to this doctrine and would never consider the possibility that a coercive interrogation without physical violence is illegal, much less hold an interrogator accountable for conducting a coercive interrogation. Even mild physical pressure is generally considered acceptable. A small minority of countries (including, notably, the United Kingdom) find the opposite to be true: they believe that all forms of coercive ver-bal interrogation strategies are unethical and violate the rights of the detainee. Therefore, the law proscribes these type of interviews and considers them unacceptable as an investigative or probative tool.

Police manuals reflect the belief that interrogation and torture are entirely separate spheres. There are no precedents in which an officer or other legal official has been indicted for inducing a false confession or for conducting an interrogation that went beyond the limits of an ethically acceptable procedure.[1] However, an interrogation *per se* – according to the UN Convention – could be considered psychological torture if it induces severe psychologi-cal suffering or pain for a purpose stated in the Convention. In many cases, this is not far from the reality of how interrogations are conducted.

Mapping the field

Eliciting information: interviews and interrogations

Traditionally, police manuals divide processes for obtaining information from others into two categories: the interview, and the interrogation.

The **interview** is a conversation between a law enforcement, military or related official that seeks information with a *cooperative* suspect, a witness, or someone who has valuable information. It is a kind of trust game, based on cognitive abilities and dialogue. There are manuals that teach interview techniques (e.g. Schafer and Navarro, 2010), which explain con-versational and environmental strategies to maximise the information obtained from coopera-tive sources. The interview is a seemingly benign encounter in which any non-coercive tactic is allowed (including mild trickery and deception).

The **interrogation** is a process in which the investigator aims to extract information from an *unwilling* person, and therefore resorts to techniques that can break the interviewee's resistance. This includes different kinds of aggressive techniques. The exact interpretation of what consti-tutes an 'aggressive' technique depends on the perspective of the author or government involved.

Some authors prefer to speak of **cognitive interrogation** – highlighting the idea that the core process involves questioning and purely verbal techniques – as opposed to **coercive interrogation** where mild force, threats, psychological pressure, deception and trickery are used (Gudjonsson, 2003).

The Intelligence Science Board,[2] a task group established by the US National Intelligence Services to provide evidence-based scientific tools for proper interrogation of terrorist suspects, proposed the expression **educing information (EI)**. The Task Group considered it preferable to 'interrogation', which, in their view, is a term with overly negative connotations for the public (Intelligence Science Board, 2006, 2009).

In their unconventional terminology, EI includes three aspects:

- *Elicitation of information*, defined as engaging with a source in such a manner that he or she reveals information without being aware of giving away anything of value
- *Strategic debriefing*, defined as systematically covering topics and areas with a voluntary source who consents to a formal conversation
- *Interrogation*, defined as an interaction and exchange with a source who appears initially unwilling to provide information

Educing Information implies that there is a team of people building a 'system' of gathering information about and from a source, and includes not only the interviews, but also the use of technology, construction of complex scenarios and other techniques that involve many different professionals.

The objective and framework of the interrogation

The techniques used in an interrogation depend on its purpose. There are three main objectives (Intelligence Science Board, 2006, 2009):

1. *Preventive interrogation.* The interrogator has very little information on the suspects. They have supposedly been detained for a specific connection or reason, but there are no concrete facts or data on background, activities or any other relevant factors. The interrogator 'explores' what the detainees know and what kind of information they can provide. As long as the target is not clear, **the objective of the interrogation is to obtain submission or cooperation.** The interviewer must use open questions and work through 'softening techniques' and threats (submission), or empathy and good rapport (cooperation).
2. *Intelligence Collection Interview.* Conducted by army officers, **the objective is to obtain concrete, specific valuable information** from sources who may or may not have such information. The final objective is to break the resistance of the subjects and to get all of the information they can through coercive and non-coercive methods. In some cases, the goal is to transform them into cooperative people who can serve as collaborators in the future (and participate in activities ranging from obtaining information to recruitment).
3. *Law Enforcement Interview.* Conducted by the police, **the objective is to obtain a confession from the suspect**.

Each objective employs different techniques. As Kleinman (2006) states, 'The confession that can be such a monumental achievement in the law enforcement world is often of little interest to the Intelligence Community.' He believes that being proficient in one kind of interrogation may cause problems when conducting another kind of interrogation, 'like being good in one sport can be a problem for practicing another'.

Law enforcement officials must adhere to federal and state laws pertaining to rights of the accused (including legal representation and the right to remain silent), standards of evidence, investigative parameters established by the prosecution and limits on the duration of custody.

In contrast, the activities of intelligence officials are governed by international and federal guidelines pertaining to the treatment of prisoners, priority intelligence requirements, the need to manage a potentially long-term process of exploitation of sources and the pursuit of actionable information, or information that corroborates or contributes to intelligence data gathered from other sources.

Classification of interrogation techniques

Meissner (2014) proposed a distinction between '*information-gathering methods*' and '*accusatorial methods*' (see Table 13.1), a classification that is more closely related to the overall goal and strategy than to the specific techniques used.

For the purposes of this book, and based on literature that directly addresses the connections between interrogations and torture (Gudjonsson, 2003; Kleinman, 2006) we have differentiated cognitive Interrogation from coercive interrogation[3] (see Table 13.1).

In cognitive interrogation (CogI), the interrogator is expected to create *a climate of cooperation and closeness*. In this regard, an arrogant attitude towards the suspect or attitudes that provoke anger or suspiciousness reduce success because they push the detainee into a position of psychological reactivity and defensiveness (Meissner and Russano, 2003; Semel, 2013). The dialogue becomes a confrontation and the interrogator must resort to ever-increasing pressure. The detainee is also less receptive to the suggestions offered by the interrogator and it is more difficult to convince him or her to provide information. Success is linked to building trust and cooperation, obtaining information and corroborating it by triangulation with other sources.

In coercive interrogation (CoerI), the basic principle is to create an *atmosphere of tension and fear* from the beginning that convinces the uncooperating person that everything has already been discovered and that he or she has no other option than to confess.

There are many intermediate options. In particular, we could consider the Confrontational Interview as a middle point between the Coercive and Cognitive paradigms: in the Confrontational Interview there is a direct accusation, while at the same time there are limitations to deception and trickery (see Tables 13.2 and 13.3). The second and third options in Table 13.2 would be deemed illegal in some countries (such as the UK under the Police and Criminal Evidence Act (PACE, 1984)), although all options listed are overtly or covertly employed by interrogators everywhere.

TABLE 13.1 Methods of interrogation: information-gathering versus accusatorial methods

Information-Gathering Methods	Accusatorial Methods
Establishes rapport	Uses direct, positive confrontation
Establishes control	Uses psychological manipulation
Employs open-ended, exploratory questions	Employs closed, confirmatory questions
Primary goal is elicitation, focuses on cognitive cues and dialogue	Primary goal is confession, focuses on anxiety cues that suggest tension, doubts or contradiction generated by the interrogator's maneuvers and tries to take advantage of this to obtain a confession

TABLE 13.2 Cognitive versus coercive interviews: overall strategy

Cognitive Interview (The UK under PACE legal protection of detainees)	Confrontational Interview (e.g. FBI, law enforcement officials with official restrictions)	Coercive Interview (e.g. Reid Technique / sections of the KUBARK Manual)
<ul><li>Establish rapport</li><li>Ask general questions</li><li>Highlight contradictions between facts and evidence</li><li>Summarise</li><li>Acknowledge cooperation</li><li>Obtain contact information for follow-up</li><li>Cross-check information in the following days</li></ul>	<ul><li>Establish rapport</li><li>Assume suspect's guilt</li><li>Confront suspect with evidence</li><li>Interrupt denials, insist on evidence</li><li>Use rationalisation (suggest a justification), projection (blame others) and minimisation (trivialise importance, consequences, responsibility)</li><li>Incriminating choice question</li><li>Summarise main points</li><li>Acknowledge cooperation</li></ul>	Includes all strategies used in the Confrontational Interview, plus:<ul><li>Maximisation, manipulation, and minimisation techniques</li><li>Mild 'softening' techniques (emotional and psychological exhaustion, control – but not deprivation – of basic needs such as food, sleep, water, isolation and others)</li></ul>

Increasing coercion

TABLE 13.3 Cognitive Interrogation versus Coercive Interrogation: basic strategies

	Cognitive Interrogation (CogI)	Coercive Interrogation (CoerI)
Basic components	Building 'confidence' Creating a climate of cooperation and closeness	Fear Omniscience Omnipotence
Starting point	Documentation Careful preparation of script and questions	Pre-interrogative interview (Behavioral Analysis Interview) in which the interviewer collects all basic information regarding the detainee's biography, actions and alibi, and decides whether the person is guilty or potentially guilty. Interrogation. The interrogator is no longer interested in obtaining information, but on breaking down resistance and making the suspect confess.
Style	Dialogue Empathic and active listening Listening is more important than asking Confronting the person with evidence Detecting incoherence	Fast, successive, constant questions using different styles. The suspect is frequently interrupted when trying to answer, questions are repeated, and themes are constantly changed. The only acceptable answer is the answer that the interrogator wants to hear.

	Cognitive Interrogation (CogI)	*Coercive Interrogation (CoerI)*
Types of questions	Open: asking for an account of events	Leading: implies the answer in the question ("and then you . . ., didn't you?").
	Closed: asking for concrete details	Hushed and lowered tones (emotional).
	Normal tone	Hostile – aggressive tone, interrupting, swearing (intimidating).
	One question at a time allowing time to answer	Multiple questions or multiple assertions in only one sentence.
	Rational use of brief silences to allow the suspect reflect on the answer	Multiple interrogators asking questions one after another without giving the suspect the opportunity to reply.
		Mindless echoing of the last few words of the suspect's reply.
		Indiscriminate use of long silences (9 seconds or more).
Summary	The interrogator explores the suspect's involvement. The focus remains open at all times. The interrogator uses broad questions and cross-checks later with evidence.	The interrogator wants the suspect to confirm his or her pre-interrogation conclusions. The focus is closed from the beginning and questions related to this focus are repeated.

The stress of interrogation. Interrogation is a stressful experience in itself. The subject usually feels high levels of anxiety and fear because of the conditions of detention (even if they are not harsh conditions), isolation (including being alone with one's thoughts), lack of control and uncertainty about what will happen next, how long the situation will last and the potential consequences. This can clearly impair the subject's ability to remember, to think clearly and logically, and to make proper decisions. Thus, the experience of interrogation is not a neutral encounter between two persons, even under normal conditions.

The Reid Technique: nine steps

Since the 1960s, the Reid Technique has become the most well-known coercive interrogation paradigm. It was originally published in 1945, then updated and structured by Inbau and Reid (1963) and extended and re-edited in successive versions for more than fifty years (Inbau et al., 2011). Most military and police interrogation manuals used in the Western world and LMIC under its direct influence come from the US; they are essentially modified versions of the Reid technique[4] (King and Snook, 2009; Neequaye, 2011; Neuman and Salinas-Serrano, 2006; Simcoe, 2006; Singh, 2008).

All of these manuals (as well as the original by Inbau and Reid) are based on the experiences of the authors, and none of the techniques proposed in the method were tested for efficacy against other models at the time. Since then, there has been some preliminary experimental research that we will review below.

Table 13.4 presents the nine steps of the classical Reid Technique, as presented to interrogators in Inbau and Reid's texts.

TABLE 13.4 The Reid Technique: nine steps of coercive interrogation

Step 1. Direct – Positive confrontation

Directly accuse detainee without any doubts, present the available evidence and suggest that there is much more (even if you, the interrogator, have none). Observe the detainee's behavioural reaction and insist again on the direct accusation.

Step 2. Theme development

Show understanding and sympathy with the accused to gain his or her trust.

Use with emotional subjects, prone to moral reasoning and feeling guilty:
- Theme 1. *Everybody would probably* . . . Sympathise with the suspect by saying that anyone else in his or her position would have done the same thing.
- Theme 2. Reduce the suspect's feeling of guilt by minimising the moral seriousness of the offense.
- Theme 3. Suggest a motivation for the offense that appears morally acceptable, or assume there is a morally acceptable reason for the offense.
- Theme 4. Sympathise with the suspect by condemning others.
- Theme 5. Appeal to the suspect's pride by using flattery and expressing approval and recognition.
- Theme 6. Point out possibilities that his or her involvement in the events has been exaggerated, that there has been exaggeration on part of accuser or victim, or that they have exaggerated the nature or seriousness of the event itself.
- Theme 7. Point out, especially for first-time offenders, that there is an opportunity to discontinue these activities and avoid problems in the future. Explain the grave consequences of continuing with criminal behaviour.

With non-emotional subjects:
- Focus on a specific lie or contradiction, and insist on repeatedly questioning this point while refusing to believe subject's responses.
- Insist that there is sufficient evidence to convict the detainee, and that the only point of the interview is to give him or her the opportunity to give his or her version in case there are mitigating circumstances.
- State that any other person involved has already confessed and held the detainee responsible for the events.

Step 3. Handling denial
- Prohibit denial. Repeated denials offer the suspect a psychological advantage and opportunity for self-reinforcement: do not allow them. Order the detainee to listen.
- Treat any denial as a lie and interrupt it. Repeat the same question endlessly to the suspect.
- Discourage any answer that does not go in the desired direction.
- Introduce the 'friendly – unfriendly' tactic (two interrogators with different personalities or one interrogator with alternating attitudes) to make the detainee more responsive to the friendly questioning, seen as a window of opportunity.

Step 4. Overcoming objections

The suspect stops repeating denials and tries to make objections to the arguments presented. This means that the subject is moving towards recognising involvement and trying to mitigate it. Recognise the objection, reward it and sometimes use it against the detainee. Do not allow the detainee go back to the denial phase.

Step 5. Procurement and retention of a suspect's attention

The detainee might feel tired and trapped and can resort to no answer or a passive attitude. Remain attentive and avoid this by forcing eye contact, working in a small environment with no distractions, and employing body language that does not allow the suspect to avoid confrontation with the interrogator. Additional important actions may include: changes in arm and leg position, eye contact or facial expressions.

Step 6. Handling the suspect's passive mood

Return to an emphatic tone, focus the discussion on the central topic and try to foster remorse and guilt in the subject, for instance by making him or her aware of the harm suffered by the victim. Other tactics include pointing out similarities between the victim and the suspect's wife or children, and appealing to the suspect's sense of honour or religion. Try to make the suspect cry or become emotionally blocked and silent.

Step 7. Presenting an alternative question

Present the suspect with two questions. Both are incriminating. One in a severe way, while the other appears to be a benign or face-saving option. Present one act as a repulsive, intentional crime, and the other as a fatal mistake. The suspect must choose between these two self-incriminating options, and is allowed to explain his or her justifications for the 'mistake'.

Step 8. Making the suspect recite various details of the offense

Once the detainee has made an initial admission, no matter how weak, go directly into details and provoke a full-blown confession.

Step 9. Converting an oral confession in a written confession

Make the detainee write his or her confession down in order avoid the possibility that he or she might later claim he or she confessed under pressure, and deny the charges.

The Reid Technique pushes the limits of what is ethically admissible. Inbau and Reid claim that physical violence ('the third degree'), and falsely promising that the attorney will not prosecute or the judge will not convict the detainee if he or she confesses, are both unethical.[5] However, they find any other method (including exhaustion, manipulation of environment, deception and lies) acceptable:

> We are opposed to the so-called third degree, even on suspects whose guilt seems absolutely certain and who remain steadfast in their denials. Moreover, we are opposed to the use of any interrogation tactic or technique that is apt to make an innocent person confess. We are opposed, therefore, to the use of force, threats of force, or promises of leniency. We do approve, however, of psychological tactics and techniques that may involve trickery and deceit; they are not only helpful but frequently indispensable in order to secure incriminating information from the guilty or to obtain investigative leads from otherwise uncooperative witnesses or informants. (Inbau et al., 2011, p. xii)

Other authors find fault with many aspects of the technique; a selection of key issues is included below.

The interrogator:

- Only accepts the possibility that the detainee is guilty and does not accept anything that goes against this hypothesis. This has been decided in the fact-finding phase and pre-interview. The interrogator does not want to listen to what the detainee has to say, only to lead him or her to recognise his or her responsibility.
- Tells the detainee that he or she has 'absolute certainty' that the detainee committed the alleged offense and that there is sufficient incriminating evidence (or confessions by witnesses or other detainees). If necessary, the interrogator lies.

- Does not allow the person to make any denials and cuts off interventions that do not go in the desired direction. The detainee is only allowed to talk in the approved manner. Exhaustion, argumentation, emotional manipulation or any other tactics deemed necessary are employed.
- Uses different 'acting' approaches (*friendly/unfriendly*, among others), in theatrical strategies to manipulate the detainee's will.
- Exploits personal information and detection of potential feelings of shame and guilt related to the detainee's social network or to personal matters.
- Presents an alternative question in which both options are incriminating once the person is extremely tired and desires to end the interrogation at any cost. This core technique, in Inbau and Reid's opinion, results in the most 'successful' confessions if used at that exact moment. This means that it is used following hours of interrogation and when the person is tired and confused.

Interrogation techniques taxonomy

Kassin (2001) classifies Reid techniques of deception in two categories: maximising (which exaggerates evidence, data, responsibility and consequences) and minimising (which alleviates responsibility and guilt). When maximising, which Inbau et al. recommend for non-emotional suspects, the interrogator frightens the suspect into a confession by exaggerating the strength of evidence against him or her and the seriousness of the offense. In minimisation strategies, recommended for remorseful suspects, the interrogator tricks the suspect into a false sense of security – and ultimately into confessing – by offering sympathy, providing face-saving excuses, partly blaming the victim or circumstances for the alleged offense, and minimising the seriousness of the charges.

This is similar to the tactics classified in an observational study on the actual practices of British police in the 1990s (Pearse and Gudjonsson, 2003) in which the authors organised tactics into six categories according to a factorial analysis.[6] Also in the 1990s, Leo (1996a, 1996b, 2008) conducted an observational study based on three North American police stations, recording a total of approximately 500 interrogations. He identified 24 interrogation tactics (which were not necessarily coercive).[7] The four most successful interrogation tactics for obtaining a confession used strong emotional manipulation but did not include trickery, deception or lies (the success rate for each tactic is in parenthesis): (1) appeal to the suspect's conscience (97 per cent); (2) identify contradictions in suspect's story (91 per cent); (3) use praise or flattery (91 per cent); and (4) offer moral justifications/psychological excuses (90 per cent). In addition to these two studies, there are lesser-known classifications that are based either on self-reporting or qualitative analyses of recorded interviews.

Kelly, Miller, Redlich and Kleinman (2013) recently proposed a taxonomy of interrogation methods. They conducted a review of research and grey literature and collected a list of more than 800 interrogation tactics. Then they began to collate, resume and group these tactics in successive rounds of consensus among experts, including researchers and US interrogators.

They concluded that the different classifications proposed in the scientific literature could be collapsed into two large categories: one including *minimisation, information-gathering, humane* and *rapport-based* categories and another *maximisation, accusatorial, dominant* and *control-based* categories, although they do not propose a name for these two groups.

Within these two groups, they propose a list of 6 domains and 71 techniques. The authors believe that all known interrogation techniques fit within their proposal, that the six domains cover all possible techniques, and that new techniques can easily be classified according to this rubric. The classification is a theoretical construct (though it arises from a small-group consensus) and requires validation through further research.

Table 13.5 presents the domains and some examples (see also Appendix 3).

TABLE 13.5 Taxonomy of interrogation methods

Domain	Definition and examples
Rapport and Relationship Building (14)	Working relationship between operator and source based on a mutual understanding of each other's goals and needs, which can lead to useful, actionable intelligence or information. Based on a respectful relationship between two humans. Examples of rapport-based techniques include finding common ground with the source, demonstrating kindness and respect and meeting the basic needs (e.g. food, water) of the source.
Context Manipulation (11)	Altering the physical and temporal space in which the interrogation occurs to maximise the probability of a successful outcome. Any technique that does not possess an interactional quality or interpersonal dynamic that occurs between the operator and the source. Examples of this include the Army Field Manual techniques of solitary confinement, or 'change of scenery', where the source is moved from a formal interrogation room to a more neutral location in an effort to reduce the stress of the source or conducting the interview in a small, windowless, room.
Emotion Provocation (12)	Techniques specifically designed to target the source's raw emotions (anger, anxiety, fear, guilt, hope, love, pride or sadness). The techniques include appealing to the source's self-interest, conscience or religion; capitalising on the stress of being captured or other periods of heightened stress; and exaggerating or alleviating the source's fear (for instance, employing the Army Field Manual approaches of 'fear up' and 'fear down').
Confrontation / Competition (19)	The operator asserts authority and control over the subject to gain compliance, and the relationship becomes a zero-sum game in which the operator wins and the subject loses. May include the operator challenging the values of the source; expressing impatience, frustration or anger; obscuring the fate of the source; or employing deception in order to induce cooperation or techniques, such as good cop/bad cop; repeated and rapid-fire questions; expressing authority and expertise; and challenging the values of the source.
Collaboration (7)	Offering rewards in exchange for information: including tangible rewards (food, water or amenities such as a pillows, extra blankets, candy or cigarettes) and intangible rewards (promises of better treatment while detained, or reduced punishment for cooperation).
Presentation of Evidence (8)	Presenting the source with actual evidence of the source's guilt, or possession of information that would be of use to the operator 'for gaining cooperation or compliance; for testing veracity or detecting deception; and/or exploring the source's level of knowledgeability'.

Adapted from Kelly, C. E., Miller, J. C., Redlich, A. D. and Kleinman, S. M. (2013).

Many of the tactics were used in combination, with several interrogators typically beginning by confronting the suspect with the evidence against him or her, followed by implying his or her guilt and then undermining his or her denial of involvement in the offense, while identifying contradictions in the suspect's story or alibi, appealing to his or her self-interest and conscience and offering moral justifications and psychological excuses for the subject's behaviour. This suggests a combination of tactics, which resulted in 41.8 per cent of the suspects making admissions (i.e. admitted at least to some of the elements of the crime), and an additional 22.5 per cent providing self-incriminating statements.

This is the most comprehensive proposal to date and a key point of reference for future research in the field.

From ethics to science: experimental studies comparing interrogation styles

An increasing number of field and experimental studies have compared research using cognitive or coercive interrogation. Some of them test the efficacy of a particular technique.

In a survey among Canadian interrogators, King and Snook (2009) found that 34 per cent of the interrogators used the Reid Technique and 27 per cent used techniques that could be considered 'coercive' according to Leo's (1996a) criteria. Confessions were somewhat associated with the proportion of core Reid components, the number of influence tactics and the number of coercive strategies observed. A recent similar online survey among 152 military and federal-level interrogators from the US on the frequency of use and perceived effectiveness of interrogation methods indicated that most people used various methods depending on the context, although rapport and relationship-building techniques were employed most often and perceived as the most effective, particularly compared to confrontational techniques (Redlich, Kelly and Miller, 2014).

In laboratory research there are two main paradigms. The 'Alt key' paradigm (Kassin and Kiechel, 1996)[8] and the 'Cheating' paradigm (Russano, Meissner, Narchet and Kassin, 2005).[9]

In a recent meta-analytic review (n=32 studies) (Meissner et al., 2014; Meissner, 2012) the authors concluded:

1. *Confessions.* Both the use of information-gathering methods ($g = 0.86, z = 2.04, p < .05$) and accusatorial methods were associated with a significant increase in confession rates ($g = 0.90, z = 3.43, p < .001$). As expected, when compared with a control group, accusatorial methods obtained more confessions than information-gathering methods.
2. *False confessions.* Accusatorial methods yielded a significant increase in the frequency of both true confessions ($g = 0.46, z = 2.24, p < .05$) and false confessions ($g = 0.74, z = 3.75, p < .001$). Information-gathering methods yielded a greater frequency of true confessions ($g = 0.67, z = 2.02, p < .05$), but did not significantly influence the likelihood of eliciting false confessions ($g = -0.23, z = -0.60,$ ns.).

Evans et al. (2013) have recently introduced a modification of the Cheating paradigm to simulate a Human Intelligence Collection (HUMINT) context. In their study, they assessed not the per centage of true or false confessions, but the amount of information that could be gathered from students in an interrogational simulation exercise. The study showed that an information-gathering approach yielded more critical details and resulted in a more talkative interviewee than an accusatorial interrogation strategy. Furthermore, a greater frequency of admissions was secured during information-gathering interrogations relative to accusatorial interrogations. In accusatorial interrogations the subject felt more anxious, adopted a defensive attitude and provided less information to the experimenter.

False confessions

False confessions are a serious ethical and legal problem. Some authors report that up to 20 per cent of self-indictments are totally or partially induced by the interrogator (Kassin et al., 2009). An analysis of DNA exonerations of innocent but wrongly convicted criminal defendants revealed that false confessions were a major cause of wrongful convictions, accounting for 24 per cent of the total (Costanzo and Gerrity, 2009). Drizin and Leo (2004) identified 125 proven false confessions over a 30-year period, primarily in cases involving murder and rape.

There are excellent reviews on the vulnerability factors for false confessions (Kassin, Gudjonsson and Kingdom, 2004; Kassin et al., 2010; Lassiter, 2004). The main factors are related to suspect characteristics (e.g. adolescence, intellectual disability, mental illness and certain personality traits related to suggestibility), interrogation tactics (e.g. excessive interrogation time, presentation of false evidence and minimisation), and not following legal procedures that inform detainees of their right not to declare against themselves.

In addition to inadequate interrogation procedures, erroneous convictions based on false confessions occur because once the person has made a self-incriminating statement, it is almost invariably accepted as unquestionable proof by judges and juries. In an experimental study, Forrest and Woody (2010) showed that allegations of deceptive interrogations did not influence juries' decisions to convict or the length of sentences assigned. Juries tended to disbelieve allegations of coercive or pressured interrogation. This is mainly due to what Leo (2008) describes as the 'myth of psychological confession': few jurors understand the degree to which police interrogation is a manipulative form of persuasion; observers find it hard to believe that suspects would go against their own self-interest by confessing to something they did not do. Moreover, jurors 'know' that they would never falsely confess. Forrest and Woody (2010) found that research participants suggested false confessions might be possible for others (87 per cent) but rarely for themselves (32 per cent).

There are no clear conclusions regarding which interrogation techniques elicit more false confessions. A desk review concluded that the vast majority of documented cases involved used *false-evidence* ploys (Kassin et al., 2010, p. 12). There are many forms of false-evidence ploys. Leo (2008) grouped them in three categories: testimonial ploys (e.g. a claim to have eyewitness or video evidence), scientific ploys (e.g. a false claim to have DNA, footprint or other scientific evidence), and demeanour ploys (e.g. a false claim that the suspect's behaviour indicates guilt).

Gudjonsson's (2012) review of interrogation tactics concludes that likely the most dangerous part of the Reid Technique is *being pressured to choose between two incriminating alternatives*, one with very serious consequences and the other with more ambiguous, and by implication, less serious consequences (e.g. the interrogator suggests that the act was unintentional, accidental or in self-defense).

Conclusions: are manipulation and deception torture techniques?

Surprisingly, in the introduction to their proposal for a comprehensive taxonomy of interrogation techniques, Kelly et al. (2013) advise the reader that they have only included *interrogation* techniques, but not any *torture* techniques. They cite Colb (2009) to argue that torture is 'a different thing', but, as the evidence we have reviewed thus far in this book reveals, that is inaccurate. The line between interrogation and torture should be based on the selection of ethically acceptable techniques.[10] The distinction between interrogation and torture based only on the use of certain techniques without considering the context does not make sense. Some, if not all, of the techniques used in the Enhanced Interrogation program (which has been found to constitute torture) appear on their list. As the testimonies of survivors in Chapter 2 remarked, the most benign interrogation procedure can destroy a person when he or she has been subjected to a 'softening' period (e.g. he or she has been kept in isolation, without access to a toilet or food, or after undergoing sleep regulation for days, without being informed of the reasons for detention). The underlying assumption when reading their work is that all the interrogation techniques described in their taxonomy would not be considered torture because they are not 'physically abusive techniques'.

The presence or absence of torture is defined not by technique, but by *the context and the way in which techniques are applied*. This is not linked to the amount of physical pain.

In his groundbreaking research Leo (2008, 1996a) proposed, for instance, that an interrogation should be deemed 'coercive' when at least one of ten conditions was present. These included, among others, failure of the police to issue the Miranda warning, the use of threats and inducements, unrelenting and hostile questioning, an interrogation lasting more than six hours and the suspect's will being overpowered by some other factor or combination of factors.

The most extreme examples of the difficulty determining the limits of what is admissible in interrogation are the use of deception and lies, and the cognitive manipulation of the suspect. Coercive interrogation related to police deception has been defined by interrogators both as an art that, when used properly, gives unparalleled results (Buckley, 2000), and as a danger to the profession (Arrigo and Wagner, 2007; Intelligence Science Board, 2006). Accordingly, as Forrest (2010) reviews, legal scholars argue for a variety of positions, ranging from eliminating police deception outside of severe circumstances (e.g. Paris, 1997), increasing the rigor of the limits on police deception (e.g. Slobogin, 1997, 2007; Thomas, 2007), avoiding deception prior to Miranda warnings (Mosteller, 2007), or leaving current limits unchanged, provided there is no overt physical violence (e.g. Magid, 2001).

Some manuals suggest that using deception and lies is preferred by most agents, though they know that method is dangerous because it can be easily detected by the subject. According to ethnographic research, this is because it is more difficult to train officers to build positive rapport and confidence, which requires a greater amount of empathy, patience, energy and time when compared to faster, more coercive methods (Neuman and Salinas-Serrano, 2006). There have been many reviews, opinions and academic papers on the subject in the fields of military intelligence (Intelligence Science Board, 2006), policing (Culhane, Hosch and Heck, 2008), legal rulings (Kageleiry, 2007), as well as social and psychological fields (Borum, 2009; Costanzo and Gerrity, 2009; Evans et al., 2013; Kassin and Fong, 1999). Many of these sources reject the use of deceptive techniques in interrogation for both pragmatic and ethical reasons; some feel the US should adopt provisions similar to the British PACE to prevent deceptive techniques from being employed. There are demands that judges increase their commitment to applying the Exclusionary Rule, which states that evidence collected or analysed in violation of the defendant's rights (especially under ill-treatment or torture) is inadmissible for a criminal prosecution in a court of law.

Others defend deception as powerful tool and merely propose modifications, including: additional negotiation strategies (Dotson, 2009); improved training (including caution with vulnerable populations); cross-checking all information obtained before presenting it as valid in order to avoid false confessions (Adcock, 2012); updating the 'themes'[11] (Copes, Vieraitis and Jochum, 2007); or increased sensitivity with specific populations like children and adolescents (Kostelnik and Reppucci, 2009). As Slobogin (1997), a professor at the Stanford School of Law put it: 'I have argued that police deceit during interrogation is permissible when: (1) it takes place in the window between arrest and formal charging; (2) it is necessary (i.e., non-deceptive techniques have failed); (3) it is not coercive (i.e., avoids undermining the rights to silence and counsel and would not be considered impermissibly coercive if true); and (4) it does not take advantage of vulnerable populations (i.e., suspects who are young, have mental retardation, or have been subjected to prolonged interrogation)' (p. 17).

In spite of available documentation regarding the dangers of accusatorial and coercive interrogations, and the experimental studies showing that information-gathering methods obtain better results, most governments fail to ban unacceptable methods and conditions for interviewing suspects.[12] The problem is that in the minds of interrogators, judges and most public opinion, coercive interrogation *works*. Moreover, interrogators are often under pressure to get results, and resort to techniques that appear less time consuming. A former interrogator in Guantanamo wrote that unit members had to produce an average of 20 to 25 reports weekly that were expected to have 'actionable' information, and that they were pressured by commanders (who were in turn pressured from Washington) if the results were not 'satisfactory'. Any information, however banal, could produce a 'report' (Pardo, 2014). Similar situations were described by Uruguayan interrogators in Chapter 3. Under such pressure, in most cases the interrogator will go back to the 'easier' methods of verbal and physical aggression, simply because they are *less* demanding and the interrogator does not need to employ strict emotional regulation or self-control (a challenge in stressful environments).

The data reviewed in this chapter show that coercive interrogation works slightly better than cognitive interviewing in getting confessions, but that such results come at the expense of an unacceptable increase in false confessions; coercive interrogation is also less effective for gathering information from a source (Meissner et al., 2014).

Being trained in the Reid Technique produces a strong distortion in the perception of its dangers, resulting in a kind of self-fulfilling prophecy. For example, Kostelnik and Reppucci (2009) have shown that police officers using deception with adolescents tend to see them as more mature and more capable of withstanding an 'adult' interrogation than they truly are. In an experimental study, Simcoe (2006) found that compared to controls, police officers trained in the Reid Technique had highly significant distortions in their perception of the honesty of 'sources', and tended to perceive many more 'lies' and 'deceptive answers' than were actually present.

This helps explain why judges rarely apply the exclusionary rule (Mendez, 2013), tend to accept confessions obtained under high-stress conditions and dismiss allegations of false confessions based on the use of coercive techniques – even when expert testimony is given (Behan, 2009; Elsea, 2004; Forrest and Woody, 2010; Kageleiry, 2007).

In sum, according to the UN Convention, an interrogation *per se* could be considered psychological torture if it induces severe psychological suffering for the purpose of obtaining a confession or for the purpose of debasing, humiliating or punishing a person. But the interrogation is also a central part of the process of building a torturing environment. Language is used to create confusion and impair the detainee's judgment in order to extract information from an otherwise *unwilling* person; interrogators resort to techniques that can break the interviewee's self and identity. The interrogator only accepts the possibility that the detainee is 'guilty' and does not accept anything that contradicts this hypothesis. The interrogator does not want to listen to what the detainee has to say, only to lead him or her to confess by using exhaustion, argumentation, manipulation of emotions or whatever other methods are deemed necessary. Experimental data show that this encourages confessions – especially when certain techniques are used, such as false-evidence ploys or having to choose between two incriminating alternatives in a state of exhaustion. Still, these methods increase the number of false confessions and ultimately gather less information.

Certain countries provide some legal guarantees (such as the Police and Criminal Evidence Act in the UK [PACE, 1984]), though all governments, when menaced or pressed for results, overtly or covertly accept coercive techniques despite the fact that even senior interrogators have rejected such techniques for both pragmatic and ethical reasons. False confessions are not only a serious ethical and legal problem, they are also a practical problem that causes confusion and additional work for those seeking the truth.

Interrogation techniques can amount to torture and should be integrated into a general schema on how torture works. The fact that this is one of the more neglected aspects in the research on psychological torture makes it all the more important.

Notes

1 Gudjonsson (2003) offers a description of a verdict that reveals a rare exception: a local US judge found that 'the continued and persistent challenges and verbal assault on the veracity of the suspect's replies had a marked and deleterious effect on the defendant's willpower and resistance (. . .). A relentless refusal to entertain the suspect's point of view was bound to undermine the most resolute of defendants and amounted to "oppression"' (p. 82).

2 The Intelligence Science Board worked from 2002 to 2010 for the US National Intelligence Services. Surprisingly, the group worked in a transparent manner and immediately released most of their material to the public through the Federation of American Scientists website. Its members, mostly professionals working for the army with strong links to universities, had a liberal perspective and defended overhauling the way intelligence is gathered. The group proposed a 'third generation' of intelligence-collection work which would bring out the 'human' side of interrogation based on scientific research. Their position was that there was no evidence or data supporting the assumption that harsh coercive interrogations lead to better results in terms of actionable information, and that there was enough data to suggest the opposite. They advocated for a 'measured' and 'scientifically controlled' use of coercive techniques, appealing to efficiency and vague ethical concerns. They tried, unsuccessfully, to draw a line between what was and was not acceptable. Their rhetoric was so appealing that even anti-torture groups surprisingly greeted them as 'colleagues' (see, for instance, the IRCT Secretary General Brita Sydhoff's public statement from 23 January 2007). A careful reading shows that, in fact, the group (again, composed mostly of military employees) supported 'controlled' coercive techniques (even harsh ones) as a necessary, lesser evil in the fight against terrorism, but argued that interrogations should be less discretional and more evidence-based, with respect for the Geneva Convention. The ISB was ultimately an innovative exercise in transparency with civil society on the part of the US Intelligence Services; it tried to create change from within the system. Unfortunately, it was quickly dismantled, apparently due to budgetary constraints. It is likely that the Board was simply renamed, and that some of their most liberal members removed while the work was reformulated in less progressive ways, and results and reports became classified.

3 Gudjonsson (2003) proposes using the expression 'Pressured Interrogation' to avoid the legal connotations of the term 'coercive'.

4 The Federal Bureau of Intelligence (FBI) uses the Direct Accusation Approach, which is a slightly modified version of the Reid Technique. Training materials from the FBI teach agents to show all the evidence from the beginning, interrupt any attempt at denial by the suspect, and repeatedly acknowledge the subject's participation in the crimes, while asking questions about motivations or

circumstances of 'proven' actions. The process is described as a long process (on average, three to four hours of monologue and persistence in using rationalisation, minimisation and emotional and moral discussion). They support all Reid techniques, including *god cop/bad cop, two incriminating choices*, and others, though they emphasise trying to build a positive rapport with the suspect and not resorting to physical violence (Neuman and Salinas-Serrano, 2006).

5 The expression 'third degree' is a euphemism for police torture (the 'inflict[ion] of pain, physical or mental, to extract confessions or statements'). It classically defined the use of physical violence to extract confessions from alleged criminals, and was considered routine procedure. It was banned in the US in 1931 after the Wickersham Commission. The Reid Technique is seen by many as simply a psychological version of the third degree.

6 Factor 1: <u>Intimidation factor</u>: emphasising the serious nature of the offense, maximising the suspect's anxiety, manipulative use of or reference to others, highlighting the experience of the officers, manipulating self-esteem, manipulating details, multiple assertions, and use of silence; Factor 2: <u>Robust challenge</u>: claiming that the suspect was lying, highlighting inconsistencies, interruptions, and continuing to dispute their version of events; Factor 3: <u>Manipulation factor</u>: minimising the serious nature of the offense, minimising the suspect's responsibility, offering incentives, use of themes or scenarios; Factor 4: <u>Questioning style</u>: leading questions, closed questions, echoing answers, multiple questions; Factor 5: <u>Appeal factor</u>: appealing to the suspect's good character, telling them to tell the truth, reassurance, suggesting that it is in the suspect's interest to confess, use of silence; Factor 6: <u>Soft challenge</u>: introducing the witness' version of events, using a low tone of voice, introducing evidence, using tactics aimed at shame reduction.

7 The total sample was comprised of robbery (43 per cent), assault (24 per cent), homicide (12 per cent), burglary (12 per cent) and various other crimes (9 per cent). The great majority (87 per cent) of the suspects had previous criminal convictions and therefore had some prior experience with the criminal justice system. A very low percentage of interrogations were in fact coercive. The 12 most commonly used tactics and the percentage of cases in which they were used were as follows: appeal to the suspect's self-interest (88 per cent), confront suspect with existing evidence of guilt (85 per cent), undermine suspect's confidence in denial of guilt (43 per cent), identify contradictions in suspect's story (42 per cent), any Behavioral Analysis Interview question (40 per cent), appeal to the importance of cooperation (37 per cent), offer moral justifications/psychological excuses (34 per cent), confront suspect with false evidence of guilt (30 per cent), use praise or flattery (30 per cent), appeal to the detective's expertise/authority (29 per cent), appeal to the suspect's conscience (23 per cent), minimise the moral seriousness of the offense (22 per cent).

8 Subjects take part in a reaction–time task using a computer keyboard. They are told not to press the Alt key or the computer will crash. Suddenly the computer crashes and the subject is accused of pressing the prohibited key. Half the subjects are then presented with false evidence in the form of a bogus computer printout showing that they had pressed the key they were warned not to touch. All subjects are innocent, and all are prompted to sign a confession. Across distinct replications of the study, between 30 per cent and 70 per cent of participants sign the self-incriminating statement and accept paying for the repair.

9 Subjects are paired with a confederate for a problem-solving study and instructed to work alone on some trials and jointly on others. In the guilty condition, the confederate sought help on a problem that was supposed to be solved alone, inducing a violation of the rules of the experiment; in the innocent condition, the confederate did not make this request to induce the crime. The experimenter soon 'discovered" a similarity in their answers, separated the subject and confederate, and accused the subject of cheating. The experimenter tried to get the subject to sign an admission by either (1) overtly promising leniency (research credit in exchange for another session without penalty), (2) making minimising remarks ('I'm sure you didn't realise what a big deal it was'), (3) using both tactics, or (4) using no tactics. This paradigm enables researchers to assess the diagnosticity of various interrogation techniques. In the original study, the confession rate was higher (1) among guilty subjects than innocent, (2) when leniency was promised than when it was not, and (3) when minimisation was used than when it was not.

10 However, Kelly et al. risk giving the false impression (to those who don't know that the authors have taken a clear, public stance against torture (e.g. Kleinman [2008]) that torture can be avoided by using only certain methods (echoing the positions of those who seek to justify practices that amount to torture – e.g. Rumsfeld, 2003).

11 In coercive interrogations the interrogator adopts a monologue or discourse that attempts to convince the detainees that they should confess for their own good. 'Themes' are the different kinds of arguments, adapted to the presumed crime and the psychological characteristics of the person being questioned. There are hundreds of themes (see, for example, Senese [2014], *Anatomy of Interrogation Themes* (John E. Reid and Associates), in which the author describes 70 different themes). In the US Army field manuals there is a list of 19 themes which are officially approved and authorised as part of the Enhanced Interrogation Techniques [see Table 14.1]. A theme can be developed for up to two or three hours. For example, in Ego Down, the theme focuses on showing the detainee that he or she is worthless, a criminal who can do nothing useful other than confess. In the case of the Futility theme, the discourse involves repeatedly insisting on the uselessness of resistance and negation [see the analysis of Mohammed Qahtani's log interrogation in Chapter 14].

12 Opinions regarding the limits of interrogation, coercive interrogation and torture depend on one's perspective: each actor involved faces different priorities and concerns. A forensic psychiatrist knows how easily a person can assume a submissive and compliant behaviour under any kind of authority, or how easily he or she can be induced to make a false confession. A lawyer worries about his or her clients making self-incriminating statements when the law clearly protects them against this situation. An interrogator reads the situation in terms of efficiency and professionalism (measured by the percentage of reports or confessions obtained), and faces pressure from all sides to get new information and confessions from suspects. A 'source' who is interrogated harshly for the first time will remember the experience as one of the most perplexing, shameful, difficult and traumatic he or she can go through. A judge must decide whether an interview was abusive and apply the exclusionary rule when there is little alternative evidence. A politician worries about the pragmatic elements of national security more than about abstract ethical concerns. A human rights defender attends to the global landscape of civil rights and the dangers that emerge when the limits of what democracies can accept are crossed. This is why this is a delicate issue that requires strong ethical convictions from those who make decisions and define policies.

14

INTERROGATION PROCEDURES IN MILITARY INTELLIGENCE GATHERING

US Army Manuals: drawing the line between interrogation and torture?

Most of the recent debate regarding torture comes from the legal debate in the US concerning what is admissible in interrogation of suspects of terrorism, and the questionable concept of Enhanced Interrogation. This debate stems from a long tradition coming from the time of the School of the Americas (SOA) in the 1980s. Here we map the evolution of contemporary US military intelligence collection procedures.[1]

Comparing FM2-22.3 and the Reid Technique

In the language of the US Army, interrogation is part of Human Intelligence (HUMINT) and an interrogator is known as a HUMINT collector. The army regularly publishes manuals with guidelines for each strategic area, including manuals for HUMINT collectors. The first manual was FM 34.52, released in 1987 and updated in 1991. It described how to conduct effective interrogations in line with US and international law. Human Intelligence Collector Operations (FM 2-22.3) superseded it in 2006[2] (US Army, 1992, 2006) (for a detailed review of the legal battle see endnote 2).

The surprising fact is that FM 2-22.3 is intended as a guide for interrogators deployed in war zones, and thus it provides directions for the interrogation of enemies, including 'terrorists'.[3] According to these HUMINT Manuals, most of the Reid Techniques (which we reviewed in the previous section), *are absolutely proscribed and considered illegal* in the Geneva Conventions and the ethical codes of the army.[4] In Table 14.1 we detail interrogation procedures authorized in FM 2-22.3 and compare them with the Reid Technique. The table speaks by itself. While some techniques are allowed (A), for most of them there are Restrictions (AR), are Not Recommended (NR) or simply Prohibited (P). We will not discuss whether these HUMINT Manuals are the actual guidelines for US interrogators deployed in war zones, or if they are manuals written for a wider audience. In the introduction FM 2-22.3 clearly states that 'the doctrine in this field manual is not policy (in and of itself)', but is '. . . a body of thought on how Army forces operate. . . . [It] provides an authoritative guide for leaders and soldiers, while allowing freedom to adapt to circumstances' (p. 8). But the fact is that it draws a clear

TABLE 14.1 US Army Field Manual FM 2-22.3 and the Reid Technique

'Softening techniques'	
Fear / threats Allowed in a moderate way if it does not include threating with measures that would violate the Geneva Conventions.	AR
Hooding / duct tape or adhesive over the eyes	P
Blindfolds / earmuffs	A

Isolation
1. Under special authorisation by commander
2. Restricted to resistant sources with potential important information when other techniques have not been successful
3. Limited to 12 hours after capture (to prolong the shock of capture) and prevent communication with others
4. Limited to 30 days (special permission needed to allow an extension)
5. Care should be taken to protect the detainee from exposure (in accordance with all appropriate standards addressing excessive or inadequate environmental conditions) to:
  – Excessive noise
  – Excessive dampness
  – Excessive or inadequate heat, light or ventilation
  – Inadequate bedding and blankets
	A

Sleep deprivation The detainee must have 4 hours of continuous sleep per 24-hour period.	A
Restriction of food or water Restriction of access to toilet/shower facilities Temperature manipulation Poor cell conditions Improper clothing	NS
Stress positions	NS
Building 'trust'/creating a climate of cooperation and closeness	SR
Direct accusation	NR
Repetition and rapid-fire questioning (asking successive, fast questions with different styles, including interruptions, repetition and quick switching of styles)	A
Silent approach technique (using long silences)	SR
Leading questions (implying the answer in the question, e.g 'and then you. . ., didn't you?')	NA
Multiple questions or multiple assertions in only one sentence Hostility – using an aggressive tone, interrupting, swearing (intimidation) Multiple interrogators asking questions one after the other without giving the suspect the opportunity to reply	A
Maximisation 1. Fear-up and fear-down approaches (maximising anxiety; threats) (must not include threats that would violate the Geneva Convention) 2. File and dossier technique (suggesting evidence; showing a large, false 'file') 3. Emotional love approach and emotional hate approach (direct appeal to the subject's conscience, emotions or feelings)	A SR SR

'Softening techniques'	
4. Deception (mentioning possible comrades who have already confessed)	SR
5. Establish your identity technique (challenging everything the detainee says)	A
Manipulative techniques – use of deception and lies	
1. Manipulation of details	NR
2. Emotional-pride, ego-up and ego-down approaches (manipulating self-esteem, attacks on the personal emotional well-being or moral stature of the detainee)	SR
3. Mutt and Jeff technique (good cop/bad cop) (requires special permission; it must not include any kind of violence or unlawful physical contact by the 'bad cop')	A
4. False flag technique (creation of scenarios; theater; the interrogator simulates being an intelligence agent from a country akin to the detainee)	SR
5. Elicitation	A
Minimising techniques	
Part of the emotional hate, fear-down, and ego-up approaches, the emotional futility approach (the interrogator minimises the serious nature of the offense; the interrogator minimises the suspect's responsibility; the interrogator emphasises the responsibility of the victim or a significant third party (face-saving excuses); confession is in the best interest of the detainee; shame reduction)	A
Incentive approach (offering deals: the detainee may be offered money; privileges, including food, tobacco and contact with relatives or others; or transfer to other locations)	A
Control (part of the emotional futility and we know all techniques) (showing omnipotence and omniscience)	A

A: Allowed; AR: Allowed with restriction; P: Prohibited; NS: Not specified (assumed allowed) SR: Strongly recommended; NR: Not Recommended.

Source: Author

line defining what is acceptable and what isn't when interviewing enemies, according to the experts from the army. Reid techniques (which are applied to civilians in time of peace and non-combatant civilians, which would be protected by the Geneva Conventions) are clearly at stake.

An analysis of FM 34-52 under the Geneva Conventions

The Congressional Research Service (CRS) is an entity working exclusively for the United States Congress, providing policy and legal analysis to committees and members of both the House and Senate, regardless of party affiliation. In 2003 they were commissioned to develop a legal analysis of the lawfulness of interrogation techniques described in FM-34.52 under the Geneva Conventions (Elsea, 2004).

The Geneva Convention Relative to the Treatment of Prisoners of War (GPW) 6 Article 17, Paragraph 4, provides the general rule for interrogation of prisoners of war[5]: 'No physical or mental torture, nor any other form of coercion, may be inflicted on prisoners of war to secure from them information of any kind whatever. Prisoners of war who refuse to answer may not be threatened, insulted, or exposed to unpleasant or disadvantageous treatment of any kind.'

Common Article 3 states the following obligations:

1. 'Persons taking no active part in the hostilities, including members of armed forces who have laid down their arms and those placed hors de combat by sickness, wounds, detention, or any other cause, shall in all circumstances be treated humanely, without any adverse distinction founded on race, color, religion or faith, sex, birth or wealth, or any other similar criteria.'
2. 'To this end, the following acts are and shall remain prohibited at any time and in any place whatsoever with respect to the above-mentioned persons: (a) Violence to life and person, in particular murder of all kinds, mutilation, cruel treatment and torture; (b) Taking of hostages; (c) Outrages upon personal dignity, in particular humiliating and degrading treatment.'

Civilians are protected by the Hague Convention, which states in Article 31 that '[n]o physical or moral coercion shall be exercised against protected persons, in particular to obtain information from them or from third parties'.

Table 14.2 summarises the recommendations of the CRS regarding the legality of FM 34.52 (Elsea, 2004). Overall, even when taking into account the so-called softening techniques (restrictions in food, sleep, control of temperature, isolation, etc.), the CRS believes that the problem is not any one technique in itself, but the accumulated effect of techniques. Prolonged and repeated interrogation, interrupted sleep and narrow cells with poor conditions cannot be considered ill-treatment; they are all part of a normal interrogation procedure. The extreme combination of these elements might constitute ill-treatment or torture.[6]

TABLE 14.2 Analysis of Interrogation Army Manual FM 34-52 under the Geneva Conventions

- **Coercion.** Proscribed by the convention. The pertinent question appears to be whether the person subject to treatment designed to influence his or her conduct is able to exercise a choice and complies willingly, or has no choice other than to comply. Some authorised techniques may violate the convention.

Manipulation of environment
- **Dietary manipulation.** Not allowed if it is intended as coercion.
- **Manipulation of environment.** Not allowed if it is intended as coercion.
- **Sleep management** (reversing sleep cycle day/night, sleep deprivation, Sleep disruption). Not allowed if it is intended as coercion.

- **Isolation for up to 30 days.** Not allowed unless it is for the safety of the detainee.
- **Sensory deprivation.** Not specified. Possibly constitutes ill-treatment or torture.

- **Stress positions (4 hours every 24 hours).** Criteria defining the limit for allowed suffering or humiliation not firmly established.

- **Use of drugs.** Alerts that not all drugs are banned, only those which 'induce lasting and permanent mental alteration and damage'. Most drugs will not do that, but will severely impair the detainee's will.

Interrogation techniques
Some of the techniques might be considered coercive for the purposes of a criminal prosecution, and would likely be inadmissible were they used to elicit statements from an accused soldier prior to a court-martial.

- **Direct approach.** While it may be acceptable to exploit a detainee's initial shock upon capture to obtain information, exploiting a detainee's suffering by interrogating a wounded prisoner would be more problematic, and could constitute a breach of the obligation to provide medical treatment.
- **Incentive / incentive removal.** Admissibility depends on whether or not the 'incentive' is covered by the Geneva Convention.
- **Emotional love / hate.** Legal if it does not include direct threats to relatives or loved ones.
- **Fear-up harsh / mild.** Legal.
- **Fear-down.** Legal.
- **Pride and ego-up / down.** The approach could contravene the Geneva Convention's prohibition of insults and degrading treatment.
- **Futility.** Extreme treatment designed to induce a feeling of overall futility could cause mental suffering severe enough to raise questions under the Geneva Conventions.
- **We know all.** Legal.
- **Establish your identity.** The technique appears to involve trickery that may be acceptable under the Geneva Conventions, but could conceivably be applied in a threatening or coercive manner.
- **Repetition.** Taken to extremes, for example, during prolonged interrogations, it might be said to induce mental suffering.
- **Rapid-fire questioning.** Legal.
- **Silence.** Legal.
- **Change of scenery.** Extreme conditions might be unacceptable under the Geneva Convention. It is not clear how such extreme conditions are defined.

Other conditions
- **Forced nudity.** Forced nudity without threats or sexual assault may not rise to the level of an 'outrage upon human dignity', but would probably be considered inhumane and degrading.
- **Removal of comfort or religious items.** The removal of religious items could entail a violation of GC Art. 27, providing that protected persons are entitled to respect for their religious convictions and practices; or GPW Art. 14, respect for the person of the prisoner of war.
- **Threats: use of scenarios designed to convince the detainee that death or severely painful consequences are imminent.** Violate the Geneva Conventions, because they constitute coercion, threats and possibly psychological torture.

Source: Congressional Research Service – Elsea, 2004.

The standards and their interpretation

Though there is an official shift towards a third generation of interrogation procedures in which non-coercive methods are supposed to become the norm (see note 2 on High-Value Interrogation Group), it is unlikely that coercive interrogations – or torture – will disappear any time soon. Increased concern about the prohibition of abusive interrogation procedures is important, but each manual has its own interpretations and all norms contain grey areas which can be 'understood' freely by interrogators. Furthermore, detention centres are closed spaces that escape public scrutiny, and they are increasingly being outsourced to third-world countries.

Mullenix (2007), a long-time trainer of Reid Associates and an interrogator, has repeatedly offered his version of how to apply the Reid method to suspected terrorists. His 'interpretation' of the rules goes far beyond what the FM 2–22.3 permits, suggesting a model in which the detainee is assumed guilty and forced into confession through methods based on mental confusion, exhaustion, lies, undue pressure and leading questions. In a recent review of the

KUBARK Manual commissioned by the Intelligence Science Board, Kleinman (an army intelligence official and campaigner against the use of torture in interrogations) concluded that there were positive elements in the Manual; techniques that violated the Geneva Conventions (according to the CRS report) were deemed acceptable in Kleinman's review (Kleinman, 2006). He and others (Kelly et al., 2013) have recently proposed a model to integrate interrogation techniques into a conceptual model; they argue that 'Context Manipulation' is an essential part of any technique.

Although there were formal compromises under the Obama Administration to end the use of torture in Guantanamo Bay and other locations, independent reports show that widespread torture continues (Center for Human Rights and Humanitarian Law, 2009).

From coercive interrogation to psychological torture

FM 34–52 and the FM 2-22.3 highlight the debate about which interrogation procedures are officially admissible. Both manuals constantly refer to the Geneva Conventions and US domestic law, and make clear statements about which situations would be considered degrading treatment or torture. Both expressly prohibit 'acts of violence or intimidation, including physical or mental torture, threats, insults, or exposure to inhumane treatment as a means of or aid to interrogation', and name only 19 authorised interrogation techniques – most of which are based on the Reid Technique. They expressly forbid any kind of 'softening' techniques. Due to lack of success, the Bush Administration reportedly[7] approved additional psychological techniques.

Enhanced Interrogation Techniques (EIT) are a group of techniques that combine several of the well-known 'softening methods' (isolation, stress positions, sleep disruption, etc.), with some limitations (see Tables 14.1 and 14.3); EITs also propose additional 'themes' for interrogation. To date, EITs are considered the most refined methods of coercive psychological interrogation; they are designed based on the expert advice of psychologists, SERE experts and experienced interrogators (Rumsfeld, 2003). They adhere to the principles of trying to convince detainees to cooperate without using physical violence or defeating them through unbearable pain or suffering.

An analysis of Case 063

Mohammed al-Qahtani (file 063), a Saudi Arabian citizen, was the first detainee in Guantanamo officially recognised by the US Government as a victim of torture (Center for Human Rights and Humanitarian Law, 2006) by Susan J. Crawford. She was the Convening Authority for the Guantanamo military commissions, appointed by the Bush administration on February 7, 2007.[8] Crawford belonged to the most conservative sector of the army legal system, and had absolute power in deciding which detainees were transferred for military trial under which charges. When she interviewed Qahtani, she saw a destroyed man. The detainee showed behaviour consistent with extreme psychological trauma (talking to non-existent people, reportedly hearing voices, crouching in a corner of the cell covered with a sheet for hours on end) (Gutierrez, 2008).

Crawford later declared,[9] 'We tortured Qahtani. His treatment met the legal definition of torture. And that's why I did not refer the case [for prosecution] . . . The techniques they used were all authorised, but the manner in which they applied them was overly aggressive and too persistent. . . . You think of torture, you think of some horrendous physical act done to an individual. This was not any one particular act; this was just a combination of things that had a medical impact on him, that hurt his health. It was abusive and uncalled for. And coercive. Clearly coercive. It was that medical impact that pushed me over the edge [to call it torture].'

Her definition is perfect. The techniques used were all authorised, and according to the Geneva Conventions, they did not include any kind of 'horrendous physical act', but the manner in which those techniques were applied made them amount to torture. Independent reports from the FBI (FBI Review Division, 2008) and CIA (Office of Professional Responsibility, 2009) acknowledged that the abuses amounted to torture. The charges against Qahtani were dropped in January 2009, because the evidence had been obtained through torture and was inadmissible in court.

What were the tactics used in case 063 that qualified 'undoubtedly' as torture by an official who supported the use of Enhanced Interrogation Techniques, the FBI and the CIA? The case is documented in several reports (Gutierrez, 2008) which show that after his arrival in Guantanamo, Qahtani was placed in isolation for three months. FBI agents, who used standard techniques, initially interrogated him. In December 2002, Secretary of Defense Rumsfeld authorised, in writing, the use of 17 <u>enhanced interrogation techniques</u> on Qahtani. Someone at Guantanamo leaked the log of the interrogation from late November 2002 to early January 2003, written in daily diary entries. On March 3, 2006, *Time* magazine published the log (Anonymous, 2006). It is a unique, first-hand account of how Enhanced Interrogation Techniques (which are an extreme version of the basic Reid Technique) worked in practice, at least with prisoners considered to be of 'high value'.

The log details coercive techniques and interrogation themes. Table 14.3 offers a content analysis of the log focused specifically on interrogation methods.[10] Though the details may at first appear monotonous, reviewing the log is incredibly revealing. It shows how allegedly innocuous techniques can easily fall into ill-treatment or torture, even from the perspective of those who initially endorsed it. Such no-touch treatment is now presented as something from the past, a product of trial-and-error experimentation based on the recommendations of two cognitive-behavioural psychologists with no experience in interrogation (Kleinman, 2006). This kind of interrogation takes the army manuals' recommendations (which supposedly adhere strictly to the Geneva Conventions) to their limits, twisting their words to reinterpret them in an entirely different spirit. This type of 'interpretation' will repeat itself in the future whenever a government deems it necessary.

TABLE 14.3 Interrogation log of Guantanamo detainee Qahtani: content analysis

Total hours of interrogation: 49 days × 20 hours per day (on average)= 980 hours of interrogation		
Approach / theme *(names given by interrogators and used in the log)*	**N**	***Objective pursued by the theme***
Direct approach. (Simple questions)	1	–
Silence. The interrogator sits in silence in front of detainee for as long as necessary.	1	Increasing need to talk

(continued)

TABLE 14.3 Interrogation log of Guantanamo detainee Qahtani: content analysis (*continued*)

Total hours of interrogation: 49 days × 20 hours per day (on average)= 980 hours of interrogation

Approach / theme *(names given by interrogators and used in the log)*	N	Objective pursued by the theme
Love of brothers in Cuba. Alone and isolated from others. He can be with other detainees (transferred from X-Ray to Delta camp) if he cooperates.	9	Need for belonging
Detainee's family theme. Detainee is reminded of his family. He probably will never see the again. They are probably disappointed by him.	6	Need for belonging
9/11 theme. The detainee is confronted with 9/11 either by having to see videos of the attacks, or the victims, pictures (especially of wounded children), hearing the narrative of victims. Detainee forced to listen to others presenting arguments supporting the right of the US to defend the lives of its citizens.	14	Guilt and remorse
Global War on Terrorism (GWOT). Interrogator talks to the detainee about the GWOT and the right of US to defend itself against terrorism.	2	Guilt and remorse
Level of guilt. Maximising responsibility / enhancing guilty feelings.	8	Guilt and remorse
Guilt reduction. Minimising responsibility to calm down and increase rapport.	1	Anxiety control
You can make this stop / 'self-inflicted suffering' theme. The person is the only one responsible for what is happening to him.	4	Self-inflicted pain
Good Muslim / Bad Muslim / judgment day. Al-Qaeda destroyed Islam and the detainee's life had been spared. It was now his jihad to tell the world about how 9/11 was wrong, and help rebuild Islam / Al-Qaeda members are bad Muslims / If he does not confess, when he dies he will be sent to hell for killing innocent people.	4 2 2	Identity – Religion
Muslims in America. Because of his association with the al-Qaeda organisation, he was a part of the cause of attacks on Islam and Muslims in America.	7	Guilt
Saudi support for US approach / betrayal by Saudi government approach/ you can never go home. Saudi Arabia supported the fight against terrorists and is a friend of the US. Saudi Government is corrupt and does not care about its people / Saudi Government had abandoned him / Showed pictures of Saudi Arabia and said he would never see his country again.	6 2 2 2	Need for belonging

Total hours of interrogation: 49 days × 20 hours per day (on average)= 980 hours of interrogation

Approach / theme *(names given by interrogators and used in the log)*	N	Objective pursued by the theme
Futility approach. Telling detainee it is useless to resist. Nothing except 'telling the truth' will be useful to make this stop / It does not matter what the detainee says or does, the only way to stop interrogation way is 'confessing' / 'No hope of ever being believed'/ "Life is hopeless for you' Especially used linked to the Manchester Document theme	38	Lack of control Hopelessness
Detainee has no hope of being found innocent. (Variant of futility approach)	4	Hopelessness
You will be here forever. (Variant of futility approach)	1	Hopelessness
Manchester Document Theme. The detainee is read, shown or told about a document found in Manchester attributed to al-Qaeda explaining how to resist an interrogation. The detainee is accused of knowing and using the strategies described, told that this confirms he belongs to al-Qaeda and that it is useless to attempt to use these strategies.	19	Confusion Hopelessness
Pride and ego-down approach. 'The questioner attacks the subject's intelligence, abilities, appearance, or any other perceived weakness in his self-image or identity.'/ 'Detainee was reminded that no one loved, cared [about], or remembered him.'/ 'Detainee was forced to look at a family of rats and was told that they were better and enjoyed more freedom than him.'	35	Humiliation Identity
Arrogant Saudi approach. A variant of pride and ego approach	2	Humiliation Identity
'You are a failure' approach. He has failed in everything in life: his family, country, and his mission. He is good for nothing / 'Control writes the Arabic words for "liar", "coward", and "failure" on the wall'/ 'Explained how the words liar, stupid, weak, and failure apply to detainee.'	8	Humiliation Identity
Captured and talking approach / Mission approach. (Likely variants of 'You are a failure' approach)	2 1	Humiliation Identity
Mohammed the slave. (Likely a variant of ego-down)	1	Humiliation
Invasion of personal space / Invasion of space by a female. The interrogator remains very close to the detainee. A female interrogator conducted most of these interrogations. 'He stated that he would rather die at my hands than to be subjected to my invasion of his personal space. He stated that this is unbearable to him, my being in his personal space.'	6	Breaking Taboos Identity Humiliation

(continued)

TABLE 14.3 Interrogation log of Guantanamo detainee Qahtani: content analysis (*continued*)

Total hours of interrogation: 49 days × 20 hours per day (on average)= 980 hours of interrogation

Approach / theme (names given by interrogators and used in the log)	N	Objective pursued by the theme
National anthem. The detainee is forced to stand and hear the US National Anthem. Once with his hand over his heart.	4	Identity Humiliation
Al-Qaeda falling apart approach. Al-Qaeda used him and now they don't care about him anymore. Talking is his opportunity for revenge.	18	Supposed sense of belonging and group identity
Al-Qaeda is against Islam. A good Muslim should go against al-Qaeda. Al-Qaeda used Islam (1) / Al-Qaeda destroyed Islam (2) / Al-Qaeda 'raped' the Koran (1) / Al-Qaeda members are cowards (2) / Al-Qaeda 'raped" Islam (1)	7	
Student teacher approach. The detainee must listen to the interrogator talk about different themes. He is later asked for details. If he fails, the lesson begins again.	3	Forcing acceptance of new ideas
Attention to detail approach. He is forced to see pictures of women in underwear (which he strongly rejects and tries to resist) and memorise the details. He must later give an accurate description of each one or he will have to begin again.	9	Submission Humiliation
Drill Instructor Approach (Unclear)	4	
Control approach. Usually associated with interrogators changing shifts. The new interrogator demonstrates, with his or her voice, attitude or words, that he or she has absolute control from now on. 'Detainee was berated harshly' / 'Ordered to sit and stand several times to reinforce control' / 'Drink water or wear it' (if he does not drink the water he is offered, its poured on him) / 'He was told that [the] interrogator was in control of everything that happened to him.'	14	
Rule of the Day approach. Interrogator says how the detainee must behave during that day's interrogation, e.g. remaining silent at all times.	5	Submission Lack of control
Rules have changed. Interrogator says that things will get worse and that the rules have now changed.	8	
Respect approach. The detainee is said to be disrespectful by not answering questions. He is threatened in a loud voice, told to be respectful and obey orders.	13	
Big Brother approach. (Not clear. Probably similar to We know all approach.)	1	

Total hours of interrogation: 49 days × 20 hours per day (on average)= 980 hours of interrogation

Approach / theme *(names given by interrogators and used in the log)*	N	Objective pursued by the theme
Fear-up approach. The interrogator induces fear through attitude, voice, hitting or throwing objects, or making direct threats to the detainee.	9	Submission Fear
Holes in cover theme. The interrogator says that cover story is a lie, and asks for details which are cross-checked with answers to the same questions given in other interrogations.	6	Confusion
Circumstantial evidence theme. The interrogator repeatedly recites all of the circumstantial evidence against the detainee, and says over and over again that there is enough material for a full sentence.	52	Confusion Memorising confession Hopelessness
What we know theme. The interrogator draws a timeline with previous statements by the detainee and asks him to fill in the holes. Situations are suggested that directly involve the detainee (like being in al-Qaeda meetings).	5	Confusion Inducing false memories
Cards and minds. The interrogator plays cards. Guesses the card of the detainee. He says that he can also read his mind. This creates extreme confusion.	1	Confusion Control
Leniency. Telling 'the truth' as a means of obtaining a milder sentence.	3	Inducing false confessions
Other relevant elements		
Loud music / 'white sound'. The detainee was forced to hear rock music (which he thought was forbidden by Islam). A variety of musical selections were played to agitate the detainee.	39	Identity Confusion

Detainee was mocked. The interrogator ridiculed the detainee:
  a. by making him dance (twice);
  b. making him dress grotesquely (3 times);
  c. with puppets (once);
  d. by hanging pictures of swimsuit models around his neck (4 times);
  e. by taping pictures 9/11 to his body/face (twice) ('Lead taped picture of 3-year-old victim over detainee's heart').
	12	Humiliation

Head shaved. (Forced into shaving)	3	Identity Humiliation Control
Injection of serum via IV. The detainee did not drink enough water and became dehydrated due to heat conditions. Sometimes he went on strike. A doctor came to see him almost daily. He was forced to accept IV serum.	25	Control

(continued)

TABLE 14.3 Interrogation log of Guantanamo detainee Qahtani: content analysis (*continued*)

Total hours of interrogation: 49 days × 20 hours per day (on average)= 980 hours of interrogation

Approach / theme (names given by interrogators and used in the log)	N	Objective pursued by the theme
Naked / stripped / cavity search. Detainee was naked in front of the female interrogator. /Detainee was stripped. / Detainee was searched despite the fact that he had no contact with the outside world.	6	Identity Humiliation Control
Consequences		
Crying. The log reflects that the detainee cried and says he cannot take it anymore.	24	
Anger. Detainee tried to resist the guard, despite being secured (handcuffed) and the fact that there were Military Police everywhere. Uncontrollable anger.	6	
Confusion. The log recognises the detainee is almost asleep or looks very confused. He is awakened and the interrogation continues. / Most self-incriminating statements are given in this condition, and the following day the detainee denies them, saying that he either does not remember or was confused.	9	
Forced exercise. Detainee is told to exercise for 5 to 10 minutes. Sometimes this clearly means squatting but generally it is unclear whether this is considered rest or punishment.	46	

The detention log reveals that:

1. Qahtani underwent 900 hours of interrogation in 49 days, including:
   - Approximately 20 hours of continuous interrogation per day conducted by pairs of interrogators who rotated every 6 hours, with a 4-hour rest period each day (according to what was authorised).
   - Occasional 30–60 minute naps when the detainee was too weak or tired to pay attention to the theme.

   However:
   - The log shows a shift in sleeping hours. Initially the detainee was allowed to sleep from 00:00 to 4:00 AM. Three weeks later, he was allowed to sleep from 7:00 AM to 11:00 AM, a schedule which was maintained for the rest of the 49 days of interrogation.
   - The log shows that on 34 occasions the detainee was awakened during a session and forced to go to the bathroom, drink water or exercise for 10 minutes. On 6 occasions, the interrogators allowed him to sleep only to awaken him shortly thereafter. When taken together, these actions reveal a pattern of shifting sleep hours and interrupting sleep that nevertheless *does not violate official rules.*

2. According to the names given to each theme in the log, the interrogators introduced 42 different themes, subthemes and approaches. They used the *direct approach* (which was initially recommended) on only one occasion. The log shows that the interrogator devoted between 20 minutes and 3 hours to a given approach (or combination of approaches) before changing. There were 3 shifts of interrogators (sometimes from different institutions) who took turns, on average, every 6 hours. Over the course of 49 days, this amounted to 351 changes in themes, subthemes and approach, averaging 7 changes per day. In some cases an interrogator would start with one theme and then switch to another, and after changing shifts, a new team would return to the initial theme. Qahtani was flooded by all kinds of themes, which were constantly changing.

Figure 14.1 summarises the log into a conceptual map in which the size of each circle is proportional to the importance of each approach, theme or subtheme. Elements linked to the manipulation of primary needs, attacks on sensory perceptions, and manipulation of environment have been excluded because they are considered part of the process of disorganisation and confusion that was simultaneously taking place. Figure 14.1 focuses specifically on the interrogation. The interrogators' questions did not have a clear focus, nor did they know exactly what they were looking for; all actions were directed towards making the detainee recognise affiliation with al-Qaeda. In theory, once this was achieved, then the objective would have been to engage him as a stable, long-term collaborator who could provide potentially unknown but useful intelligence information.

The interrogators elaborate on their tactics every day. The log explains that approach/theme is decided daily, and sometimes a session is interrupted to discuss and redirect the approach.

Most of their energy was devoted to **Emotional Manipulation Tactics**, mainly Humiliation (71 times); Instilling Hopelessness (66 times); Submission, Dependence and Compliance (62 times); and Guilt (24 times). This is likely the reason why there were relatively few **Cognitive Manipulation Tactics**. From the very first moment, and increasingly as days pass, approaches were used that directly attacked **Identity Structure**: Self, Self-Worth (55 times); Family Identity (6); and Social Identity (29).

The interrogators designed this process to demolish the prisoner's identity structure, a practice that is strikingly similar to what the KUBARK Manual referred to as inducing a process of 'regression'; it is also similar to the colloquial term 'brainwashing', used by Lifton (1961) and Biderman and Zimmer (1961) when analysing Chinese and communist methods.

The end result is that no harsh physical violence has taken place. Moreover, when analysed individually, the interrogators could be said to have used a standard Reid Technique – reinforced by some additional special measures – that an inspector with no direct access to what was happening would view as respecting army regulations in the Field Manuals, the Geneva Conventions and domestic law. But, as the Convening Authority for the Guantanamo military commissions who *supported* this type of psychological interrogation ultimately had to accept, 'the manner in which they applied them was overly aggressive and too persistent. (. . .). This was not any one particular act; this was just a combination of things (. . .) that (. . .) was abusive and (. . .) clearly coercive.'

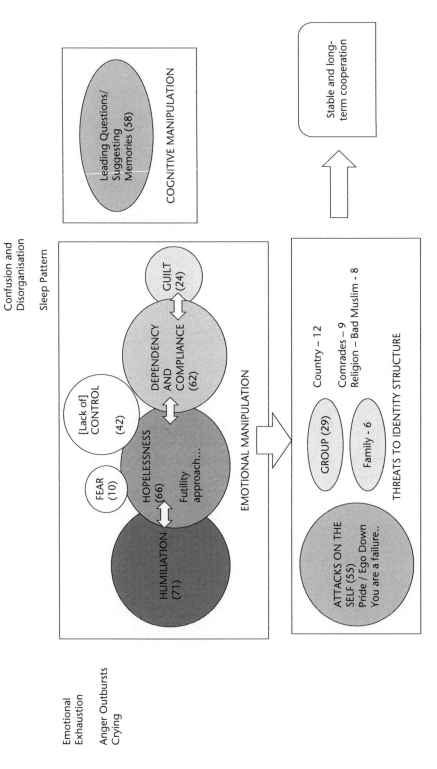

Emotional
Exhaustion

Anger Outbursts
Crying

Confusion and
Disorganisation

Sleep Pattern

COGNITIVE MANIPULATION

Leading Questions/
Suggesting
Memories (58)

GUILT
(24)

DEPENDENCY
AND
COMPLIANCE
(62)

[Lack of]
CONTROL
(42)

FEAR
(10)

HOPELESSNESS
(66)

Futility
approach....

HUMILIATION
(71)

EMOTIONAL MANIPULATION

Stable and long-
term cooperation

Country – 12

Comrades – 9
Religion – Bad Muslim - 8

GROUP (29)

Family - 6

ATTACKS ON THE
SELF (55)
Pride / Ego Down
You are a failure...

THREATS TO IDENTITY STRUCTURE

FIGURE 14.1 Interrogation of Qahtani: use of themes.

The hybrid paradigm

For 18 years, Guiora, a former Israeli judge now living and teaching in the US, was involved in the interrogation of Palestinian prisoners accused of terrorism. He believes that there should be a balance between human rights and national security. He argues that torture and coercive interrogation are different things, and though he maintains that torture is inadmissible, he considers coercive interrogation to be necessary. In his view (Guiora, 2008), coercive interrogation is an intelligence-gathering process that includes situations that may not be comfortable for detainees, but that do not violate their constitutional rights – whether they are US citizens or not:

> Coercive interrogation measures might be used only to facilitate a specific interrogation provided that less coercive measures have proven unsuccessful. (. . .). Detainees, even if [they are] not American citizens, are entitled to basic constitutional rights. (. . .). Torture as an interrogation method is illegal, and the so-called ticking time bomb exception is not to be condoned or adopted. (p. 160)

Guiora considers the following to be basic rights of the detainee: '(1) Lawful coercive interrogation of a suspect granted [Miranda rights] (the right to remain silent and the right against self-incrimination); (2) remand hearings before a court designed to prevent indefinite detention (. . .); (3) the right to counsel of the suspect's own choosing' (p. 9). He states that 'military commissions are illegal', and that all interrogations should be under 'active judicial review' by the United States Supreme Court (p. 161).

He believes that what happened in Guantanamo and Abu Ghraib was a consequence of vague rules and a lack of adequate supervision of the interrogators. In a violent context, the absence of clear rules causes torture to become the norm. A crucial point in his argument is what he refers to as the 'lawful coercive interrogation', understood as 'the imposition of moderate methods – in a highly controlled environment – that although causing detainees discomfort does not cause them severe mental and physical pain' (p. 86). He adheres to the 'severe suffering' paradigm, and proposes that moderate suffering (which he calls 'discomfort') is permissible.

In his interpretation of US law, he argues that the limits of acceptable treatment are:[11]

1. Solitary confinement, which he finds unacceptable on any grounds based on the evidence that it produces severe mental suffering and may produce permanent damage.
2. Unlawful threats. He discusses lawful versus unlawful threats, and argues that if an interrogator threatens a detainee to break his or her will, that should be considered unlawful regardless of whether or not that threat specifically produced fear in the interrogated individual. Examples of unlawful threats include direct threats to family members or threats of physical pain or death. Admissible threats are mentioning a possible prison sentence for obstructing justice if the detainee is uncooperative.
3. Cumulative mistreatment. Guiora states that cumulative mistreatment occurs when law enforcement officials either hold a detainee for an extended period of time and subject him or her to seemingly endless interrogations, or deprive the detainee of his or her basic needs for a significant period of time. He does not specify how time limits should be defined. 'Cumulative mistreatment can be identified by asking whether the continuousness and cumulativeness of the interrogation was the specific factor that broke down

a detainee's will' (p. 93). He gives the example of the *Anderson v. United States*[12] (1943) case, in which the petitioners were held in custody and questioned by federal agents intermittently over a period of six days during which they saw neither friends, relatives nor legal counsel. That interrogation produced incriminating statements from six of the petitioners. He considers cumulative mistreatment to be 'the lengthy and cumulative use of sleep deprivation, stress positions, isolation, hooding, sensory deprivation and use of dogs to induce fear' (p. 97).

Bearing these limits in mind, he proposes distinguishing 'torture methods' from methods that produce an 'uncomfortable' situation, and considers the latter to be admissible. The practices he considers admissible include (Guiora, 2008):

1. The use of uncomfortable chairs (i.e. stress positions)
2. Modification of room temperature
3. Sleep deprivation (according to the Geneva Conventions, detainees are to be ensured eight hours sleep in a twenty-four hour period; however there is no requirement that the eight hours be continuous)
4. Playing loud, cacophonous music
5. The placing of hoods over the detainee's head

The use of these five methods would require written authorisation from the head of the relevant security agency (which means that the senior command would be accountable for any mistreatment) and written authorisation from an on-site physician who is not in the chain of command, does not have a dual loyalty dilemma and is held liable in the event that the detainee is harmed.

In brief, a modified version of the British Army standard procedures that were considered ill-treatment by the European Court of Human Rights and "probably torture" in subsequent sentences.

Conclusions: clear regulations for cumulative ill-treatment

This hybrid paradigm represents a step forward in distinguishing coercive interrogation from torture in that it stresses the need for authorities to provide strict, clear rules on accepted procedures *before* interrogation; such authorities must then, of course, be held responsible for what happens during interrogation. Vagueness should be avoided because it leaves decisions about whether a situation would be considered torture to a post-facto assessment that depends on the discretionary opinion of juries, judges and the interrogation unit's commander. This means that interrogators in the field, not those who truly give the orders, are the ones who end up being held responsible and accountable for hypothetical acts of abuse because they are the weakest point in the chain of command.

The problematic point is why these five techniques are considered permissible while others are not. There is no justification for this selection beyond Guiora's own experience as an interrogator and a review of selected cases in US jurisprudence. Some of the techniques he proposes as 'safe' can be considered damaging, especially when used in combination. Prolonged stress positions combined with room temperature modification can be lethal. Guiora does not specify what the time limit should be when applying the five acceptable techniques (leaving one to wonder whether their indefinite application would be permitted); nor does he specify at what intensity or in what combinations these techniques become illegal (Should certain combinations be allowed? What about combining all five 'acceptable' techniques?).

Thus, while the idea of strong and clear pre facto regulations is a step forward, the distinction between 'torture' and 'discomfort' appears to be a semantic one. If an interrogator twists a detainee's will, what difference does it make whether the outcome was achieved through 'discomfort' or through 'torture'? Such coercion clearly violates the detainee's Miranda rights and the constitutional rights that Guiora claims are non-negotiable.

The idea of holding the commander and an appointed medical physician fully accountable for any damage inflicted on the prisoner is important, and would offer greater protection from abuse. Although there were actually similar provisions in Guantanamo. The case of Mohammed al-Qahtani (file 063) provides strong support for the idea of considering cumulative mistreatment a keystone in any future proposal on the limit between coercive interrogation and torture. Evaluating the combined effects of multiple techniques is the basis of our proposal regarding torturing environments at the end of this book and should be the new paradigm of analysis of torture in the coming years.

Notes

1 Most of the international debate occurs in the US and focuses on US methods. Unfortunately, we cannot conduct a similar review of other armies that have used similar tactics. There are testimonies and images available on the Internet of ill-treatment and torture of similar severity at the hands of Israeli, British, Canadian, Spanish and Italian forces deployed in Iraq, Afghanistan, Somalia and The Democratic Republic of Congo – to cite just a few examples among Western democracies. Much of what we do know comes from US army manuals; other countries should also provide public access to official army manuals to increase transparency.

2 The manual established safeguards for detainees that prohibited practices being used in Afghanistan, Iraq and Guantanamo. To overcome this difficulty, the Bush administration used different strategies: employing civil interrogators (who are not subject to the same rules as military interrogators); employing interrogators from civil agencies (like the Central Intelligence Agency); identifying suspects as 'irregular combatants' and proposing that they were not subject to the Geneva Conventions; and finally, issuing a special memorandum that authorised the so-called 'Enhanced Interrogation techniques'. As Secretary of Defense, Donald Rumsfeld authorised the use of techniques that were far beyond F34.52. These 'extended techniques' were the core interrogation practices during the Bush administration. There was intense debate inside the US and in the international arena. On July 25, 2005, the Republican Senator and former Presidential Candidate John McCain, who opposed these practices, submitted an amendment (called the Detainee Treatment Act) intended to restrict all US government interrogators (including civilian interrogators working for US intelligence services and the CIA) from using interrogation techniques not authorised in F34.52. After long disputes and several different drafts, on September 6, 2006, the US Army announced the publication of Field Manual 2-22.3, *Human Intelligence Collector Operations*, which specifically prohibits many of the controversial Enhanced Interrogation techniques (including mock executions, hooding, sexual harassment, <u>waterboarding</u> and others) but only for the military interrogators. On January 2009, President Obama finally restricted all interrogations by civil or military personnel to the limitations of FM 2-22.3. In April 2010 he created the High-Value Interrogation Group (HIG), an elite team that includes linguists, cultural specialists, analysts and a selection of interrogators from the CIA, FBI

and Army under direct Presidential control that is activated in special cases (according to official data, 14 occasions in its first two years). The group has raised serious concerns. It works mainly overseas, sometimes in military ships anchored in international waters. According to public statements, their work strictly adheres to, and even surpasses, criteria authorised in FM 2-22.3; moreover, they stated that they abandoned some of the strategies allowed in that manual after an assessment from (unnamed) Geneva Convention experts (Ackerman, S. Meet the High-Value Detainee Interrogation Group. *The Washington Independent*. 24 August 2009). The HIG is presented as a new generation of experts employing a non-coercive interrogation style, with a multi-professional team and a personalised approach to each detainee based on internationally approved human-rights standards.

3 For F34-52, this included scenarios in Vietnam, Granada and Panama; for FM 2-22.3 Afghanistan, Iraq and Guantanamo Bay.

4 Point 8.80, p. 159 states: 'US HUMINT collectors are obligated to treat all detainees in accordance with applicable law and policy. Applicable law and policy include US law; the law of war; relevant international law; relevant directives including DOD Directive 3115.09, "DOD Intelligence Interrogations, Detainee Debriefings, and Tactical Questioning"; DOD Directive 2310.1E, "The Department of Defense Detainee Program"; DOD instructions; and military execute orders including FRAGOs. Detainees and, in particular, EPWs are guaranteed certain rights and privileges. The HUMINT collector may not take any action to remove, state that he will remove, or imply that he will remove any guaranteed right if a detainee fails to cooperate. Under the GPW, EPWs cannot be denied their rights or their privileges accorded them by rank as guaranteed by the GPW. Privileges afforded to them, however, which are not guaranteed by the Geneva Conventions or other applicable law or agreements, may be withheld.' (See Appendix A, Section I.)

5 Additionally, Article 13 provides, in part, that '[p]risoners of war must at all times be humanely treated' and they 'must at all times be protected, particularly against acts of violence or intimidation. . . .' Furthermore, it describes '[a]ny unlawful act or omission by the Detaining Power causing death or seriously endangering the health of a prisoner of war in its custody' as a 'serious breach'. Article 14 states that '[p]risoners of war are entitled in all circumstances to respect for their persons and their honor'. Article 25 states that, regarding living conditions, 'Prisoners of war shall be quartered under conditions as favorable as those for the forces of the Detaining Power who are billeted in the same area. The said conditions shall make allowance for the habits and customs of the prisoners and shall in no case be prejudicial to their health. (. . .) The premises provided for the use of prisoners of war individually or collectively, shall be entirely protected from dampness and adequately heated and lighted, in particular between dusk and lights out.' Article 22, regarding solitary confinement affirms that 'Subject to the provisions of the present Convention relative to penal and disciplinary sanctions, prisoners of war may not be held in close confinement except where necessary to safeguard their health and then only during the continuation of the circumstances which make such confinement necessary.'

6 Cohen (2001) is quoted as saying: 'a prisoner subjected to prolonged, intense questioning, perhaps after a sleepless night on a narrow prison bed, while seated in an uncomfortable chair [is probably not suffering torture, or even] being treated inhumanely, given the fact that interrogations inherently tend to employ some measure of physical discomfort. However, extreme applications of a combination of these factors – prolonged lack of sleep, being forced to stand for unreasonable periods of time with arms held to the front at shoulder level, being denied food and use of a lavatory for extended periods, culminating with concentrated questioning and verbal threats of future abuse could be considered torture, although any one of these activities by itself might not be severe enough to constitute torture per se'.

7 Six years after prisoners were first taken to Guantanamo, more than 500 of the 774 detainees had been released without charges and considered 'not an enemy combatant', after an average of three years in detention. It became self-evident that the main reason for the lack of success of the interrogations was that the people detained had nothing useful to say. As became well known years later, most of the detainees had been sold in Afghanistan to get the reward that the army offered for suspects (anywhere between 3,000 and 5,000 dollars).

8 http://en.wikipedia.org/wiki/SU.S.n_J._Crawford#Guantanamo_discussion.

9 Bob Woodward (14 January 2009). 'Detainee Tortured, Says US Official: Trial Overseer Cites "Abusive" Methods Against 9/11 Suspect.' *The Washington Post.* p. A01.

10 The log was analysed using Atlas.ti 6.0 software.

11 He suggests the application of the *totality of the circumstances* and *voluntariness test* in order to accept a self-incriminating statement given during an interrogation as valid evidence in Court. In the totality of circumstances test, the Court examines all of the factors surrounding a confession to independently determine its validity. The voluntariness test examines whether the defendant independently chose to confess. He dismisses the 'shock the conscience' standard that establishes that deception is inadmissible when it 'shocks the conscience' of the Court.

12 https://supreme.justia.com/cases/federal/us/318/350/.

15

THE PSYCHOLOGICAL MANIPULATION OF IDENTITY

'Brainwashing': the myth and reality of identity manipulation and its application in the definition of psychological torture

Brainwashing is a sensationalist, not scientific, term. Etymologically, it suggests being able to erase the contents of a person's mind and introduce new content that conforms to the will of the perpetrator. Medically speaking, this is impossible. However, the term has gained popularity because of its impact in the media and as a way of selling popular books (e.g Taylor, 2004). It has been said that the word was coined by an American journalist, Edward Hunter (1951), who studied 're-education' programs applied to American prisoners in North Korean concentration camps. Hunter claimed that 'brainwashing' is a translation of the Chinese phrase *his nao*, which was (according to his informants) how the Chinese referred to similar re-education programs. Lifton (1961) argues that this was soon applied by extension to the methods (purportedly) used by any communist country to indoctrinate its citizens, interrogate political dissidents and convert enemy spies into allies. The term gained popularity and was incorporated into jokes and folk psychology, and other media such as an educational film that dramatically portrayed the way a prisoner was treated in the USSR and the way he was 'brainwashed' to follow communism (see Chapter 10).

Persuasive coercion vs. coercive interrogation

Schein (1960) affirmed that, contrary to popular belief, Chinese indoctrination practices were completely unrelated to Soviet interrogation tactics. China developed a program to *shape* the population's perspective (especially dissidents) through changes in identity and worldviews using persuasion and collective pressure without resorting to physical violence. This included three stages: (1) Unfreezing: preparing the person for change by a process of reflection and self-criticism that lead to a rejection of 'past errors', distancing from the past, and preparation for the future. (2) Changing: The slow introduction of a new set of behaviours, thoughts and emotions, shared with the group and society. Creation of new routines and assimilation of the collective goals and the revolutionary mystique. (3) Refreezing: Providing new purpose in life and new activities that create a sense of fulfillment, rejecting the 'old' self and making a voluntary commitment to the new self (even changing one's name and residence). Subjects were also involved in spreading the word and reeducating other people.

This process of coercive persuasion is completely different from interrogation procedures of detainees in the USSR. Though neither coercive persuasion nor interrogation use direct physical violence (the detainee is not beaten or ill-treated), during Soviet interrogations detainees were isolated and subjected to an exhausting regime of repeated interrogations (combined with the manipulation of the environment, sensory exhaustion, sleep manipulation and the creation of a mixture of fear and emotional dependence with the interrogators).

These early texts divide what could be considered *techniques of persuasion* (more closely related to the folk concept of 'brainwashing' and the indoctrination of torturers, child soldiers, or that which occurs in destructive cults) from *techniques of coercive interrogation* (more closely related to the ideas of *breaking the self* and *torture* as we understand them today).

From a psychological point of view, these terms merge very different techniques and phenomena (which are not so different in their inner mechanisms) that have one thing in common: the subject suffers radical *changes of identity* (either by imposition or by persuasion). We will briefly review these terms and explore the connections between major identity change and contemporary torture.

Targeting identity

Identity is the idea one has of oneself and one's role in the world. Starting in childhood, it is built through a dialectic process between the subject and his or her environment rooted in daily experiences. Identity is created in a self-reflective, introspective process of awareness.

Identity is not who we are, but who we think we are. It is how we define ourselves. It includes individual identity (more developed in individualistic societies) and collective identity (when a person naturally incorporates a group in defining him or herself and cannot properly define him or herself without making reference to the group).

Therefore, identity is a diverse (and usually small) set of more or less accidental elements that a person thinks defines him or herself. Identity includes roles (mother, son, lover); professions (farmworker, anthropologist) and hobbies (body builder, painter); physical characteristics (tall, handsome, disfigured); traits or attributes (funny, loyal, insecure); beliefs and worldviews (left-wing, Muslim, vegetarian); collective identities (Kurd, Canadian, Roma); and groups to which one belongs (fan of a sports team, member of a violent gang), among other elements with which a person may identify.

This patchwork of elements constitutes a person's mental map – which is not a comprehensive definition, but rather a collection of snapshots of relevant elements that the person considers key to his or her understanding of who he or she is.

A person develops his or her identity in a process that combines two elements:

Unconscious processes. The person absorbs information about relevant aspects of him or herself from the way others treat and refer to him or her in different environments. Influence from family (parents, siblings or other caregivers) or primary groups (school, friends, etc.) is especially relevant.

Conscious processes. The subject develops a personal narrative in every environment in which he or she interacts with others. This narrative is based on introspective processes, thinking and making decisions about who he or she wants to be, what his or her ideal self is like, what he or she thinks is his or her actual self, and ways to change and improve.

During the very early years of life, initial interactions become the core foundation of identity: groups with which one identifies, one's cultural milieu, physical and psychological traits, and many other aspects of one's self are formed. Depending on the pattern of inter-action (attachment) and the way the key aspects of identity are (or are not) reinforced by relevant figures, the person can develop in one way or another. At one extreme are people with a rigid or strong sense of self, usually rooted in fixed, dogmatic concepts; at the other are people with fragile identities, who often have a confused, vulnerable self-image and feel ambivalence towards themselves and others. In the middle of these two extremes is a person with a balanced identity: he or she can, in normal conditions, maintain a positive self-image without abandoning critical thinking or distance toward negative aspects of him or herself or others.

Thus, identity is not an intrinsic attribute, but rather a dialectic process between the individual and the world (Goffman, 1959) which is slowly and constantly being confirmed and re-created. Identity depends on context. Although basic traits may be constant, in every milieu people observe themselves and react by adapting to particular environments by expressing themselves in different ways.

In sum, identity is the conscious or unconscious understanding that every person has of his or her own place in the world; it determines how one interacts in it, the meaning that one assigns to the groups to which one belongs and the multiple roles that one plays in each of those groups. Childhood and adolescence are key moments of identity development.

Elements and methods of identity modification

Instead of employing the folk concept of *'brainwashing'*, we can focus on the concept of *radical identity changes*. As we have seen, the creation of identity is a multifaceted process that includes many individual and contextual elements, all of which can be manipulated. Therefore, the possibilities of inducing a radical change of identity are almost infinite. We have classified the elements involved in 16 categories (see Figure 15.1) related to Context, Interaction, Cognitive Processes and Installation of the new identity. There are two main pathways to identity change (marked in the figure): isolation and collective pressure (which can occur simultaneously).

The 16 elements involved, to a greater or lesser extent, in situations of identity manipulation are:

1. **Isolation.** Cutting contact with others who might help the person have a different perspective and be aware of or question the changes; inducing forced integration into the new reality.
   - Isolation from human contact.
     - The external world is either dangerous, impure or evil, or part of a past that should be avoided (e.g. cults).
     - Contacting the outer world is forbidden and punished (e.g. trafficking)
     - Removing alternative sources of information. No access to books, newspapers, radio or the Internet. Only authorised sources of information are permitted.
     - Immersion in the new context.
2. **Fully-controlled environment.** Totalising institutions are those in which all elements of daily routines are planned, organised and controlled externally, allowing minimal space for a person to exercise his or her will. Over time the person adjusts to the environment and changes him or herself in order to fit within it. Prisons, long-term facilities

at psychiatric hospitals, geriatric residences or cloistered convents are examples of totalising institutions. The so-called 'institutionalisation syndrome' appears in people who have been in closed institutions for years: apathy, lack of will, apparent cognitive deterioration, emotional and affective numbness, and regressive and childish attitudes as a response to an environment that patronises people and overturns their identities. The difficulties of "deinstitutionalisation" show how deep these changes are and how difficult it is to recover past aspects of identity.

3. **Disorientation – being stunned.** The person may be blindfolded, handcuffed or otherwise restrained, and he or she may be locked in a closed space (e.g. room, cell, box, etc.). Any input that would allow for temporal or spatial orientation (e.g. sound) is blocked. The atmosphere (including noises, lighting, etc.) fosters confusion. Threats are vague and messages unclear. Disorientation and being stunned are methods often used in kidnapping, torture and trafficking.

4. **Fear / terror.** The person is under constant tension after witnessing the torture or death of others (e.g. in the case of child soldiers, torture victims); constant threats of death (e.g. situations involving kidnapping, torture of detained/disappeared persons, violent gangs); beatings/threats of extreme pain or disfigurement (e.g. trafficking, domestic abuse); threats of rejection (childhood sexual abuse); among other situations. Fear and terror can induce dissociated states in the victim to alleviate physical and psychological pain, or induce absolute submission in an attempt to appease the wrath of the perpetrator.

5. **Power imbalance.** The perpetrator controls all decisions, and the person subjected to this process is at his or her disposal. All aspects of the detainee's life (even the right to life itself) is under external control. The detainee is in a state of powerlessness, and even the smallest detail can be used as a source of pressure. This scenario may include:
    *   Exhibiting omniscience and omnipotence.
    *   Making absurd, arbitrary decisions that show who has the power.
    *   No command can be rescinded, wrong as it might be. Power and hierarchy are more relevant than the decision itself.
    *   Punishing any attempt of the victim to gain control, or feel power, even in minor actions (such as shifting positions, drinking water, etc.).
    *   Invading intimacy / boundary dissolution. The person is stripped naked, sexually humiliated or raped as the ultimate sign that the body of the victim belongs entirely to the perpetrator and nothing escapes from his or her power and will.
    *   The person feels helplessness, powerlessness and lack of control. He or she feels that the future is unpredictable.

    These elements of power imbalance appear during torture, kidnapping, and trafficking, as well as in concentration camps.

6. **Interpersonal manipulation.**
    *   Forced pseudo-choices (lose-lose dilemmas)
    *   Misleading or deceptive information
    *   Impossible choices leading to betrayal
    *   Role-playing (e.g. good cop/bad cop), then unexpectedly reversing the roles

7. **Manipulation of affective bonds. Fostering emotional dependence.** The person is pushed into the middle of a plethora of overwhelming emotions. Isolated and scared, the person is especially receptive to emotional messages that can alleviate anguish and despair.

- Manipulation of affect. The controller, kidnapper or torturer establishes a caring relationship with the victim in the midst of a horrific situation. Affective bonds can appear (and may even be sincere); the victim (and sometimes the captor) may feel deeply engaged.
- Sudden changes in mood and affect. Kindness may be combined with disapproval and rejection, fostering emotional dependence.
- The person has feelings of ambivalence towards the perpetrator. In abuse, the controller is a source of pain and care at the same time. Torturers (or controllers) and victims may voluntarily maintain the affective relationship even after kidnapping or torture ends.

8. **Group pressure.** Human beings have a strong need for belonging. When a person feels menaced, he or she resorts to the group. Creating a shared identity with others helps individuals feel protected and powerful. Part of the process of creating a group identity is defining the boundaries of the group (who belongs and who does not belong). Powerful and well-known ways of drawing this line include:

- Defining outsiders as enemies.
- Making it very difficult to be admitted and costly to leave.
- Involving all members in shared responsibilities (e.g. committing atrocities or sharing secrets).
- Reinforcing identity through rituals, songs and other symbolic practices; valuing loyalty highly.
- Pressing others to act according internal norms or rules.
- Punishing attitudes that go against the interest of the group, and reinforcing attitudes that strengthen the group.
- Introducing the idea of reciprocity: the person is indebted to the group because of everything the group has given him or her.
- Strong positive feedback when the person assumes risky attitudes or difficult compromises that are exemplary to others (though nothing is ever enough).
- Strong internal hierarchy based on attitude and involvement.
- Reinforcing the emotional impact of the group's rhetoric and the mythology of belonging: the group represents positive values and has power and influence, and by belonging one acquires these shared traits.
- Creating uniform lives: wearing the same clothing or other external symbols (tattoos, etc.), sharing common elements (music, food, etc.) or routines (praying or other activities). Creating a shared identity and a way to define the group.
- Effectiveness: the group attains goals which are impossible for a single individual to achieve.
- Diluting responsibility: the individual is not responsible because collective responsibility justifies individual behavior.
- Consistency: if the majority does something, it means that it is the right thing to do, even if individuals do not fully understand the action.

9. **Breaking with the past.** The person undergoes a process in which everything that was part of his or her previous life is questioned and considered problematic – it represents the past and what is wrong or evil. It is possible to enter a new age, but the person needs to detach him or herself from this past. They must try to reflect upon and detect internal remnants of the past in order to eliminate them and prepare to become part of the new era. This may also mean convincing, rejecting, avoiding or killing those

with differing ideas about the truth or the future, people who are still attached to the past. These attitudes and actions can appear in cults working with dissidents, in military training or as part of affiliation with extremist groups.

10. **Breaking assumptions and beliefs.**
    - Irreversibly changing one's perception of human beings
    - Challenging the belief in a benevolent, just world
    - Breaking ideas of trust and confidence in others
    - Questioning personal values and ideology
    - Questioning, distancing and doubting the people in one's social network and life, and their values

    Breaking assumptions and beliefs is part of the process of breaking identity in child soldiers, torture survivors, concentration camps and situations of human trafficking.

11. **Questioning basic values.**
    - The person's inner world and core moral ideas become confused. The person may ask him or herself, *what is the difference between right and wrong? Is evil relative?*
    - Past ideology and commitments are questioned as useless, childish or wrong.
    - Involving the person in wrongdoing provokes guilt, shame and the need run from one's past.

    Questioning basic values is associated with training torturers, as well as with domestic abuse and violent gangs.

12. **Self-conscious emotions: guilt and shame.** The person is involved in processes that instill deep feelings of guilt and shame. Guilt is associated with acts that are deemed immoral because they violate the person's internal values or norms:
    - Perpetrating cruel or atrocious acts against others to survive
    - Making decisions that deceive people who are important to him or her (their partner, relatives, children, figures they respect, etc.)
    - Doing shameful things (competing with other victims for, or depriving other victims of, food, clothes or shelter)
    - Cooperating with the perpetrator or having thanked them at some point, especially if it was in public
    - Accepting intimate relationships with the perpetrator

    Shame is linked to the introjection of humiliation and to breaking one's self-image (see Chapter 5). It can appear after:
    - Being publicly debased (naked, dirty, confused, weak, etc.)
    - Feral treatment; being treated as subhuman
    - Being teased or ridiculed in front of others (e.g. domestic abuse)

13. **Installing an identity.** Human beings are affected by others, especially those whom they trust or those who have special influence or power. This means that there are many ways in which one's identity can be altered, including:
    - Introduction of the new paradigm, new values and meanings; process of self-reflection and adjustment to the new expected behaviours.
    - Intensive 'critical' reflection (individual or group): readings, discussions groups, lectures, etc. (seen in situations involving cults, re-education, military training). Only one source of information is allowed.
    - Blocking and criticising all reflection by prioritising 'action'.
    - Surveillance and control of behaviours and attitudes by the leader or group; internal systems of control.

- Promoting public sharing of wrongdoings, confessions and publicly committing to the new goals or identity.
- Accomplishment of objectives; hidden or unexpected tests of loyalty.
- Adapting to please the other: being connected to a religious leader or a hierarchical superior may depend on talking, thinking and behaving in a similar way (even on the subtle level of body gestures or manner of dress).
- Rewarding positive outcomes and decisions in the 'proper' direction. The person receives love and affection when he or she thinks or acts according to the (expected) wishes of the figure of reference or the new ideology, and is ignored or punished when he or she does the opposite. For example, a very religious mother shows love and devotes extra time and interest to her son when he exhibits religious thoughts and attitudes, and she is distant when he does not. Or, a military leader may express confidence and friendship to a loyal torturer, and be distant or cruel when his inferior does not meet expectations.

In addition, the process of installing the new identity involves procedural elements:

- Involving the person in new and perhaps violent actions or activities as soon as possible to produce cognitive dissociation that will likely be resolved by adjusting his or her thoughts to justify actions.
- Making the person rush into certain actions. Prohibiting reflective thought, pushing forward in a frantic process in which there is no turning back.
- The person feels that they are in an unreal state in which he or she is not even fully aware of what he or she is doing (e.g. child soldiers, human trafficking).

These strategies for installing new identities are seen in situations such as cults and domestic abuse. Lifton (1961; 1987)[1] reviewed their use in processes of indoctrination in China.

14. **New self-serving adaptive worldviews.** The victim questions his or her previous worldview following the trauma of torture or abuse. He or she may develop a new attitude towards the world that is adaptive for survival and functional to the abuser.

- *Pragmatic view of self.* 'I am happy. Things are not so bad. I can say I am happy in spite of everything.' 'Ideology is stupid. Others are always using you.' 'Suffering is useless.' 'Surviving is the only rule. We'll see what happens later.'
- *Others as indifferent bystanders or as enemies.* 'Life is a jungle where only the strong survive. The weak or soft-hearted disappear.' 'No one cares.' 'Everybody uses me, I have the right to defend myself.' 'Everybody tries to take advantage of me. Trusting others only brings pain.'
- *The world as an evil place.* 'The world is unfair. It is better to take care of myself.'
- *The world is unsafe.* 'I need protection.' 'If I do not do anything wrong, everything will be all right.'
- *Reject control / accept destiny.* 'Life is uncontrollable. The wisest thing to do is to accept things as they are . . . do it the easy way, and try to be happy.' 'Acceptance leads to peace, calm, and joy.'

These changes may be permanent or temporary. When the rules change, there is a natural tendency to adapt. When the traumatic situation disappears, some of these adaptive worldviews might disappear and the person might even wonder how he or she could have seen the world that way. In his sociological studies, Martín-Baró (1990) described how people in El Salvador changed during wartime: how fear, demonisation of the enemy, and polarisation and distrust towards the state, media and others were the norm. He showed that this was an interactive process between the individual and society: both were changing. Society during wartime affected individuals, and the sum of individuals with these defensive worldviews produced a fragmented and polarised society. Thus, both individuals and society developed adaptive *war identities* in which they saw the enemy everywhere. Some of these collective and individual traits receded at the end of the war, but others lasted for generations. People adapt similarly to prison. Changes may be temporary, but if people are forced to maintain these changes over long periods of time, they can become permanent. Someone who has been in prison for years incorporates strong changes in the way he or she relates to other people and to the world, changes which may have been useful adaptations at the time, but remain long after they have served their purpose.

Examples of such situations include people who have experienced war, child soldiers and victims of domestic violence.

15. **New adaptive emotions.** The emotional world is reduced and adapts to the context. Emotions (both positive and negative) are dangerous. They make the person weak and vulnerable to others, and they make survival more difficult. Only certain emotions are allowed, while the rest must be suppressed. It seems best not to think too much, not to feel, to try to live in the new world on a day-by-day basis.

The person adapts to a new identity with:

- Lack of emotional responses, either because they are consciously suppressed or as side effects of the broken self and broken ideals and worldviews.
- Dissociative states, secondary to chronic trauma. The different selves play alternative roles with contradictory emotions and changes of mood and behavior.
- Emotional detachment, cynicism, lack of empathy towards others.
- A distrustful, defensive, and sometimes paranoid attitude.
- An unconsciously suicidal attitude. When the perpetrator makes demands, the victim responds by assuming risks and dangers without questioning.
- Nihilism.

This is an adaptive mechanism in torture survivors or child soldiers.

16. **Normalising the abnormal.** The person adapts to almost any environment, develops new routines, and assumes this is 'normal'. At the end of World War II, when the concentration camps of Auschwitz and Buchenwald were liberated, there were many accounts of what was called 'the anguish of liberation'. People who had survived in the camp for more than two years and had adapted to that life perceived liberation as a menace and feared its consequences. In another example, a patient who had been trafficked for three years was liberated by the police and sent to a protected, anonymous shelter where all her needs were met and where she received psychiatric attention. The patient, who was dissociative most of the time, renounced all assistance after one month. She voluntarily returned to the place where she was held and explained that wanted to reassume 'her job'. The harsh – but familiar and routine – conditions of her second identity were preferable to the anguish of trying to return to the person she was seven years prior.

These methods do not work as isolated procedures, but in combination. Table 15.1 maps the role these different mechanisms play in some instances of identity manipulation (grey cells indicate when a given mechanism is involved; cells marked '+' indicate a decisive mechanism).

TABLE 15.1 Attacks on identity: selected cases

	I	FC	D	FT	P	IM	ED	GP	BP	BA	QBV	GS	II	AW	NE	NA
Psy-TORTURE Breaking detainee and cooperation	+	+	+	+	+	+	+			+	+	+	+			+
Training a torturer								+		+			+	+		+
Genocide								+			+		+	+		+
Child sex	+	+	+		+	+	+									+
Child soldier				+	+					+	+	+	+		+	+
'Mara'/juvenile gang		+					+				+					+
Cult	+	+				+	+		+				+	+		
Stockholm syndrome	+	+	+	+	+											
Domestic abuse	+					+	+					+				
Trafficking	+	+		+	+				+	+					+	
Re-education of dissidents	+	+		+			+	+					+	+		
Military indoctrination					+		+						+			
Paramilitary groups							+					+				+
Prolonged imprisonment	+	+											+			
Concentration camp		+		+	+							+		+	+	+

[1] Isolation (I). [2] Full control (FC). [3] Disorientation (D). [4] Fear / Terror (FT). [5] Power imbalance (P). [6] Interpersonal manipulation (IM). [7] Emotional dependence (ED). [8] Group pressure (GP). [9] Breaking with the past (BP). [10] Breaking assumptions and beliefs (BA). [11] Questioning basic values (QBV). [12] Guilt / Shame (GS). [13] Installing an identity (II). [14] New self-serving adaptive worldviews (AW). [15] New adaptive emotions (NE). [16] Normalising the abnormal (NA).

Breaking down this analysis according to the main human rights violations involved in breaking or changing the identity of the victim, we find:

1. Normal citizens can **become torturers** by training them in a harsh, fully-controlled environment; keeping them under the influence of a strong leader who uses rewards and punishment; instilling basic ideas about ideology, purpose and the importance of their mission; subjecting them to strong group pressure; or making their own survival depend on adapting to the environment in which they must torture (Haritos-Fatouros, 2003; Scarry, 1985).

2. Even political activists can end up **cooperating with their torturers** if they are immersed in a fully-controlled environment with inhuman conditions in which every detail in their lives depends on the interrogator's decisions. Cooperation may occur after constant humiliation, debasement and weakening of the ego, or if victims are offered a chance to regain their humanity by siding with the winners. They may also end up cooperating if they are convinced of the supposedly humanitarian goals of their torturers, or of the possibility of saving their comrades by helping capture them. Small acts of betrayal or cooperation with torturers are magnified and revealed to other detainees so as to isolate the victim, break social bonds and support and instill the idea that there is no turning back (see the description of 'co-operators' in Mario Villani's testimony in Chapter 2, and the biographical memories of Marcia Alejandra Merino [1993] and Luz Arce [1993]).[2]

3. **Genocide** may result from a combination of several factors: pre-existing conditions that create a milieu (social inequalities, historical 'offenses'); social polarisation of groups seen as antagonistic (distrust, fear, ideological or racial extremism); justifications for violence (being the victim, claiming just motives for aggression, stereotyping the enemy as representing evil, annihilating the enemy as the solution to all problems); and group pressure (using symbols that provide social cohesion, a sense of belonging, and combat fear, or being involved in group violence and solving cognitive dissonance by justifying such violence) (Baum, 2008).

4. Teenagers can come to participate in **child pornography** or **prostitution** if they live in inhuman conditions in which receiving affection depends on complying with the wishes of the person who controls them. Compliance is rewarded with gifts or positive bonding. This installs a positive identity centred around an uncritical submission to the wishes of others. (Epstein, Schwartz and Schwartz, 2011).

5. Following abduction, the process of training **child soldiers** includes: creating extreme fear through the constant feeling of being near death, unpredictable behavior from the perpetrator, absurd ill-treatment, killing of other children or villagers, provoking grotesque behavior and omnipotence. This increases the likelihood that the child will attempt to manage the perpetrator's reactions through absolute compliance. Terror is instilled in the children through unpredictable outbursts of violence and capricious enforcement of rules, forcing the children to commit crimes or using them as sex slaves. The effect is to convince the child that both the perpetrator and the group *are* everywhere, *see* everything, can *do* whatever they want, and, ultimately, to force the child to join the group. Being the cruelest of the cruel is a way to feel powerful and safe (Wessells, 2009). Victims exhibit insolence, violence and even cruelty with people who are lower in the hierarchy, and absolute submission and annihilation of their own identity with people who are higher up in the hierarchy. The perpetrators force their victims to violate their basic moral rules and betray connections with relatives, friends and other humans. After being forced to see others being hurt, survival depends on dehumanising others and blocking any possible affection (Bandura, 1999).

6. Victims of **kidnapping** may develop strong positive feelings towards their captors (the so-called Stockholm syndrome) that may persist beyond release. This results from a combination of a perceived threat to their physical or psychological survival at the hands of the abuser(s), inescapability, perceived signs of kindnesses from the abuser to the victim and adopting the perpetrator's perspective as an unconscious survival strategy. People

identify with their aggressors, introject their values and adopt a position of regression by identifying with their captors as a helplessness child might accept an authoritative parent's decision (and ask for his or her protection). Cognitive dissonance is resolved by magnifying the virtues and legitimacy of the torturer, captor or kidnapper, and justifying siding with the captor by telling themselves that it is the only way to keep themselves safe (Cantor and Price, 2007).

7.   People may become members of a **destructive cult** as a result of psychological domination through isolation from the environment (family, friends); prohibiting contact with the outside world (news, organisations, groups); focalisation of attention (prayers, meetings, exhausting tasks and activities related to the cult, periods of 'meditation'); deceptive ideals and superior goals; involving others (especially sons and daughters) in the cult; creating confusion; enforcing strict rules; inducing guilt; making affection dependent on compliance; giving gifts and other actions to make victims feel special; intimate dependence (sometimes including sexual activities among members or with leaders); group rejection if norms are broken; creating an atmosphere of secrecy; sharing pieces of information among several people to create rumors and division; and instilling fear while simultaneously promoting the moral duty to express peace, joy and happiness to others.

8.   People subjected to **domestic abuse** are slowly pushed into a situation of debasement, humiliation and inferiority. Perpetrators convince them that they cannot make decisions because they always make mistakes. Psychological or physical ill-treatment is seen as a consequence of pervasive errors and inability to improve. Violence is normalised (the 'all husbands beat their wives' paradigm). Leaving the family group is not to be taken lightly, and circumstances may force children or women to accept subordinate status and abuse. The battered wife cannot resort to friends or relatives and is progressively isolated and forced to adopt the abuser's perspective. When she threatens to leave, the abuser may increase psychological pressure, or, alternatively, may apologise and promise to change. Once forgiveness is achieved, the cycle begins again. The process is cross-cut by feelings of guilt: guilt towards the perpetrator for not fulfilling his expectations, guilt towards the children for having to suffer violence and humiliation, guilt towards relatives or therapists who disapprove of the relationship and press for separation (or, alternatively, who pressure her to work things out), guilt before society and guilt for not being able to overcome all the fear and guilt, resolve her ambivalence, break free from the problems that trap her and make decisions.

9.   In **trafficking**, victims are offered a job and a future. Sometimes they are confined physically, but more often they become trapped via: (1) the payment of a huge debt for being transported from the country of origin to the country where they are trafficked; (2) documentation (passport) in the hands of the captor; (3) death threats to family in country of origin if the victim tries to escape; (4) magical claims regarding rituals and the power to psychologically manipulate a victim if they do not obey (seen in some cases involving victims from Nigeria and other African countries). A trafficked woman may slowly be involved in prostitution by at first having to control other women, and later being forced to 'service' a client. Alternatively, she may be violently gang-raped and abused for several days until she is helpless and frightened to death; this creates such terror that she may see obeying orders and accepting prostitution as the only way to avoid future torture. In trafficking, the women require some freedom to see

clients, so they must be coerced and subjugated to create a parallel self that can work in prostitution 24 hours a day as an automaton, often in an almost dissociative state (Hopper and Hidalgo, 2006). This is exacerbated by physical exhaustion and confusion due to working night shifts and long hours in clubs or other spaces with constant artificial light. Ultimately, over time (sometimes over the course of several years), the person gets used to sex as an automaton, without any emotional involvement. Running away is too risky and difficult to even be considered. The woman accepts having a passive attitude, being treated as an object, complying with external instructions and being malleable to any demands, and suffers an impaired ability to act or decide autonomously. Victims are obliged to accept a distorted sense of reality, one in which the exploitation and control of women is naturalised. Once the captor relies on the slave, a paternalistic relationship evolves in which the trafficker is a source of safety and kindness and even affection. A victim may declare to the police that she was voluntarily working for the network, and it may take a long process of therapy to uncover the truth.

Figure 15.1 shows some of the key aspects that repeatedly appear in cases of identity change linked to trauma: *isolation, power imbalance, questioning basic values* and *normalising the abnormal*. Also frequent are *total control, interpersonal manipulation, fear, group pressure, breaking assumptions and beliefs, guilt and shame* and *installation of a new ideology*. In specific situations we also find *disorientation, emotional dependence, breaking with the past* and *new adaptive worldviews and emotions*.

Process vs. crisis, modification vs. substitution

Progressive changes. Changes in identity can occur rapidly. Some experiences that entail overwhelming emotions can induce a 'transformation' within the person (usually someone who already has a weak or confused identity) causing him or her to vehemently embrace new ideas in a very short time. Though this scenario is possible, it is uncommon. More often, the process is slow and gradual, and may take months or even years. The process of becoming a member of a cult or a torturer requires time and certain predisposing conditions (conditions that experimental social psychology has studied since the Milgram and Stanford experiments).

Identity modification and identity substitution: structural dissociation. In all of these processes, the identity is not substituted, but rather displaced and changed. It is not possible to erase an identity, only to induce changes that make the person more compliant. However, there are some exceptions: under extraordinary circumstances (especially in children under four years of age and very vulnerable adults), it is possible to induce multiple dissociated personalities, and that one or more of these personalities are fully compliant (Lacter, 2011). This is achieved through a process of inducing multiple, unbearable traumas in the person, which are impossible to understand or assimilate by an immature identity. The only way to deal with them is to split and create a dissociated self. For instance, children who have been recruited by paramilitary groups are involved in, and witness to, atrocities from a very young age. They see other children being killed or tortured or have to do it themselves, and they are sexually abused, beaten or suffer hunger or strenuous physical exertion. Sometimes they are forced to kill their own relatives to show compliance and loyalty. This reality is impossible to process, and the person develops

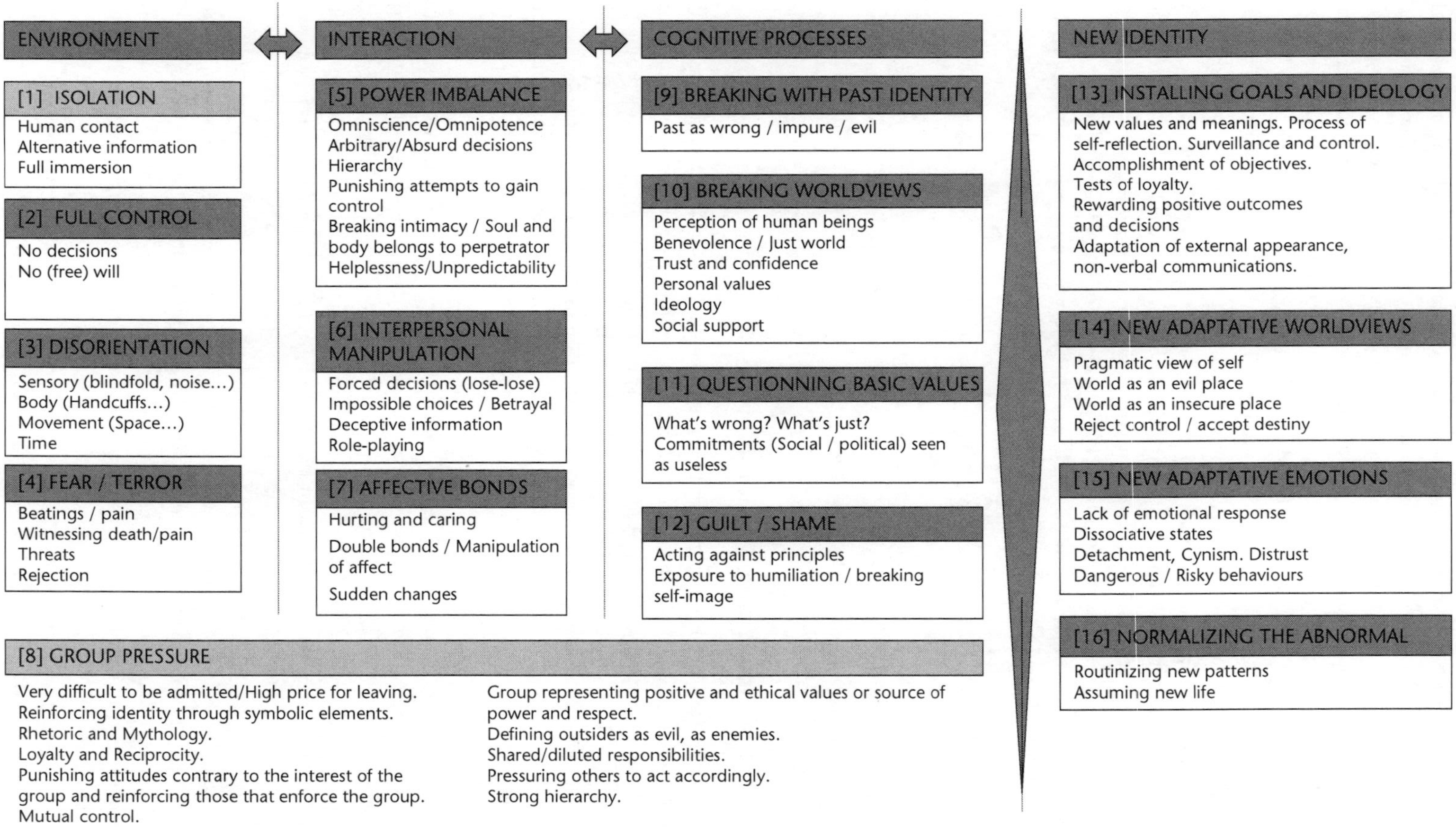

ENVIRONMENT

[1] ISOLATION
Human contact
Alternative information
Full immersion

[2] FULL CONTROL
No decisions
No (free) will

[3] DISORIENTATION
Sensory (blindfold, noise...)
Body (Handcuffs...)
Movement (Space...)
Time

[4] FEAR / TERROR
Beatings / pain
Witnessing death/pain
Threats
Rejection

[8] GROUP PRESSURE
Very difficult to be admitted/High price for leaving.
Reinforcing identity through symbolic elements.
Rhetoric and Mythology.
Loyalty and Reciprocity.
Punishing attitudes contrary to the interest of the
group and reinforcing those that enforce the group.
Mutual control.

INTERACTION

[5] POWER IMBALANCE
Omniscience/Omnipotence
Arbitrary/Absurd decisions
Hierarchy
Punishing attempts to gain
control
Breaking intimacy / Soul and
body belongs to perpetrator
Helplessness/Unpredictability

[6] INTERPERSONAL MANIPULATION
Forced decisions (lose-lose)
Impossible choices / Betrayal
Deceptive information
Role-playing

[7] AFFECTIVE BONDS
Hurting and caring
Double bonds / Manipulation
of affect
Sudden changes

Group representing positive and ethical values or source of
power and respect.
Defining outsiders as evil, as enemies.
Shared/diluted responsibilities.
Pressuring others to act accordingly.
Strong hierarchy.

COGNITIVE PROCESSES

[9] BREAKING WITH PAST IDENTITY
Past as wrong / impure / evil

[10] BREAKING WORLDVIEWS
Perception of human beings
Benevolence / Just world
Trust and confidence
Personal values
Ideology
Social support

[11] QUESTIONNING BASIC VALUES
What's wrong? What's just?
Commitments (Social / political) seen
as useless

[12] GUILT / SHAME
Acting against principles
Exposure to humiliation / breaking
self-image

NEW IDENTITY

[13] INSTALLING GOALS AND IDEOLOGY
New values and meanings. Process of
self-reflection. Surveillance and control.
Accomplishment of objectives.
Tests of loyalty.
Rewarding positive outcomes
and decisions
Adaptation of external appearance,
non-verbal communications.

[14] NEW ADAPTATIVE WORLDVIEWS
Pragmatic view of self
World as an evil place
World as an insecure place
Reject control / accept destiny

[15] NEW ADAPTATIVE EMOTIONS
Lack of emotional response
Dissociative states
Detachment, Cynism. Distrust
Dangerous / Risky behaviours

[16] NORMALIZING THE ABNORMAL
Routinizing new patterns
Assuming new life

FIGURE 15.1 Identity changes linked to trauma.

different selves (one might be fragile, childish and frightened, the other cruel and sadistic, or numb and cold). This is not 'brainwashing', because the old self is still there. Instead, multiples identities are created. If the child is so young that their self-conscious identity has not yet formed, the fragmented and submissive/sadistic self might be the only apparent one.

Notes

1 Lifton listed eight components of creating a totalitarian ideology: '*Milieu control* (control of an individual's communication with the external world, hence of his or her perceptions of reality); *Mystical manipulation* (evoking certain patterns of behavior and emotion in such a way that they seem to be spontaneous); *The demand for purity* (the belief that elements outside the chosen group should be eliminated to prevent them contaminating the minds of group members); *The cult of confession* (the use of and insistence on confession to minimise individual privacy); *Sacred science* (viewing the ideology's basic dogmas as both morally unchallengeable and scientifically exact, thus increasing their apparent authority); *Loading the language* (compressing complex ideas into brief, definitive-sounding phrases, or "thought-terminating clichés"); *The primacy of doctrine over person* (the idea that a dogma is more true and more real than anything experienced by an individual human being); *The dispensing of existence.*'

2 Merino and Arce were left-wing activists who were tortured and became collaborators of the intelligence service of the Pinochet dictatorship for nearly 15 years. These books describe the ambivalent and complex relationship that they had with their torturer, Coronel Krasnoff Marchenko. Merino, for instance, describes how over time she began to see her torturer as handsome, and how the situation of deprivation and fear combined with small indulgences (a cigarette, some chocolate or a more comfortable cell) undermined her psychological resistance early on. With time she was released and allowed to live on her own, and she kept working for the DINA as a paid contractor. She couldn't imagine the possibility of breaking the relationship of dependence with the torturer. Years later, she was surprised to find that Krasnoff Marchenko was short, ugly and spoke awkwardly, and she couldn't understand how she had ever admired or been seduced by him.

16

TECHNOLOGICAL RESEARCH AND PSYCHOLOGICAL TORTURE

One of the central problems facing interrogators during coercive interrogations is that they are confronted with too many doubts. They must decide in a short period time who is a 'high value' or 'low value' detainee, usually with only limited information about the detainees. As we saw in Chapter 10, the old French school of torture would enclose an entire area or village and torture people one by one until someone helped build an initial list of 'suspects'. This approach was also used in British colonies and Vietnam. After 9/11, US intelligence services paid local people to turn in 'terrorists', who were then sent to Guantanamo.[1] Over time, the majority of those detained were shown to be innocent.

An initial screening process classifies people willing to cooperate and people who resist, people who potentially have information and those who do not. The screening process is not without risk. The interrogator may be faced with a person who remains silent or provides nonsensical information in spite of being subjected to physical or psychological suffering. Is this person a resilient combatant or an innocent farmworker? In Guatemala and other Latin American countries, their armies' intelligence services followed the French model and responded to this problem by torturing and killing everyone detained – combatants or not, there would be no 'errors'. It is possible to create hell on earth: a place where large numbers of people are held captive without knowing whether they are actually involved in the events under investigation, where teams are overburdened with unnecessary harsh interrogations and do not know when to stop a 'procedure', or even to what extent they can truly say that someone is guilty or innocent.

The last 20 years have seen the emergence of biomedical research on biological markers sensitive to interrogation procedures. These procedures imagine a future in which a group of suspects could be subjected to a series of verbal or sensory stimuli associated with the events under investigation, and then screened and classified according to their involuntary bodily responses. In this scenario, interviewers could monitor via computers how successive queries impact the involuntary bodily reaction of the subject, and identify when the interrogator touches upon relevant information. In an ideal world, this would make torture unnecessary. In the real world, this would supposedly result in a better selection of whom to interrogate (the procedure does not provide 'answers') and whom to torture, if 'necessary', and thus involves entering into complex ethical terrain. We will briefly summarise the technical and ethical challenges presented by technological advances in this chapter.

Monitoring interrogations with the aid of technology

There have many unsuccessful attempts to detect involuntary signs of deception and lies and develop interviews that help assess the credibility of the accused or of witnesses. In practice, very few techniques actually work (Porter and Brinke, 2010) – not even coercive and deceptive interrogation techniques (Kassin, 2009).

Classical texts on interrogation devoted ample space to the polygraph as an aid in obtaining information from a resistant person. The polygraph was once called the 'machine of truth'. It was announced as a device that could reliably measure the psychophysiological responses of a person during interrogation, distinguishing truth from lies. Different reviews have concluded that the percentage of success in detecting deceit is close to 50 per cent (Lewis and Cuppari, 2009) and very few courts in the world accept it as evidence in tribunals.

However, medical science, neuroimaging and recording of the brain's electrical activity has developed remarkably over the last 30 years, and now offers possibilities that were previously unthinkable. Currently, much civil and military research is dedicated to finding alternatives to the polygraph. Table 16.1, summarised from Heckman, Mark and Ballo (2005), shows some of these investigations. An official report by the National Research Council (2009) concluded that because of challenges which remain, these technologies are not to be used in the immediate future; nonetheless, there is evidence of their use (Marks, 2007).

TABLE 16.1 Technological detection of deception: potential uses and current shortcomings

Device	Psychophysiological basis	Detection of lies or deception	Shortcomings
	Psychophysiological measures		
Electrogastrogram (EGG)	Electrodes uniquely sensitive to mental stress are placed on the surface of the abdomen and measure electrical waves or pulses.	Significant decrease in the percentage of normal gastric slow waves when the subject lies associated with significant increase of heart rate.	CBS RAT
Radial Vital Signs Monitor (RVSM)	Remotely measures psychophysiological motion processes (heartbeat, breathing, blinking) using electromagnetic waves.	It is non-invasive, portable and remote. This means that it can be used without the subject being aware of it. Too sensitive to body movements of the subject.	CBS ARF
Monitoring Facial Expressions	Non-intrusive ongoing automatic facial expression recognition system. It detects micro-facial expressions. Handles non-frontal poses and moderate head movements.	It classifies the expressions of the suspect into seven basic emotions: happiness, sadness, surprise, disgust, fear, anger and neutral. It is non-invasive, remote (subject not aware) and works in real time. It only requires a video recording and a portable computer.	Basic emotions are not synonyms of truth or lies. Difficult interpretation.

(continued)

TABLE 16.1 Technological detection of deception: potential uses and current shortcomings (*continued*)

Device	Psychophysiological basis	Detection of lies or deception	Shortcomings
Psychophysiological measures			
Measuring Ocular Movements (Blinking, Saccades and Fixation)	Subject's blinking patterns distinguish between relevant and irrelevant images showed to them. Similar to measuring saccades.	The type of movement is irrelevant, but an increase in time the eye remains fixed after hearing the question ('thinking time') correlates low to moderately with deception.	RAT CBS UNS
		Non-invasive, remote (subject not aware). Currently does not work in real time.	
Voice Stress Analysis (VSA)	Detects trembling in the subject's voice under stress.	Commercialised as a lie detector, it was discarded by the US Army as a non-reliable measure.	UNS
Thermal Imaging	Detects changes in microcirculation in the body (especially the face). Radiometric infrared cameras can detect in vivo real-time images of thermal changes in the body.	Real-time automated non-invasive recoding. Only requires a thermal camera and a computer. Can record images for later analysis.	
		Analysis unclear. Can detect sweating, embarrassment and other psychophysiological responses with thermal implications. The US Army has a classified line of research using this technology.	
Neurological mechanisms			
Electro-encephalography (EEG)	Measures changes in the electric potential of an electric field by means of electrodes placed on the surface of the scalp. Detects specific waves called event-related potentials.	Small, portable equipment. The results are promising but still unspecific. There are several different lines of research.	CBS UNS
Magneto-encephalography (MEG)	Distance recording of magnetic fields on the surface of the scalp associated with brain activity. Frequently used in studies on memory.	Preliminary data show that familiar and novel stimulus generate different patterns of brain activation. It is non-invasive.	RAT ARF

Device	Psychophysiological basis	Detection of lies or deception	Shortcomings
	Neurological mechanisms		
Positron Emission Tomography (PET)	A radiolabeled positron is injected into the person. The PET scanner can detect radioactivity and produces a three-dimensional image of functional brain activity.	Preliminary results show that deceit may be associated with activation of the anterior cingulate cortex. Very invasive and non-portable. Clear ethical impediments.	RAT UNS ETH
Functional Magnetic Resonance Imaging (fMRI)	The fMRI produces strong magnetic fields that are echoed differently by oxygenated and deoxygenated hemoglobin. It can form a dynamic sequence of images of the brain indicating areas in which there is an increase in neural activity in real time.	Results are unclear and depend on the experiment's design. Preliminary results suggest higher brain activation associated with lying. Invasive; requires sophisticated and very expensive equipment. Occasional secondary effects.	RAT UNS ETH
Functional Near-Infrared-Spectroscopy (fNIRS)	Measures changes in the concentration of deoxygenated and oxygenated hemoglobin during functional brain activity on the surface of the brain. It only allows exploring activity in the cortex.	Preliminary results suggest that levels of hemoglobin oxygenation are higher during a 'lie' task, coincident with fMRI studies. The results are promising but still unspecific. Different lines of research continue. Minimally invasive, inexpensive and portable device.	UNS
Transcranial Magnetic Stimulation (TMS)	A coil on the surface of the scalp produces a high-intensity magnetic field during microseconds, which interrupts normal functioning. It can excite and inhibit specific cortical areas, allowing the elucidation of causal relationships between external stimulus (including cognitions and behavior) and brain activity.	Preliminary results suggest increased cortical activity during deception. The results are promising but still unspecific. Different lines of research continue. Non-invasive, portable device. Occasional secondary effects (headaches). Requires technical expertise to interpret the results.	UNS

RAT. Requires advanced technology and equipment. Hospital device. ARF: Artifacts. Contaminated by other sources of body signals (e.g. movement). CBS: Contaminated by other sources of stress. False positives. UNS: Unspecific. No clear association with lie detection. ETH: Unacceptable ethical implications.

Adapted from Heckman, K. E., Mark, H. D. and Ballo, J. R. (2005).

Functional magnetic resonance imaging (fMRI)

Functional magnetic resonance imaging (fMRI) produces a dynamic sequence of images of the brain indicating areas in which there is an increase in neural activity in real time, by creating strong magnetic fields that are echoed differently by oxygenated and deoxygenated hemoglobin. When the person is confronted with a series of statements or with a narration of events, the device highlights different areas of the brain that become activated. This, in turn, is associated with a higher probability of either true or false statements.

An early review by Heckman et al. (2005) found that fMRI was a useful technology for experimental purposes, but unreliable, expensive and unpractical in real life. Since then, further arguments have emerged which discourage its use:

- **Images are not objective, hard measurements.** In a recent review, Marks (2010) showed that fMRi images are the product of human decisions about scanning parameters and extremely subjective criteria for deciding the level of statistical significance in comparing (1) the parameters with control groups together with (2) subjective acts of interpretation and representation of the images. The review showed that the results often represent the pre-conceptions of the researchers.
- **Group versus individual.** There are important differences among studies regarding the exact areas of the brain potentially involved in deception and lies (Luber et al., 2009). In general, and across studies, these areas do not reach 70 per cent specificity (Monteleone et al., 2009). In other words, they can be activated by many potential factors unrelated to deception. Additionally, when we focus on the analysis of individual cases, there is great variability among subjects (Luber et al., 2009). The predictive capacity for individual cases is, thus, clearly insufficient to support a conclusion with certainty.
- **Countermeasures.** In a recent fMRI study (Ganis et al., 2011) participants were trained to use countermeasures such as slightly moving their fingers or toes immediately after answering, without being noticed by the researchers. Among subjects trained in these countermeasures, deception detection accuracy decreased from 100 to 33 per cent.
- **Deception is a complex cognitive act.** Lying in an experiment while following instructions from a researcher is not comparable to being in a real situation in which there are many emotional and cognitive process involved in deciding whether or not to deceive the interrogator (Sip et al. 2008). Experimental studies do not take into account the most important issue in real-life situations: the reason why the person tries to hide the information, and the context in which the process takes place. In real life there is a deliberative process that involves five elements: (1) managing information that one has provided during the interrogation to avoid contradiction; (2) predicting the amount of information that the opponent has, and their degree of certainty; (3) guessing how the interrogator would feel, think and react if he or she knew about the deception; (4) handling nonverbal signs, showing or hiding empathy and building trust with the interrogator, and changing one's attitude according to the opponent's body language; and (5) conducting a risk analysis of when the benefits of deception exceed the risk of being caught, and looking for an alternative strategy if things do not go well.

This cognitive and emotional process is far from the typical experimental design, in which subjects are taught to lie about whether or not a certain date (like their birthday) is known to them. There are some early studies in natural environments. For instance, in one experimental paradigm, the subject tries to summarise a text in front of an audience, and tries to trick them. He or she is rewarded by his or her level of success. Such studies indicate that there are other areas of the brain related to the limbic system and the system of emotions involved in deception, and that the analysis of real-life data is far more complex and unreliable that what lab designs suggest (Hakun et al., 2009).

- **What exactly does fMRI tell us?** The test, in its standard form, tells us if a person actually recognises a stimulus presented to him or her (a word, an object, a picture, etc.) in spite of what he or she says. The conclusion does not tell us whether the person is lying, because different witnesses confronted with the same situation will always remember different things. The most we can conclude is that, for instance, a person claims that he or she was not in contact with a stimulus, while the fMRI tells us that he or she was (Sip et al., 2008). There may be dozens of explanations for such an outcome, and obviously the machine cannot distinguish among them. The fMRI can only detect objective facts (the person saw this before), not subjective states (the person wants to lie).
- **Quality of research.** Much of the relevant research has not been published in peer-reviewed journals. It has been produced and financed by interested scientists connected with companies that are already selling this technology as a brain-reading machine, such as CEPHOS or No Lie MRI (Schauer, 2010).

fMRI technology currently in use

Law enforcement procedures

In law enforcement processes, some authors believe it is unimportant that the information provided by fMRI is not 100 per cent reliable. A judge would not expect perfect reliability, and may see the fMRI as an aid in gaining an overview of the credibility of the suspect or the witness; he or she may feel that when combined with other evidence, the fMRI helps make better decisions. The danger is that it is difficult for a judge or jury to avoid succumbing to the supposed veracity of a series of pictures of the human brain of a detainee, especially when a forensic expert claims that the colors moving in real time prove that the accused is lying (Schauer, 2010).

Interrogation of suspects

The US Army, through the Defense Advanced Research Projects Agency (DARPA), part of the Department of Defense (DoD), has financed basic research on the use of fMRI in interrogation since 2004[2] and is currently financing research on portable fMRI devices as well as innovative methods of distance nuclear magnetic resonance using QORS (Quantum Orbital Resonance Spectroscopy). In the near future, the army expects to have portable and non-invasive devices that can be deployed in areas of conflict as an aid to interrogators (Albu and Grier, 2010).[3] There are different lines of research regarding remote neural monitoring and imaging using wireless near-infrared technology. According to Jonathan Marks (2007), a human rights bioethicist, the US Army has already used fMRI in Iraq. Citing first-hand declassified information, he writes that suspects were exposed to certain trigger words (like 'SEMTEX', the name of a common explosive used in many countries for civil and military purposes) while having their brain scanned at the same time. The device helped classify suspects into different degrees of 'suspiciousness', according to their reaction to the word. This is one clear example of how fMRI was not employed to prevent torture, but rather to select subjects for more 'intensive' interrogations.[4]

Brain Fingerprinting: event-related potentials (EEG–ERP)

The second technology already in use is event-related potentials, marketed as Brain Fingerprinting by the first company to commercialise the method. Reports suggest an 86 per cent success rate with the Guilty Knowledge Test (GKT) using event-related EEG-evoked potentials measuring the P300 wave (Abootalebi, Moradi and Khalilzadeh, 2009). In the Guilty Knowledge Test, the subject is asked many multiple choice about the details of the crime (e.g. 'Which was the murder weapon: (a) the hunting knife, (b) the baseball bat, (c) the rifle, or (d) the pistol?'). There is only one correct choice (called 'the proof'), and when it is mentioned to the guilty subject (who denies the correct choice), the largest physiological response is expected in comparison with their responses to the other choices (called 'the irrelevants'). Initial studies showed that the test was sensitive to measures of dissimulation (Rosenfeld et al., 2004). New protocols showed ways to overcome these countermeasures (Labkovsky and Rosenfeld, 2012) and, according to authors, even detect when the suspect is trying to deceive the machine by using a new index, reaction time (RT). ERP does not require the subject to answer questions; he or she merely reacts to the *recognition* of stimulus. While fMRI supposedly shows cortical areas activated by true versus deceptive answers, ERP shows an increased P300 wave when the person is exposed to stimuli (visual, auditive or other) with which they he or she has had previous contact.

Brain Electrical Oscillation Signature testing (BEOS), a variant of ERP, is already in use in forensic proceedings in India.[5] In 2008, a court accepted a BEOS test as proof for convicting a suspect accused of murdering her fiancé with arsenic[6] (Church, 2012). During the test (which she accepted voluntarily), she heard a description of the supposed acts in first person, involving her as the main person responsible. According to the expert (who had links to the seller of the device) the BEOS showed that she 'already knew' about the 'acts' she was hearing (Giridharadas, 2008). This could mean that she remembered being there, or that she simply remembered having heard the same story from another person before. But the experts (from a private company) considered that the first option 'was the most likely'. The sentence was strongly criticised,[7] especially in the scientific community. There have been at least two other similar cases in India, and currently Israel, Singapore and Spain are among the countries that are also considering permitting these types of tests in law enforcement processes (Church, 2012).

There are two main objections to this new technology:

1. The device only detects that the brain had 'previous contact' and that it reacts to a certain stimulus. This does not prove much regarding the memory or how it was formed. Marks (2007) explained that as an Irish resident, he heard often heard talk on the news about SEMEX, an explosive used by the Irish Republican Army (IRA). If his brain was scanned, he would have been classified as a potential terrorist.
2. There is an increased risk of a false positive result in people who have experienced torture or who suffer from PTSD. Neuroimaging studies show that torture victims present changes in areas of the brain near areas deemed significant in the lie detection test (Mirzaei et al., 2001). Paradoxically, people who have been captured in stressful circumstances and interrogated using traumatic techniques can easily produce a misleading result that would seemingly 'confirm' that they are lying, and that they deserve further interrogation.

Use of drugs

Drugs such as sodium pentothal, sodium amytal, and scopolamine have been used since World War II to encourage detainees to cooperate against their will during interrogation. As reviewed in Chapter 10, MK Ultra tested the use of LSD and other psychotropic drugs for interrogative purposes.

Keller (2005) reviewed the legal framework of 'truth serums' and if their use qualifies as torture. She found that – according to case law – the compulsory injection of truth serum *per se* would not be considered torture because the pain inflicted by an injection is minimal, whereas the *threat* of using truth serum would be considered torture because it could create high levels of anxiety that may be considered mental suffering. She disagreed with this illogical reasoning and pointed out the lack of clear legislation.

The Istanbul Protocol mentions the use of drugs as a separate category of torture techniques. Principle 21 of the *Body of Principles for the Protection of All Persons under Any Form of Detention or Imprisonment* forbids the use of 'methods of interrogation which impair the capacity of decision or judgment'. Additionally, the participation of doctors in administering drugs violates the World Medical Association's ban on cooperation with interrogation processes. In some cases, the use of drugs may infringe on the International Chemical Weapons Conventions, which outlaws 'any chemical that can cause death, temporary incapacitation, or permanent harm to humans or animals" (Organisation for the Prohibition of Chemical Weapons, 1997).

Oxytocin and the new 'truth serums'

Classical 'truth serums' are drugs that make the person feel happier and more talkative, with a variable degree of amnesia following the interrogation. They do not guarantee that the information provided has any connection to the 'truth'. A new generation of studies have recently focused on the use of different hormones and neuropeptides – and specially oxytocin – that increase emotions of empathy and closeness (Macdonald and Macdonald, 2010). Oxytocin is a hormone produced in the human brain that helps to create bonds among humans. It is involved in mother–child interactions and in fostering social relationships. Preliminary data show that after its use, the person feels closer to and friendlier towards others, with a greater tendency to be influenced by and acknowledge others' opinions.[8] This would make oxytocin the ideal interrogation drug. It would substitute pain with positive emotions. Instead of a good cop/bad cop schema, only the good cop would be necessary.

From a technical point of view, its use might in fact be more complex than it first appears:

1. It is unclear whether oxytocin increases empathy or increases *awareness of others' emotions* (both good and bad). In a study, intranasal oxytocin was compared to an intranasal placebo in a random sample of major depressive patients (Cardoso and Ellenbogen, 2013). The protocol demanded that experimenter be 'neutral' and not show special concern or empathy towards the patient. This provoked an important increase in anxiety responses in the depressed group, which was more sensitive to this 'neutral' attitude from the interviewer. Thus, oxytocin seems to be an interactive drug, or at least appears to have a non-linear, contextual-dependent effect on subjects.

2. In a study on oxytocin and trauma, an international group of researchers compared the willingness to share traumatic events in a sample of volunteers, randomised to intranasal oxytocin and placebo (Lane et al., 2013). The results showed that oxytocin did not make

people more 'talkative', but rather more willing to 'connect' and 'share' the traumatic event. There were no differences in 'the facts'; when using oxytocin, no additional details were added. Oxytocin made people more willing to share the *emotions* experienced during the traumatic events and the emotions experienced during the interview.

It is not clear that oxytocin will work for every detainee or that it would be useful in obtaining more information during an interrogation. It would probably allow the interrogator to conduct an interview more centred on emotions than facts. In the long term, it would likely facilitate the emotional manipulation of the subject by the interrogator. However, if the subject has strong negative feelings towards the interrogator, it is possible that these feelings would be increased, impeding emotional manipulation.

In addition to clarifying oxytocin's effects, available research also mentions the existence of other methods of taking the hormone that are less obvious than intranasal methods like drops or sprays. Studies also seek to further define the contextual factors that influence results.

Ethical concerns related to new technologies

We are entering an era of biometrics which poses unprecedented legal and ethical challenges. Authorities can measure a detainee's fingerprints and irises, take nonconsensual DNA samples using saliva or hair, or spray a detainee with oxytocin to facilitate interrogation.

Consent issues

Currently, it is not possible to measure psychophysiological or brain activity in a way that provides true insights on a person's thoughts. But science is rapidly advancing towards developing non-invasive devices that will be able to measure external correlates of brain activity without the subject being aware of it, much less giving consent. Thermographic cameras and functional near-infrared spectroscopy (fNIRS) are just the beginning.

Should these technical developments be considered illegal methods of coercion? If we take coercion to mean forcing someone to do something against his or her will, it is unclear how these new methods for discovering the 'truth' fit that definition.

The contemporary definition torture (in the UNCAT) requires severe suffering to take place. In theory, mechanical recording of brain activity is not torture. If we allow police officers to take photographs or record video of a detainee, why not a thermal video recording? However, this simplistic reasoning does not take into consideration *the basic right of every detainee not to make incriminating declarations against him or herself*, a provision accepted in the vast majority of countries. And this is what interrogation (and in some cases torture) is all about: extracting information from an unwilling and uncooperative source.

Some argue that with the use of new technologies, painful methods will no longer be necessary. But this is not true at present. Many of these ethical and legal concerns were addressed when the first polygraphs appeared. At that time, it seemed that forensic work would never be the same. One clear, crucial difference between then and now is that polygraphs could not be used in a covert manner, and most of these new devices can.

This is an important new legal debate among judges, law enforcement agents and civil and human rights defenders, and a new ethical challenge for the medical profession. It requires our urgent attention. Used with legal provisions and adequate civil rights protections, it may be a useful aid for innocent suspects.

The debate focuses on whether an fMRI is physical evidence (like a blood or DNA test), or a signal of human thoughts. In DNA testing, a judge can order a compulsory extraction of blood or saliva. But there is no legislation regarding access to human thoughts (Luber et al., 2009). Can the same legal principles used to justify violating intimacy in strip searches be used for thought searches? The rights of the detainee would also be infringed if neuroimaging is considered a form of detecting and interpreting *communication*. Can the same legal principles applied to opening and censoring the mail of a prisoner be used for thought interception?

Privacy

In an analysis based more on science fiction than truth, Kerr et al. (2008) discussed the potential of unwanted intrusions in human minds through remote, surreptitious brain surveillance. They call this subject *Brain Privacy*. They compare the detection of brain waves with the detection of thermic changes used by police to detect people moving inside a house, and the contradictory sentences regarding whether brain surveillance technologies violate the legal right to privacy. They also compare this kind of surveillance with the use of body scan devices in airports. They coincide with Luber et al. (2009) and others in proposing the use of these image procedures under an *informed consent protocol*, in which the person accepts potential health hazards associated with the test, and authorises the invasion of privacy it can entail. The consent would also cover the delicate issue of the legal right not to incriminate oneself. Procuring consent is unlikely to occur within a torturing environment.

International conventions

Thompson (2005) has convincingly shown that the involuntary use of fMRI and similar devices in foreign detainees (i.e. people detained in third countries) would violate the anti-coercion provisions of the Geneva Conventions,[9] and would likely be illegal under International Human Rights Law[10] and the US Constitution. He distinguishes two scenarios:

The first involves neuroimaging as a tool to detect deception. In his view, this does not violate any right of the detainee. During an interview, interrogators can try to detect deception by any means (intuition, facial movements, changes in voice or semantic analysis of speech). This is done to the best of his or her ability, and is part of the process between two people on opposite sides of a voluntary conversation. Thompson believes that using a neuroimaging device is simply a more accurate way to do this, which does not undermine the rights of the detainee. The second scenario is when neuroimaging and neurophysiological tests are used to extract information from the mind of the subject against his or her will. This exposes the person to a series of stimuli that might reveal intimate aspects of his or her life, memories and wishes without his or her consent. In other words, it involves the forced extraction of cognitive contents related to self and identity.

US Army Training Manual FM 34-52 defines coercion as 'actions designed to unlawfully induce another to compel an act against one's will (. . .). *Coercion revolve[s] around eliminating the source's free will*' (paras 1–8). Under US law, a defendant is coerced if the confession was not 'the product of a rational intellect and a free will' (ibid.). Thompson (2005) argues that:

> fMRI is much more coercive than most methods of aggressive interrogation, such as the application of physical pressure. Physical pressure is coercive because it puts the subject *to a choice* between enduring more physical pressure or providing information. Under such

circumstances, a subject's decision to provide information is said to be 'coerced' because external forces have compromised the subject's ability to take a rational decision to reveal or not reveal information. (. . .) Admittedly, fMRI *does not present the subject with such a choice*. (. . .) But this makes fMRI more, rather than less, coercive. The point is not that the detainee 'chooses' to endure more coercion or to give up information, but rather that the coercive interrogation method *has robbed the detainee of his free will* to choose.

Thus, Thompson argues, neurophysiological procedures represent the most severe example of a violation of the Geneva Conventions: extracting information from a brain against the will of the subject, depriving the subject completely of agency or free will.

The need for a new generation of human rights: cognitive liberty

These advances and those to come confront society with the need to legislate a new generation of basic human rights. The first such right is **cognitive liberty**[11] (Boire, 2000; Marks, 2007). Cognitive liberty is defined as the right to control one's own consciousness. As Boire (2005, 2000) says, 'If freedom is to mean anything, it must mean that each person has an inviolable right to think for him or herself. It must mean, at a minimum, that each person is *free* to direct one's own consciousness; one's own underlying mental processes, and one's beliefs, opinions, and worldview.'[12]

The Orwellian concept of machines having access to feelings and thoughts is now close to becoming reality. The law must regulate these previously inexistent fields of human reality.

People have undeniable rights to privacy, dignity and security against arbitrary and invasive acts. But what are the limits of these rights? Some legislators would argue that this is similar to strip search procedures. The state must have some right to violate a subject's privacy and dignity for the sake of overall community security; access to the mind (and therefore to thoughts and feelings) is seen as justified in certain situations. The first step in this regard was the Universal Declaration of Bioethics and Human Rights (UNESCO, 2005), which aims to protect the rights of citizens given new scientific developments, though the declaration does not cover neuroimaging research specifically.

At the time of writing, there is no international system of rules that gives a clear answer to these problems or that determines whether a mandated neuroimaging test would amount to a human rights violation. This is undoubtedly because there is no clear definition of the rights of the human mind.

Incorporating new technologies into human rights work

Kolber (2011) proposes an experiential view of interrogation procedures. He says that new technologies increasingly permit the measurement of subjective experiences of suffering. He argues that in the near future, interrogation procedures will likely be monitored in order to *protect* the detainee. He proposes the development of easy, portable devices that can function when a detainee is interrogated and signal when the interrogator is entering into a prohibited zone of pressure. If there were sufficiently reliable technologies to measure acute distress, we could further protect those interrogated by stipulating the maximum levels of distress they are permitted to experience. Kolber believes that banning certain techniques may not be adequate, given that pain is subjective. Some people might be severely damaged by even the 'softest' coercive techniques, while others may show strong physiological and psychological endurance.

He proposes hiring psychologists in police and army departments or training technicians, and basing their assessment on objective measures of suffering strictly regulated by law.

While well-intentioned, his proposal has too many drawbacks:

1. International organisations fighting against torture have been proposing for decades that interrogation procedures be video recorded to prevent maltreatment. Different authors (Gudjonsson, 2003; Kassin et al., 2009) have insisted on audio and video recording as the best preventive measure. Currently the method does not include proper safeguards: experience shows that cameras may be turned off in critical moments, confessions may be recorded (but not the questioning) or conflicting recordings may be erased or lost. There are few – if any – cases in which a recorded interrogation at a police station could be used to demonstrate ill-treatment, because the perpetrator controls the evidence. The lack of safeguards would likely carry over to new interrogation technologies.
2. The same device proposed to 'protect' the detainee could easily be used to 'enhance' interrogation. The Milgram studies show that knowing the level of damage inflicted on a victim does not prevent the interrogator from escalating the level of pain. Moreover, it may provide a dangerous sense of scientific 'justification' for practices that amount to torture.
3. There are strong ethical concerns about the cooperation of health professionals in these types of procedures.

An alternative, and perhaps more useful, view focuses on the potential of these subjective measurements of suffering in conducting studies on the impact of torture methods; these studies could lead to banning methods scientifically proven to damage health. In other words, the debate on waterboarding or sleep deprivation cycles could end if a group of volunteers accepted being part of a controlled experiment on the subjective effects of a technique, and proper epidemiological analysis of relative risks could help make informed decisions regarding certain techniques. Human rights groups try to document the impact of torture by having post-facto measures (for instance through forensic documentation using the Istanbul Protocol), by studying the long-term sequelae of torture methods using standard clinical measures or, recently, through neuroimaging (Catani et al., 2009; Ray et al., 2006; Weierstall et al., 2011).

These studies have many methodological problems, not least the difficulty of isolating the effects of individual interrogation techniques from other traumatic experiences (previous or concurrent with the interrogation) and measuring the cumulative effect of combined techniques. The shift towards using technology to monitor interrogations goes one step further by conducting in vivo research to test the most controversial interrogation techniques and give scientific support to claims for banning them.

Although researching the use of technology in interrogation procedures presents various ethical and methodological problems, it may open a channel for human rights defenders to respond in an informed and scientific way to military investigations. One way to protect those interrogated from torture is to wage a legal fight in favour of a ban on techniques which research shows are likely to cause extreme pain or suffering.

Pustilnik (2012) has addressed this issue by proposing that neuroimages can 'objectively' measure levels of pain. After a brief analysis of the reliability of these measurements and the methodological problems yet to be solved, she reflects on a science-fiction scenario: the possibility of defining the differences between harsh interrogation, torture and inhuman treatment based on pain measurements taken from neuroimaging. In theory, this would allow interrogation procedures to be monitored and adjusted to standards of 'surmountable' pain.

Pustilnik recognises that imaging procedures will never be able to measure 'psychological pain' but argues that they will at least provide measurements of unbearable physical stress. The proposal has serious shortcomings for at least three reasons: (1) it is doubtful that technology can provide real-time pain measurements; (2) torture is not synonymous with pain (painless methods can still destroy a person); and (3) psychological suffering should not be ignored: neuroimaging procedures only measure *physical* pain, while torture is defined in the UN convention as the infliction of 'severe physical and *psychological* suffering'.

Notes

1 In other cases they were sent to torture centres operated by subcontractors in Yemen, Libya and other countries. This allowed them to avoid scrutiny in the US, while receiving reports from the subcontractors on 'information' obtained.

2 See www.darpa.mil (last consulted April 2014).

3 See www.darpa.mil/program/quantum-orbital-resonance-spectroscopy.

4 http://news.psu.edu/story/189806/2008/03/17/high-tech-interrogations-may-promote-abuse

5 It should be noted that Brain Fingerprinting has helped to free supposedly innocent people: the Iowa Supreme Court accepted its use in the case of *Iowa v. Harrington* to exonerate a person wrongfully accused of murder 25 years after the conviction, demonstrating that he had no recognition of the crime scene (cited by Kerr et al., 2008).

6 See, for instance, http://io9.com/5050009/indian-court-accepts-brain-scans-as-evidence-of-murder.

7 www.nytimes.com/2008/09/15/world/asia/15brainscan.html?_r=3&pagewanted=print.

8 Its use has been proposed in psychotherapy. According to preliminary results, it would shorten therapy, because there would be no need to devote sessions to building confidence between the therapist and the patient, and it would help treat 'resistant patients'.

9 The Convention allows the interrogation of prisoners. Article 17 of Geneva III sets forth the general rule for the interrogation of POWs. It provides that '[n]o physical or mental torture, nor any other form of coercion, may be inflicted on prisoners of war to secure from them information of any kind whatever'. In addition, POWs 'who refuse to answer may not be threatened, insulted, or exposed to unpleasant or disadvantageous treatment of any kind'. Article 13 states that no POW 'may be subjected to . . . medical or scientific experiments of any kind which are not justified by the medical, dental, or hospital treatment of the prisoner concerned and carried out in his interest'. Article 13 also provides that '[p]risoners of war must at all times be humanely treated'. The ICRC commentaries go further: 'the right of respect for the person (. . .) includes (. . .) the right to physical, moral and intellectual integrity (. . .). The right *to* "intellectual integrity" (. . .) applies to the whole complex structure of convictions, conceptions and aspirations peculiar to each individual.'

10 Under Article 44 of the Hague Convention, which protects civilian populations during war, the occupying power may not 'force the inhabitants of territory occupied by it to furnish information about the army of the other belligerent, or about its means of defense'. Similar rights are covered by Articles 27 and 31 of the Fourth Geneva Convention.

11 For an introduction to the concept of 'cognitive liberty', coined by Richard Boire and Wyre Sententia, see Richard Boire, On Cognitive Liberty, 1 *J. Cognitive Liberties* 7, 7 (2000), available at www.cognitiveliberty.org/jcl/jcl_online.html, and Richard Boire, Searching the Brain: The Fourth Amendment Implications of Brain Based Deception-Detection Devices, 5(2) *Am. J. Bioethics* 62, 62–3 (2005) (arguing that the Fourth Amendment is inadequate and too incoherent to protect cognitive liberty).

12 Boire refers to a broad set of conflicting uses: the right not to be forced to undergo psychiatric treatment without consent; the right to consume any mind- and consciousness-altering drugs (like LSD, marijuana or others); the right to have access to any kind of text or material on whatever matter; etc. He discusses 'the government appeal to a legitimate interest in "protecting" a person from him or herself'.

SECTION 6

Definition and measurement of psychological torture

17

REDRAWING THE CONCEPTUAL MAP OF TORTURE

An overview of where we stand: five definitions for the same act

Throughout this book we have examined the concept of psychological torture from all possible angles. Testimonies, studies, opinions, reports, laws and facts have helped us delve deeper into the complexities of creating a definition that takes into account the perspectives of survivors, academics, interrogators, mental health and human rights workers, judges and lawmakers. Each of these actors comes from a distinct experience and has different, sometimes even opposed, objectives.

At the end of each chapter we have summarised information from a specific perspective in order to derive conclusions that we will weave together in this chapter. Here we face the challenge of making sense of this wealth of information. Our goal is to establish a common ground from which we can continue to work towards a conceptualisation of torture.

We started out by reviewing the UN's official definition, and examining why it is so difficult to make it operational (Table 1.1). Two major problems emerged: the *severity of suffering* and the *purpose* criteria. The Inter-American Convention circumvents both problem criteria (Table 1.2). Among various international conventions and treaties, we highlighted the Geneva Conventions, which explicitly forbid torture in the context of war.

In Chapter 4 we observed the differences between Cruel, Inhuman and Degrading Treatment (CIDT), and torture from the perspective of jurisprudence, and the shift from an emphasis on the *intensity* of the suffering in the 1970s to its *motivation* in the 1990s (Tables 1.2 and 1.3).

TABLE 17.1 Legal definitions of torture

United Nations Convention Against Torture	'Any act by which (1) severe pain or suffering, (2) whether physical or mental, (3) is intentionally inflicted on a person for such purposes as obtaining from him or a third person information or a confession, punishing him for an act he or a third person has committed or is suspected of having committed, or intimidating or coercing him or a third person, or for any reason based on discrimination of any kind, (4) when such pain or suffering is inflicted by or at the instigation of or with the consent or acquiescence of a public official or other person acting in an official capacity. It does not include pain or suffering arising only from, inherent in or incidental to lawful sanctions.'

Inter-American Convention Against Torture	'For the purposes of this Convention, torture shall be understood to be any act intentionally performed whereby physical or mental pain or suffering is inflicted on a person for purposes of criminal investigation, as a means of intimidation, as personal punishment, as a preventive measure, as a penalty, or for any other purpose. Torture shall also be understood to be the use of methods upon a person intended to obliterate the personality of the victim or to diminish his physical or mental capacities, even if they do not cause physical pain or mental anguish.'
Geneva Convention	'No physical or mental torture, nor any other form of coercion, may be inflicted on prisoners of war to secure from them information of any kind whatever. Prisoners of war who refuse to answer may not be threatened, insulted, or exposed to unpleasant or disadvantageous treatment of any kind.' Serious law-breaking activity includes '(a) Violence to life and person, in particular murder of all kinds, mutilation, cruel treatment and torture; (b) Taking of hostages; (c) Outrages upon personal dignity, in particular humiliating and degrading treatment.'
Legal Boundaries	ECHR (1969/1978): There are three levels of severity of wrongdoing. Level 1 (Degrading Treatment) is about outrages to dignity; Level 2 (Cruel or Inhuman Treatment) is applicable when the case fulfils the motives but not the necessary level of mental and psychological suffering; and Level 3 (Torture) applies when there is a clear purpose or motivation and severe physical or mental suffering occurs. Accumulated jurisprudence of the 1990s and beyond: Level 1 (Degrading Treatment) is found in cases with low levels of physical or mental suffering, Level 2 (Cruel or Inhuman Treatment) when there is a lack of clear purpose or motivation regardless of severity of suffering and Level 3 (Torture) when there is a clear purpose or motivation and severe suffering occurs.

Psychological torture is slowly gaining recognition as a defined entity in the juridical world. A number of sentences have recognised 'psychological torture' as an entity with criminal implications in itself. The Inter-American Court of Human Rights has been especially clear: it specifically recognises psychological torture, even in the absence of mental suffering, if there is an attack on the psychological integrity of the person. There is case law to support that fear and threats in and of themselves can amount to torture.

We also exhaustively reviewed existing academic perspectives and found different conceptualisations of psychological torture.

In our review of testimonies in Chapter 2, listening closely to the voices of survivors revealed that over the course of 70 years – and despite very different contexts – survivors show important commonalities in their subjective perception of torture as well as in the key elements that they identify as constituting torture. The result was three cognitive maps (Figures 2.1 to 2.3, at the end of Chapter 2). In the first map there was a circle in the centre in which pain, and especially expectations of pain, fostered fear (potentially leading to anguish and terror). Torture built a scenario in which the body became simultaneously the source of support and the enemy. We also observed the cognitive determinants and battles that appear in the mind of the victim during torture, and evaluated the role of time, control, uncertainty, logic and hope. The second map showed denigration and humiliation leading to self-doubt and the eventual breaking of self-consciousness and identity. We observed the role of attacks on dignity through the control of basic physiological needs, nakedness and sexual attacks, insults, deprecation and feral treatment. Finally, we identified *Pain-Fear* and *Humiliation-Identity* as the cornerstones of psychological torture from the victim's point of view.

The lessons from the survivors' testimonies are brought together in the following definition:

> *Definition 1.* Torture is [1] the manipulation of a human being through terror [2] produced by the infliction of pain and harm, the disruption and control of bodily functions, and the manipulation of time, the environment and the senses [3] in order to break the individual, [4] to instill fear, to physically or psychologically punish, to produce information, to attain self-incrimination, or to change the detainee's identity or worldviews to accommodate the will of the perpetrator. [5] Although it is the torturer who makes the rules, torture is experienced as a physical, intellectual and emotional battle against oneself that leaves permanent marks on the individual (usually in the form of guilt, shame, recurrent memories and the inscription of pain in the body).

Next we analysed the torturers' perspective. In Chapter 3 we reviewed the accounts of torturers from different countries and contexts, and also found important commonalities. We grouped the torturers' responses into three mindsets (Figures 3.1 to 3.3). The first reflects the cognitive map of a harsh interrogator according to his or her perspective: '*Torture is a loaded word used to describe a strong professional interrogation that obtains information from an uncooperative source. 'Torture' requires training, bravery, dedication, special skills and the ability to push each person to his or her limit by finding the best method and ideal intensity. Enhanced interrogation is an art unrecognised by a hypocritical society.* The second mindset focuses on procedures: *some procedures (like nakedness, hooding, and regulation of sleep, food or water supplies) are normal routines in all detention centres. The line that separates enhanced interrogation from torture is behaving unethically (e.g. committing rape) or provoking useless suffering in the detainee.* The third cognitive mindset develops the idea of an imaginary 'safety zone' in which the interrogator sees him or herself as so wise and well-trained that he or she can confidently push the detainee without putting the detainee into an irreversibly damaged state.

We can summarise the interrogators' point of view in the following definition:

> *Definition 2.* Torture is a loaded term that should not be used to refer to coercive interrogation, which is [1] the art of obtaining information from otherwise uncooperative sources who do not comply with normal interrogation procedures [2] by finding their weak emotional and psychological points and pushing them beyond their limits, [3] so that cooperating or providing information is their best option. [4] This is achieved by (1) creating a standardised situation of strong unease and discomfort (2) using specific psychological pressure techniques tailored to each detainee, and (3) conducting a skillful interrogation that helps uncover information even against the conscious resistance of the subject. [5] Coercive interrogation is a legitimate resource for obtaining information that takes into account both detainees' rights and society's right to security and to confront menaces. It amounts to torture in cases where the interrogator uses techniques that are 'inhuman', acts unprofessionally or causes severe and permanent physical damage, or when it is done for purposes other than those mentioned above (e.g. punishment or revenge).

We examined in Chapter 5 the concepts of Dignity and Humiliation as discussed in neuroethics and philosophy, and how torture is conceptualised in a relational way. The philosophical definition of torture centre, from this perspective, on the concepts of autonomy, control and free will (Koenig, 2013; Luban and Shue, 2012; Maier, 2011; Parry, 2003; Pollmann, 2011; Scarry, 1985; Sussman, 2006). It can be summarised as:

> *Definition 3.* Torture is [1] a relationship between two human beings characterised by [2] a violation of *dignity* understood as the lack of recognition and respect, and [3] a violation of autonomy, expressed in the absolute *power, control* and imposing of *will* of the perpetrator and the absolute *lack of control, powerlessness* and *suppression of free will* of the victim. [4] The victim is often forced to play an *active role in his or her own suffering* by not only being forced to act against his or her will, but also being forced to commit self-betrayal. [5] The victim is absolutely helpless.

Classifying torture methods according to statistical or nomothetic procedures presented more challenges than advances, as seen in Chapter 7. HURIDOCS and the Istanbul Protocol emphasised physical torture, and did not provide clear insights for a definition of psychological torture. Ojeda (2008) proposed a parsimonious solution by using an extensional definition: *psychological torture is an updated list of all categories and techniques in the torture literature that are known to break a detainee.* But this utilitarian solution had significant drawbacks. We called for a teleological approach in order to link torture methods to impact on the victim, and grouped methods according to their purpose within the torturing process. But linking methods to impacts is not enough. We also learned that torture methods are rarely used alone, but are almost always used in combination; this is the idea behind the *torturing environment*, developed as an integrative proposal in Chapter 18.

In reviewing the neurobiological basis of torture, we saw that researchers strongly emphasised conditions that mainly affect human brain circuits – especially those related to fear (Başoğlu, 2009) and loss of controllability. From this we deduct the following definition.

In situations contemplated by the Convention Against Torture:

> *Definition 4.* The term 'torture' refers to an entire human and environmental context that induces helplessness, loss of control and fear. A particular stressor, or cumulative group of stressors [1] hyperactivates the circuits of fear and terror, [2] maximises helplessness and [3] maximises uncontrollability.

Thus, the distinction between torture and CIDT on the basis of the amount of pain and physical suffering has no basis. Fear, helplessness and a lack of control are not necessarily correlated with physical pain. They are indicators of mental suffering.

Finally, we must consider two additional definitions based on the concept of identity. The pioneering therapeutic work and analyses of therapists and researchers in Latin America during wartime, military dictatorships and exile laid the foundations of the modern concept of torture. Following the work of Martín-Baró on the concept of psychosocial trauma, Elizabeth Lira on the social psychology of fear and Marcelo Viñar on the analysis of prison, torture and identity, torture can be seen as the visible expression of the global machinery that targets all members of society who oppose the establishment. This can be summarised as follows:

> *Definition 5.* On an individual level, torture is any intentional process, regardless of the method or methods used, which aims to [1] destroy the core beliefs and convictions of

the victim or [2] strip him or her of the constellation that constitutes identity and to deprive the victim of his or her human condition and sense of belonging to humankind.

On a social level, [3] torture is a social institution of power and dominance. [4] The torturer or executioner is part of a torturing system that designs, orders, hides and guarantees immunity, and the victim is the representation of the whole society towards whom the message of torture is ultimately directed. [5] Torture requires the existence of those who tacitly accept the status quo and passive bystanders in society.

The first part of the above definition is very well suited to definitions based on clinical descriptions, especially those related to the concept of mental death and complex PTSD described in Chapter 9, and the definition based on the review of mind control and abuse theories in Chapter 15.

These five definitions represent paradigmatic positions and are complementary.

Definitions can have different purposes: (1) to describe the meaning or the essence of a term (essentialist definition); (2) to specify the necessary and sufficient conditions for a thing being a member of a specific category (intensional definition); (3) to operationalise attributes in a simple, measurable and specific way, reflecting current scientific knowledge (operational definition). The philosophical, legal and medical definitions of torture correspond respectively to each one of these categories. Because each definition serves a different purpose, it is not necessary (or logical) to try to merge them into one unified proposal.

Legal and non-legal definitions

There is an additional difficulty to reconciling the legal and non-legal world's definitions of torture. If we compare the table at the beginning of this chapter with the five alternative definitions that follow, we see strong differences rooted in the position of the definition's proponent and the ultimate purpose of the definition.

In Chapter 5 we saw how dignity and humiliation (which are both linked to self and identity) are key elements of almost all non-juridical definitions, while in the legal arena humiliation is a minor aspect in the overall understanding of torture, especially when compared to crude pain-producing techniques. To reconcile both positions it is important to keep in mind that:

- The only person who can qualify certain acts as torture *from a legal point of view* is a judge. We cannot expect a judge to apply mathematical procedures and scientific standards. But we can expect the politicians who create our laws to build their initiatives based on scientific and philosophical grounds, and the judges who apply those laws to be influenced by experts from forensic and medico-psychological disciplines. From a legal point of view, there is a legal definition of torture, but ultimately – and also unfortunately for the scientific, medical and academic community – torture is whatever a judge says it is.
- The preeminence of the legal world when applying sanctions does not mean that one cannot develop an operational definition from a non-legal point of view. The legal world is merely a reflection of the *real* world that fluctuates with political interests (notice, for instance, the dissimilar definitions of torture found in domestic laws of each country that recognises this crime, or the differences among countries that are signatories of the Convention Against Torture).

Debating what is or is not torture based on the subtleties of juridical terminology and historical case law is useful *for the juridical world*, but not for the advancement of knowledge and science.

Some of the disagreements come from which perspective is relevant for each definition. Health professionals work from the perspective of the victim. They empathise with the victim in order to listen and help. In contrast, a judge must evaluate the actions of the perpetrator, and give preeminence to a perspective that guarantees the rights of the accused to a fair trial and the presumption of innocence in the absence of unequivocal proof. The perspective of the victim is also relevant, but not as decisive as 'hard' proof.

From a medical or psychological perspective, a person who has been hit in a detention centre, interrogated in a coercive manner, subjected to continuous sleep deprivation and manipulation of environment (causing disorientation and confusion), debased and humiliated, and who suffers from long-lasting trauma, has suffered torture.

A health professional examining such a claimant can state beyond any doubt that he or she has suffered torture according to medico-psychological criteria (taking into account the internal consistency of allegations, the short- and long-term clinical effects, the psychosocial impact and elements of credibility analysis). A judge, on the other hand, might find that there is a lack of proof to support the claim that the perpetrator has committed the crime of torture as defined in the penal code of that specific location or country – or even if there is sufficient proof, the judge may rule that the alleged perpetrator should not be held accountable.

Too often there is a confusion between both perspectives. There are great differences between human right activists and legal actors, and when we try to define torture and psychological torture we must keep both points of view in mind. Science is not law and law is not science.[1]

An ethical and philosophical definition of torture is based on the legitimate or illegitimate character of the acts, an abstraction of what is acceptable or not in the way human beings relate to one another. It is based either on a universal system of values or on local moral principles, and can sometimes stray from the specific circumstances of the person and the acts that are being evaluated.

But concepts such as 'dignity' or 'will' are difficult to measure even for the most skilled psychologist. And ethical debates often simply mirror the ideological and political positions of individual scholars.[2]

This is where we come in. Our goal is now to move beyond ideology and put science and philosophy to work towards a better definition of torture.

Converging ideas towards a universal model of torture

We reviewed the history of torture in the 20th century in Chapter 10. We learned that there were different 'traditions' and 'schools' of torture and psychological torture, but that despite their differences, most of them began to intertwine from mid-century onwards. This involved constant exchanges between governments at all levels – from politicians and decision makers to people responsible for operations on the ground – with permanent exchanges among researchers from the UK, Germany, France and other countries, as well as intelligence reports between communist and non-communist countries. Each branch spread their preferred methods throughout the countries under their influence, but there was a general convergence of ideas and methods. Voluntary and involuntary sharing led to a common corpus of established techniques for coercive interrogation and torture.

Of course, there are torturers who still use brute force and the maximum possible production of pain – especially when their only goal is punishment and social control through fear. Moreover, pain-generating torture is probably still the most frequent. But over time governments learned that there are more socially acceptable methods that are even more efficient than brute force (even when the ultimate objective is punishment). Instead of talking about many methods of torture, we should imagine torture as a global system with local differences (which mostly lie in the *severity* of methods, the emphasis on certain *kinds* of methods and, of course, on the legal guarantees of the victims).

Over half a century has passed since the wars in Algeria, Malaysia and Vietnam, and today the practice and methods of psychological torture have been firmly established. Although there are variations, the basic building blocks are on the table. Throughout this book, we have reviewed mindsets that offered varying views of psychological torture. Now it is time to combine them into one universal model.

Fitting the pieces together in an atlas of psychological torture

A layered integrative view of torture would include three levels described in Figure 17.1. The figure does not relate specific symptoms to specific methods and outcomes (which would go against the notion of torturing environments). The specific attacks (elements of torture) in Level 1 work in a certain specific and precise combination, depending on the torturing environment, to produce one or more of the impacts in Level 2, which may have one or more of the clinical consequences in Level 3. The figure describes the mechanisms and their consequences 'as they go along'. To avoid unnecessary overcomplication, it does not include the elements modulating damage, i.e. a person's mechanisms to face the situation, personality structure, resilient strategies and contextual elements helping the person manage the traumatic experience of torture. Instead it is an analysis of damage mechanisms. However, the impact and ultimate clinical sequelae that either minimise or amplify the effects of the mechanisms described in Level 1 will be determined to a large extent by the person's resilience and mechanisms to face the situation.

Level 1. Attacks on the person according to basic human needs

The most parsimonious, practical and integrative way of classifying torture methods is using a teleological approach (one that asks, *Why is a method used? What is it for?*) and to group methods according to the *basic needs of the human beings* they target. Such a paradigm shift involves abandoning classifications based on which technique (among infinite possible methods) is used to produce pain or suffering, and focusing on a classification based on the purpose that the perpetrator seeks with the technique. As survivors and interrogators have repeated, the list of torture methods is limited only by human imagination. But all methods seek to interfere with and impact a short range of basic human functions, and to provoke an imbalance in the victim's equilibrium. The only stable, comprehensive classification that could serve as the basis for building new scientific knowledge is one built on an analysis of basic human functions and needs, and how any given torture method aims to impact these while affecting the overall structure of the human being.

Figure 17.1 could be refined by assigning different sizes to the cells to indicate its relative importance within a survivor's subjective experience, according to testimonies in Chapter 2 and the numerous lines of research reviewed throughout this book; doing so

FIGURE 17.1 Layered integrative view of psychological torture.

	Basic physiological functions [primary needs]		Relation to the environment		Need for safety	Physical integrity		Reproduction/Sexual integrity	Need of Control, Meaning, and Purpose	Self and Identity		Need for belonging, acceptance and care
Level 1 HUMAN NEEDS [ATTACKS]	Size and cell conditions	Sleep-wake rhythm	Sensory deprivation (Hooding, earmuffs…)	Handling time	Fear / Panic [witnessing, threats person, family, phobias]	Pain [beatings, blunt trauma]	Extreme pain [Burns, electric chemical pain devices..]	Forced nakedness Forced sex	Autonomy [Helplessness, Absurd orders– Forced Compliance]	Emotional homeostasis [Forced dysregulation-Exhaustion]		Isolation Solitary Confinement Incommunicado
	Food and water intake	Heat Cold Humidity	Sounds Noises Music	Light Conditions	Hope / Pain expectations/ terror [waiting, ruminations]	Forced Pain [stress positions, positional torture]	Mutilation. Organ damage	Sexual Assaults Rape	Instilling Guilt [Forced choices / Betrayal / Harm others / Themes / roles]	Instilling Shame Humiliation [Insults, Taboos, hygiene, feral treatment]		Breaking social bonds [family, social, political, religious networks]
	Urination / Defecation	Other	Mind altering methods	Other	Near death [dry and vet asphyxia, mock executions..]	Exhaustion Exercises	Brain Injury	Other	Cognitive integrity [manipulation- cognitive exhaustion – deceptive interrogationm]	Attacks on beliefs and worldviews		Manipulation of affect [Forced traumatic bonding, love/hate, random reward…]
					Other	Other	Other			Other		Other
Level 2 IMPACTS	*Brain*		*Affect and anxiety circuits*		*System of secondary emotions (social emotions)*				*Higher functions*	*Higher functions (mind) - Identity*		*Ego functions (metacognitive functions)*
	Conscience system Arousal system (tension – control)		*System of fight and defense (primary emotions)*									
	Brain damage		Confusion Unreality Emotional exhaustion	Fear Anxiety Hyperarousal Rage Hopelessness	Humiliation Guilt Shame		Impaired reasoning - Impairment of the capacity for reflection, reasoned judgment and decision			Questioning the self/identity Submissive pseudo-self (identity loss, submissive attitudes)		
Level 3 CONSE-QUENCES	Brain damage		Acute and chronic PTSD and other anxiety symptoms Permanent fear – phobias, chronic depression, dysthymia		Chronic guilt Learned helplessness Social and political demobilisation		Lasting personality changes Changes in belief systems and worldviews Complex PTSD 'Mental Death'					Modified/ changed/ grafted identity Submission Identification with aggressor/ perpetrator

would create a larger cell at the centre of the table for pain (and anticipation of pain), fear and humiliation.

We observe seven basic categories of needs that are attacked by torture:

1. **Basic physiological needs.** These needs include, among others, physical space (size and cell conditions), temperature, humidity, food and water intake, urinitation and defecation and sleep-wake rhythm.
2. **Relationship to the environment.** The conscious mind needs information from the external world to stay oriented and in control, and be able to make decisions. Torture methods that target the conscious mind include sensory deprivation (blindfolds, earmuffs, being confined to dark spaces, etc.), sensory overload (loud music or sound, noises, and especially white noise; 24-hour light; changes in circadian rhythms) or time handling (no watches, no references, changing meal times, aleatory interrogations, unlimited time for detention). Also mind-altering methods (use of drugs, pharmacological torture, white noise, visual or kinetic manipulations, monochrome environments and others). Attacks on these human needs are related to the idea of forced absorption or monopolisation of perception (Biderman, 1957).
3. **The need for safety.** Once alive and able to stay oriented, a human being has the need to feel secure. Techniques that attack the perception of security include the myriad ways of instilling fear, panic or terror. Survivors talked about the destructive power of 'waiting time', when nothing seems to happen but the mind is filled with extreme expectations and fear. We also find techniques that aim to induce the perception of imminent death: dry asphyxia (hooding, 'bolsa') or wet asphyxia ('tacho', 'submarine', waterboarding). Survivors also mentioned designing terrifying scenarios; creating expectations of insurmountable pain and situations in which detainees lose all control; threats of increasing intensity; abuse tailored to the victim; the use of phobias; and witnessing the torture or death of others.
4. **Physical integrity and bodily boundaries.** This includes the use of pain in all its forms: beatings, positional torture, exhaustion exercises. It also includes extreme pain: electrical torture, chemical torture, mutilations and dismemberment.
5. **Reproduction and sexual integrity.** As shown in previous chapters, sexual integrity is related to physical integrity, but also to identity and must be considered on its own. It includes forced nakedness, rape and other forms of sexual torture.
6. **The need for control, meaning and purpose as basic elements of self and identity.** This includes restrictions of autonomy and induction of helplessness, breaking emotional homeostasis and emotional exhaustion, instilling guilt, humiliation or shame, and attacks to cognitive integrity. This is related to being subjected to deceptive or coercive interrogation techniques, forced choices aimed to incriminate, forced betrayal of friends or relatives, or interrogators who engage in role-playing to disorient the detainee. Absurd, bizarre or grotesque rules, norms or orders.
7. **The need for belonging, acceptance and care.** Cutting off physical contact with the outside world (isolation, incommunicado detention, cultural isolation) or cutting off symbolic contact (threats to family and social networks, attacks on one's ties to their community). Manipulation of affect through actions encouraging traumatic bonding with the torturer, ambivalence feelings of love-hate, alternating rejection and providing care, 'testing' loyalty etc.

In Chapter 7, when summarising factor analytic studies, we concluded that there were strong similarities among studies, and that the seven categories proposed by Başoğlu et al.[3] (2009) in their study with survivors from Turkey and former Yugoslavia using the Exposure to Torture Scale were a useful point of departure for classifying torture methods. The first level of our schema mostly coincides with their proposal, although ours is integrated and formulated from the point of view of human needs.

Level 2. Impacts

Level 2 in Figure 17.1 links the effects of torture methods to the neurobiology of the human brain. Based on this relationship we can identify five areas of impact:

1. The **system of arousal** that regulates consciousness. The system must be working properly to maintain optimal tension and control in situations of stress. The manipulation of the environment, sensory inputs and sleep dysregulation (among other methods) provoke confusion, disorientation, misperception and the inability to distinguish what is real and what is not.
2. The system of **fight and defense** that regulates primary emotions in situations of menace. Threats, attacks to security needs and expectations, and lack of control foster emotions of rage, fear and anxiety. Sustained hyperarousal ends in exhaustion and hopelessness.
3. The system of **secondary emotions** that regulates social relationships. Emotions towards others (empathy and compassion) on one side, and emotions related to the self (humiliation, guilt and shame) on the other.
4. The system of **higher cortical functions** that permit thought associations, memory and reasoning. Exhausting activation added to the debilitation of the more basic circuits (arousal, primary and secondary emotions) leads to impaired reasoning and impaired capacity for reflection, reasoned judgment and decision-making.
5. The **conscious mind: ego functions and the system of meta-cognitions**. Techniques that attack the need for belonging, the need for respect, dignity and identity, provoke questioning of the self, identity confusion and eventually a submissive pseudo-self with submissive attitudes.

Again, impacts in Level 2 appear as a combination of one or more methods in Level 1 and there is no specific link between any single method and any specific impact. The table shows the inherent difficulties in finding neuroimage, neurochemical or neuroelectrical correlations specific to physical or psychological torture in the brain. Torture touches *all* of the main circuits, and the effects are widespread.

Level 3. Consequences

The third level shows the damage, impacts on health and sequelae of torture:

1. **Brain damage.** Not only due to direct concussions and impacts, but also the neurological damage of chronic stress, anxiety and neuroendocrine activation.
2. **Anxiety and affect structures.** Torture's impact on fear and memory circuits can lead to acute or chronic Post-Traumatic Stress Disorder, permanent fear and phobias, and other anxiety symptoms. In the circuit of affect, chronic depression or dysthymia may also appear.

3. **Higher functions – Mind.** The damage to the system of secondary emotions, higher cortical functions and ego functions can lead to chronic guilt, apathy and helplessness, enduring personality changes, changes in belief systems and worldviews, complex PTSD or mental death. In certain contexts identity may be erased and a new, modified or grafted identity may emerge which can include positive identification with the aggressor.

Figure 17.1 is a complete, but static, picture. At the end of Chapter 11 we reviewed a preliminary model of the interaction between attacks on the body, brain debilitation and vulnerability of the conscious self, on the one hand, and emotional and cognitive manipulation during coercive interrogation and torture, on the other. Figure 17.2 complements and expands upon that analysis.

Torture is a machinery that can operate at a low intensity (and exert only some pressure on a person) or at high intensity, which is devastating. The schema in Figure 17.2 shows the machine functioning at full capacity. What we usually see are only some parts of the system working at the necessary level for the intended purpose.

The two upper circles explain the initial attack on the integrity of the person. They correspond to what is euphemistically called the 'softening period' (or 'periodo de ablandamiento' in Spanish) that is described in the accounts of Villani, Gurruchaga, Liscano and Villar, included in Biderman's writing, and part of the KUBARK Manual (among other army manuals).

There are many combinations of methods for this 'softening period' (just as there are infinite combinations of the cells in Table 17.1); all of them involve severe physical and psychological suffering. Their commonalities include:

1. **Attacks on body functioning and the senses** (deprivation of food or water, sensory deprivation, strenuous exercise, stress positions, etc.) intended to make the person feel confused, disoriented and physically exhausted. There is a disorganisation of body functions that makes it necessary to concentrate all mental efforts on trying to resist and maintain a certain amount of control. Some manuals refer to this as 'forced absorption', 'attention focusing' or, as described by Villani, 'ruminated dreading', and it pushes the person over the brink of extreme exhaustion, helplessness and inner chaos.

2. **Attacks on the alert system and central emotional regulators;** these attacks cause exhaustion by provoking intense, mixed emotions (including fear and terror, and also emotional confusion, emotional blockades, hopelessness, sadness and self-pity) and rage against perpetrators, oneself and the world. Detainees are put on constant alert using silence and noise, sudden interruptions, and orders. They enter a state of hyperarousal and nervousness, sometimes alternated with isolation for endless hours, provoking shock as they are forced from one emotional extreme to the next. Detainees face different interrogators, receive contradictory messages and have no way of knowing who they can trust. It is an overwhelming situation, shifting back and forth between overstimulation and alert defensiveness to deprivation of stimuli and isolation; the final result is that resting is impossible. This process pushes the person to the point of cognitive and emotional saturation.

The attacks on body functioning, the senses and emotions (see the two lower circles in Figure 17.2) result in:

1. **Cognitive and emotional exhaustion.** The victim's body undergoes extremely harsh physical conditions. The person is disoriented, cannot remember well and has difficulty maintaining control while questioned. He or she cannot think clearly and is not even

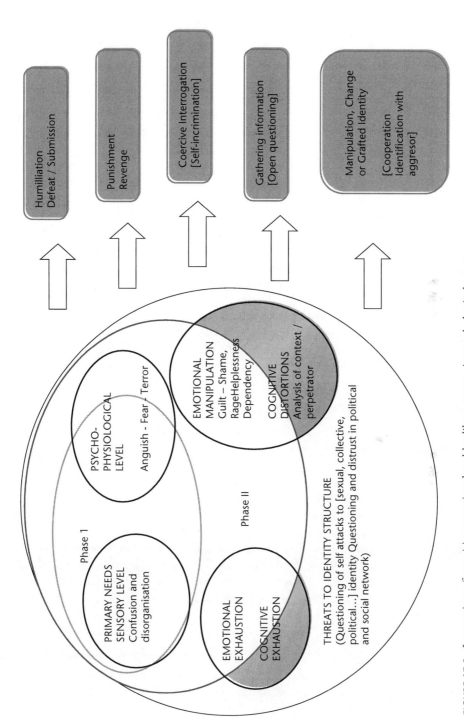

FIGURE 17.2 Interaction of cognitive, emotional and bodily processes in psychological torture.

Humilliation
Defeat / Submission

Punishment
Revenge

Coercive Interrogation
[Self-incrimination]

Gathering information
[Open questioning]

Manipulation, Change
or Grafted Identity
[Cooperation
Identification with
aggresor]

PSYCHO-
PHYSIOLOGICAL
LEVEL
Anguish - Fear - Terror

EMOTIONAL
MANIPULATION
Guilt – Shame,
RageHelplessness
Dependency

COGNITIVE
DISTORTIONS
Analysis of context /
perpetrator

Phase 1

Phase II

PRIMARY NEEDS
SENSORY LEVEL
Confusion and
disorganisation

EMOTIONAL
EXHAUSTION

COGNITIVE
EXHAUSTION

THREATS TO IDENTITY STRUCTURE
(Questioning of self attacks to [sexual, collective,
political...] identity Questioning and distrust in political
and social network)

sure which emotions are real. His or her nerves might be broken. The victim is in a situation of cognitive and emotional breakdown.

2. The person is in a position of great vulnerability to **emotional manipulation**. He or she can easily feel enraged, sad, guilty or ashamed, and it is not difficult for the interrogator to induce all kinds of positive and negative emotions in the detainee (positive in the sense of being extremely sensitive to small rewards or small signs of affection, and negative in the sense of being easily pushed to the limit with just a few manipulations).

3. The person may be sensitive to threats against his or her family or friends. He or she may also be completely vulnerable to **cognitive manipulation**. The victim may be confused, and have little capacity to understand or think; he or she may feel disoriented by a bombardment of questions with no time to answer, agonised by long silences or puzzled because the interrogator who was kind the previous day is now furious and threatening. The person might be forced to 'answer' without understanding the accusation or why he or she is detained, and try to guess. Or he or she may be unable to remember what he or she (or others) might have said, merging memories and what the interrogator claims happened. Ultimately, he or she does not know what to think, what to say or what information is or is not useful. The detainee is likely unable to do anything but try and continue to resist.

4. In addition to the intensity of this process, we must include threats and attacks on the self and identity system (represented in the wider circle). Torture is the breaking of a person. Attacks on one's sexual, collective or political identity, as well as humiliation, debasement, punishment and cruelty, all undermine beliefs and worldviews, contributing to a progressive crumbling and eventual collapse of the person. The attacks on identity have a broader impact because of the person's incredible vulnerability in this situation.

Personified versus Reified Torture

The next steps depend on the purposes of torture.

Personified Torture is a process of violence targeting a specific person because of his or her individual attributes (activism, hypothetical possession of information or other attributes). The torturer seeks to break the victim's resistance as an autonomous being by pushing him or her to his or her limits. In Reified Torture, violence is exerted against a person as an anonymous representative of a social group, not as an important individual. For example, the systematic rape of women by armed groups – classified as torture under international law – seeks to intimidate and terrorise an opposing group, annihilate rebellion, and show one's own group's supremacy while causing ethnic destruction, shame and social humiliation, as well as punishment to armed male enemies. Attacking the tortured person (her body and identity) is not an end in itself, but a means of social domination (Kivlahan and Ewigman, 2010; Mukamana and Brysiewicz, 2008).

Various interrogation purposes entail different approaches:

1. **Self-incrimination**: At this point coercive questioning can produce optimal results. If the person is guilty, he or she will probably accept responsibility for acts in which he or she has been involved, although it would be difficult to know what actually happened and what information has been distorted in the process, or what the real level of involvement is. The person has been forced to betray him or herself and make a self-incriminating declaration. If the person is innocent or knows nothing, it is probable that the interrogation will eventually obtain 'results'. In a significant percentage of cases, the detainee can be

convinced to accept responsibility for events that he or she might not actually have first-hand knowledge of, or accept an accusation that he or she does not fully comprehend – especially when confused and exhausted – if he or she is repeatedly subjected to double bind questions (lose-lose situations), deceptive information about his or her responsibility, or emotional manipulation (maximisation and minimisation strategies) in this state of weakness. All manuals recommend writing down and making the person sign a confession as soon as one is obtained, because he or she will probably reject the statement later before a judge, or even declare that the confession was obtained through torture.

2. **Gathering information** (especially names of people or places): A full disintegration of the cognitive system is not beneficial to the interrogation (O'Mara, 2016). Therefore, the attack will be mostly emotional while trying not to compromise cognitive and memory functions (O'Mara and O'Mara, 2009). The interrogator must decide where the limits are: the limits of what the detainee knows, and when he or she cannot provide any more useful information; and the limits of what he or she can endure without being lethally damaged or suffering extreme anxiety or confusion.

3. **Humiliation:** The process focuses on attacks against self-worth, denigration and annihilation of self.

4. If the purpose is **punishment**, or torture has a **function of social control**, the process extends until there are scars. Body marks and symptoms remain as a personal and social memory of harm.

5. **Reversing identity** (for instance turning the detainee into a collaborator): The process seeks to establish a *tabula rasa* and install a new, grafted identity, as we saw in Chapter 15.

These options are represented by the five squares on the right of Figure 17.2.

The 'five days is enough' paradigm: torture with and without time limits

Imagine two patterns of torture as the two ends of a continuum. On one end is **time-limited torture**. The person is in detention for a short time (limited by local laws and habeas corpus, where possible), and the interrogator has a limited period of time (ranging from 3–7 days to 1 month) before he or she must present the detainee to judicial authorities. This type of time-limited torture is associated with preventive detention or with 'incommunicado' regimes. During detention, the purpose of torture is to obtain as much information as possible, or to get a self-incriminating statement. The detainees know that eventually they will be released. The interrogator also knows this, and so they exert enough pressure to make that period unbearable. At the same time, the interrogator must not leave marks that the detainee could use as evidence. The interrogation is based on the use of techniques that maximise the *weakness and confusion* of the detainee. This pattern of torture is most commonly found in Western democracies (Table 17.2).

At the other end of the continuum is **torture as a process**, in which detainees are held for extremely long – sometimes undefined – periods of time. For example, they may be detained for an unlimited amount of time in a clandestine detention centre, usually with no official charges. The interrogator faces no time constraints, leaving the detainee completely at the mercy of the interrogators. The interrogators seek to punish detainees using as much pain as possible while first gaining full control, and later submission and collaboration. The interrogator seeks to avoid causing exhaustion and confusion (although this can be useful at a given stage in the process), utilising techniques that *maximise helplessness and progressively attack the detainee's personal identity and ego structure* (Table 17.2).

TABLE 17.2 Time-limited torture versus torture without time constraints

Time-limited torture *(investigative procedures, pretrial detention, incommunicado detention, etc.)*	*Torture without time constraints* *(clandestine detention centers, forced disappearance, etc.)*
• Maximises temporal weakness and confusion • Uses extremely coercive interrogation and pressure to achieve results • Seeks to obtain information, an accusation, or a confession	• Maximises attacks on self and personal identity • Maximises absolute control and submission • Seeks to obtain changes in identity structure, and long-term involvement and cooperation

Every situation is unique, and along the continuum between these two extremes there are as many different possibilities as there are contexts. Bear in mind that torture techniques that seek to attack the identity of the detainee will probably not be used on a short-term basis, because it will be difficult to complete the process of breaking the person. The opposite also holds true: torture as a long-term process can (and does) use techniques that promote weakening and confusion only in the initial stages, unless punishment and annihilation are the sole purpose. A permanent weakening of the person does not permit the restructuring of the core elements of the self or induce collaboration.

Time-limited torture and torture as a long-term process are characterised by dissimilar patterns of abuse, and require different frameworks of understanding and categorisation. However, it is important to remember that reality often overrides theory.

Breaking the detainee through psychological torture does not require much time; the time that it takes to break him or her depends on the degree of pressure, and the number and intensity of concomitant techniques used. With a skillful combination of attacks in the first level of Figure 17.1, one or two days can be enough for some people, and three to five days are enough for the vast majority of detainees. A few people, including those who are specially trained, activists or people with strong convictions and capacity for self-control, might endure weeks. A handful of people might even adapt and be able to resist for the duration of the interrogation, but these are very rare exceptions.

In therapy, a very young activist in an urban social movement explained that during torture a police officer once told him: 'We can have you here [in pre-trial detention] for five days. We do not need so much. You will remember things that you did not even know you knew. Not five. Three days is enough.' In therapy the patient said, in a humble voice: 'The worst thing is that he was right. Three days later, I was so confused and terrified that I would sign any paper they put in front of me'.

Most people suffer severe damage after even a few days of such treatment.

What we've learned after redrawing the map

Is all torture actually psychological torture?

Defining psychological torture does not mean defending a dualist position that separates body and mind. Our first conclusion is that torture and psychological torture are the same because *all torture is ultimately psychological*; all torture is psychological because the ultimate goal is to break a person's will and conscious mind. Pain and fear combine with other factors to target the inner self, debilitating and eventually defeating a human being. The objective is not the inanimate body, but the conscious mind. However, this is not based on a dualist position, but rather on the understanding of the human being as a living structure that has different systems which interrelate in perfect equilibrium, and when one of those systems is affected, all structures change: first they react, then they adjust. Ultimately, torture targets the foundation of the entire system: the self. Torture's battle is always fought on the field of a person's resistant self-reflective mind, the core that looks after all the systems. Pain is one of the doors to the conscious mind. So are fear, humiliation, uncertainty and lack of control. Torture is psychological, and it couldn't be otherwise.

This is what a typical intellectual position formulated within an academic department at a university would look like. When working on the ground with survivors, it is clear from the very first minute that pain is not an eidetic construction of the mind. Pain is real, *painfully real*. Jean Améry (1980) described his own torment in *At the Mind's Limits*: in torture, the human being *is reduced to a shouting body*: 'slight pressure by the tool-wielding hand is enough to turn the other – along with his head, in which are perhaps stored Kant and Hegel, and all nine symphonies, and The World as Will and Representation – into a shrill squealing piglet at slaughter' (p. 35). There is a bodily memory of pain, or, as both Scarry (1985) and survivors in Peru have expressed when recalling their suffering (Theidon, 2004): pain becomes embodied, there is a corporeal memory that appears through recurrent disease and trauma.

The idea that all torture is psychological is helpful in understanding personified torture aimed at obtaining actionable information or self-incrimination, but is insufficient if we want to understand many other expressions of ill-treatment and torture – especially torture as punishment, or as a tool for instilling terror and fostering social control. Some torturers aim to destroy the mind. Others only try to fulfil their wish to destroy the body and produce as much physical and psychological pain as possible.

Physical pain and mental pain are not torture markers

This does not mean that the severity of pain can be considered a marker of torture. Pain is not even a prerequisite for torture. If we accept that the purpose of torture is physical and ultimately psychological breakdown, then we can see that the notion *no pain means no torture* is folk concept with no scientific basis (Bellamy, 2006; Vos, 2007; Welch, 2009) which we have inherited from the images of the Inquisition and medieval torture (Flynn and Salek, 2012). We saw in Chapter 4 that the idea that *torture is not necessarily associated with pain* has already been assumed by the medical and psychological profession, and legal actors are also almost unanimously moving towards the same conclusion. From the old *UK v. Ireland* case later reconsidered in *Selmouni v. France* (ECHR, 1999), to the Israeli government's laws authorising certain techniques that 'did not produce severe pain' (later strongly rejected by the UN Human Rights Committee and the Israeli Supreme Court [Ginbar, 2009; Imseis, 2001]), to the conclusion of the Bybee Memos (now considered 'infamous' by the American General Attorney, Senate committees and the government [Lewis, 2010; Nowak, 2006; Shane et al., 2007]), today it is indisputable that pain is *not* a prerequisite for torture.

Throughout this book, we have heard agreement from the voices of survivors, interrogators, legal scholars and mental health professionals: pain does not equal torture (and torture is not equivalent to pain). For interrogators, this is even more important: for most of them, *pain is a problem*. As the *Human Resource Exploitation Manual* puts it: 'The torture situation is an external conflict, a contest between the subject and his tormentor. The pain which is being inflicted upon him [the interrogatee] from outside himself may actually intensify his will to resist.

In terms of mental suffering, the data reviewed in Chapter 9 showed that torture is one of the more devastating human experiences. The percentage of survivors with long-term sequelae is greater than that of any other traumatic experience. On average, and across studies, around 40 per cent of survivors develop lasting PTSD and one out of five manifest long-lasting impacts on their identity, belief system and worldview. However, that means 60 per cent of torture survivors cope using their own psychological resources and are resilient, and that mental harm is not a necessary condition for determining that a person was tortured.

Even if mental harm was present in all cases of torture – which is not the case – it does not manifest itself immediately. The most severe forms of mental damage can (and usually do) appear months or years after torture. This is why it is impossible to pretend that it is feasible to conduct a scientifically-based interrogation assisted by a psychologist through an instant on-site detection of mental suffering.

The mistake of searching for causal relationships instead of relative risks

The legal distinction between Torture and Cruel, Inhuman and Degrading Treatment is a particular instance within a wider conceptual error that we can call the causal fallacy. It comes from assuming that science must establish an unequivocal *causal* relationship between certain practices and their consequences (like linking Koch's Bacillus to tuberculosis) in order to determine the limits of torture. When the US Medical Services conducted secret investigations to find out whether there was a difference between applying 'enhanced interrogation techniques' simultaneously or sequentially, they assumed that their research could establish a causal relationship between certain methods and their consequences in order to maximise efficiency.

But this could not be further from truth. Some survivors are extraordinarily resilient to any kind of psychological pressure or pain and can endure the worst torture, while others are extremely vulnerable. It wouldn't make sense to focus research or legal debates on banning specific techniques based on the premise that there must be a direct causal relationship between that technique and the evidence of physical or psychological harm. This would go against the roots of epidemiological reasoning, which is the foundation of most decisions in health sciences. Medicine and psychology are sciences that involve multicausality, risks and probabilities. One might like to always have deterministic relationships, but scientific decision-making is usually based on probabilistic hypotheses implying that, *on average*, certain actions provoke certain consequences. For example, contemporary epidemiology has established that smoking increases the *relative risk* of lung cancer and cardiovascular disease. The Cuban singer Compay Segundo claimed to have smoked a big Cuban cigar daily, from his youth until his death at age 92. However, despite individual exceptions, the *relative risk* of cancer in smokers versus non-smokers is still more than enough for the authorities to impose radical restrictions and policies to deter smoking.

When medicine in general and specifically psychiatry face the issue of defining torture, they can establish practices with *a high risk ratio* of causing damage, and that this damage is of sufficient magnitude to be banned internationally. For instance, we know that absolute sensory deprivation can produce psychotic symptoms in roughly 20 per cent of volunteers in less than 6 hours and in 70 per cent in 72 hours. This magnitude is enough to absolute warrant the banning of sensory deprivation in detainees.[4] They can also establish operational (reviewable) criteria that allow a combined group of techniques to qualify as 'torture' based on the relative likelihood that these combined practices will cause physical or psychological harm.

There is no epidemiology of torture in terms of risk analysis. Of course there are clear ethical difficulties that preclude designing controlled prospective studies on the effects of torture techniques on human beings and establishing this epidemiology. However, using instruments measuring torturing environments can help build a knowledge base to decide which techniques to specifically ban.

A review of studies and available evidence using shared instruments (such as the TES presented in the following chapter) would help in this regard.

Furthermore, this avoids the risk of defining torture by creating a list of single specific techniques which might ultimately help interrogators keep their methods just within the limits of the law or find ways to circumvent it.

The main reason why a systematic review of existing literature (e.g. a Cochrane review) at this stage of our scientific knowledge would attenuate but not solve the problem of defining torture is this: the important element is not the relative risk of a given technique (given that techniques are infinite), but the way in which it is used. It is in the combination of techniques, and in the unique relationship established between torturer and victim, where torture is most destructive. This is why, again, future dialogue and research should be directed towards what we call *torturing environments* (more on this in Chapter 18).

A lack of sequelae is not tantamount to a lack of torture

If there is not a causal linear relationship, but a probabilistic one, and there are many survivors who are resilient, it follows that the absence of sequelae does not mean that the person has not been tortured. The data in Chapter 9 confirm that the presence of long-term sequelae attributable to torture supports the credibility of allegations of torture, but the absence of clinical consequences may simply be a result of processing the experience in a meaningful way and continuing to live resiliently.

Can a person's 'severity of suffering' be estimated?

A series of experimental studies in social psychology (Mcdonnell, Nordgren and Loewenstein, 2011; Nordgren et al., 2011) has shown that the perception of the 'severity of suffering' lies in the eye of the beholder. The authors asked a sample of US citizens to assess the 'severity of suffering' in three situations of ill-treatment versus torture: exposure to cold temperatures, sleep deprivation and solitary confinement. They divided the subjects into two experimental conditions. One group just read a description of the technique while the other experienced a 'mild' form of it. Then the subjects were asked about the level of pain or discomfort associated with the technique, whether its use was ethical, and whether it should be regarded as questioning, interrogation, coercive interrogation or torture. The results showed that those who experienced 'lite' forms of ill-treatment tended to assign a higher rank to the pain and suffering of the technique on the victim, consider it ethically unacceptable and more frequently label it as torture. In other words, having the possibility of minimally empathising with the victim changed the perception of the 'severe suffering' criteria.

That was a laboratory experiment. A simulated true situation yielded similar results. In 2004, British television's Channel 4 produced a documentary (*The Guantanamo Guidebook*) in which seven students from different backgrounds who were healthy, fit and had strong character volunteered to be part of an experiment. Prior to the experiment, half of the students supported enhanced interrogation. A group of retired interrogators, led by one of the people who designed Camp Delta, held them in a place that reproduced the jails in Guantanamo. For ethical reasons they were subjected to a mild, 'partial' treatment. The treatment did not include any physical beating and was purely psychological. It included being put in a small cage, being publicly exposed for 24 hours in a jail without any privacy, being naked, humiliation and harassment, sensory overload, partial sensory deprivation (earmuffs), hunger and harsh interrogation. The interrogators wanted them to confess that they were going to plant a bomb in London. *After just three days* two participants were so severely affected that they asked to stop and one had to leave. All of them were affected in some way, even after being warned and knowing that this was a time-limited experiment. In follow-up interviews, the volunteers expressed that they could never have imagined what they were talking about when they offered their first opinions on enhanced interrogation, and that the experience had radically changed their opinion of the legality of torture, even in cases of people convicted of terrorism. Two participants recognised that at different points they were eager to confess they were thinking of planting a bomb. '*It is unfair. You are assumed to be guilty and given no chance to prove the opposite . . . your only option is to confess . . . it is extremely difficult to describe how it feels. . . .*'

Both experiments show that the experience of pain is unimaginable, and that those who have not experienced it tend to underestimate it. The authors of the first experiment called this 'an empathy gap'. Being subjected to 'lite' torture diminished the gap and shifted the subject closer to the victims' experience.

It is probable that the judge who has to make a decision regarding the 'severity of suffering' of the victim (in order decide if certain actions constitute torture) has never suffered anything close to the experience of ill-treatment. Therefore, it is plausible that he or she will underestimate the real suffering felt by the victim. In any case, a judge's decision-making is subject to his or her own prejudices. This echoes Koenig's take on judges' assessment of what should be considered 'humiliating' or not, given that humiliation is a concept heavily dependent on culture.

The 'severity of suffering' criteria are unfounded in medicine and psychology

From a medical and psychological point of view, there is no correlation between the severity of the act being judged and the severity of suffering. Suffering is a bad indicator of the seriousness of the act. What happens if a woman is raped by her torturer, but she reacts with emotional distance and goes on with her life? Or what if a person subjected to endless 'waiting time' is so terrified and confused, and has such intense anticipation of pain, that tracing a ballpoint pen over his skin is enough to torture him, as Viñar explained in Chapter 2? In other words, the definition of severity is specific to each survivor and a poor indicator of the gravity of the acts being judged. The 'severity of suffering' criterion is not only impossible to quantify, it is a distraction that deepens the false assumption that pain and torture are equivalent.

How much is too much? The cumulative effect

Many authors have proposed that the impact of torture is not related to a single technique but to a cumulative effect or a combination of techniques that if used alone would not produce the same effects (Koenig, Stover and Fletcher, 2009; Reyes, 2008). As we saw when analysing the interrogation log of Qahtani in Chapter 14, a rule might indicate that the person must be allowed to sleep for at least four hours a day in order to be considered 'humane treatment', but if those four hours are distributed across midnight, then technically no rules have been broken (though in reality the person has slept only 4 hours within a 48-hour period). Combine this with constant questioning for the majority of that time by interrogators alternating in 6-hour shifts, and few could deny that this is torture.

And this is, in fact, the way torture has taken place. We saw this in Chapter 7. In one case, the *New York Times* (Shane et al., 2007) described how CIA interrogators were worried that even approved techniques had such a painful, multiplying effect when combined that they might cross the legal line. In another case, Physicians for Human Rights documented how US interrogators conducted a medical experiment under the supervision of the Office of Medical Services with a sample of 25 prisoners in Guantanamo to determine if there were differences in the sequential versus simultaneous use of 'enhanced interrogation techniques'[5] (Physicians for Human Rights, 2010).

The distinction between torture and CIDT is not supported by medical or psychological evidence although it is necessary from a legal point of view

The Convention's definition of torture makes no clear distinction between torture and cruel, inhuman and degrading treatment. Traditionally *torture*, following article 17 of the Convention, has simply been considered 'an *aggravated form of CIDT*' (Nowak and McArthur, 2006). But this lack of definition stands as one of the major elements of current controversy. It is based on a certain gradient in which excruciating pain would be at the highest level of the scale of suffering (amounting to torture), and humiliation at the lowest. We have seen in Chapters 4, 5 and 15 that attacks on identity and purely psychological torture has, on average, more devastating consequences than torture based on the production of pain. Data from qualitative and quantitative studies show that mental suffering can be deep and long lasting, and survivors' accounts in Chapter 2 indicated that fear, anguish and humiliation become imprinted in the body's memory. Once again, the ultimate purpose of any torture is to attack the conscious mind and, from a medical and psychological point of view, the legal distinctions between torture and CIDT based only on the amount of suffering infringed could easily be called into question.

This reveals an incompatibility between the legal world (which assumes a *proportionality between the act and the consequences*) and the medical–psychological world (which shows that this proportionality does not exist, and that at best there is a probabilistic relationship). Scientific research shows that the immediate consequences (suffering) and long-term consequences (sequelae) are always unpredictable. There is always the possibility that an act on the lower level of the scale of supposed severity (considered CIDT) could provoke the highest level of psychological suffering and long-term sequelae.

There are three positions, the first two legal and the third medical, to solve these problems.

Position 1. The distinction is established based on the *victim's degree of suffering*. While the perpetrator would be pursuing the same ends specified in the Convention in both degrees that the victim suffers, where there is torture, physical or mental suffering is 'severe'. This is a controversial position because, as we have seen (1) the severity of suffering cannot be measured and (2) the distinction is left to the court's culturally and ideologically subjective decision and the door is left open for certain events that could be considered 'severe' in the eyes of most observers not to be for a given court (such as in the *Ireland v. UK* case examined in Chapter 1).

Position 2. To avoid this problem, an increasing number of jurists and international institutions consider that the severity criterion should be eliminated and that what distinguishes torture from ill-treatment should be the *purpose* (as the Inter-American Convention has indeed already established). If the purposes of torture are there, then torture is as well. This comes to solve the unresolvable problem of determining the degree of suffering.

Position 3. Finally, from a medical and psychological standpoint it has been argued that the distinction itself makes no sense and should be eliminated. In the most frequently cited research, Başoğlu (2009) showed how in a broad sampling of persons tortured during the Balkan War, methods of psychological and mixed physical and psychological torture had a clinical impact that was greater in traumatic terms than sheer physical torture based on hunger or pain. It could therefore be inferred that the distinction between torture and ill-treatment made no sense. Similarly, with former Guantanamo prisoners, Alexa Koenig (2013) showed that attacks on dignity (nakedness, religion, etc.) were much more devastating than extreme physical pain.

From my personal point of view, the distinction should be maintained for the following reasons:

1. From a legal standpoint, it makes sense to establish a gradation of situations. Torture is a very grave crime that has terrible connotations in the collective subconscious. Not making nuances or using the term indiscriminately could be tantamount to trivialising or slighting it. Not everything is the same and making distinctions is advisable. Nuances are required precisely in order to describe an event in its full breadth and uphold the proportionality of the sentence.
2. There is a certain inconsistency in what it is said in Position 3, i.e. the consideration that one is talking solely of *physical suffering*. There is no doubt that Bosnian prisoners in Serbia and prisoners in Guantanamo experienced types of *extreme mental suffering* in addition to physical suffering. This is why they were so severely damaged. To propose an elimination of the distinction between torture and ill-treatment using the argument that psychological torture can be worse than physical torture is to deny the stature of psychological suffering as a cause of torture. Therefore, what should be demanded is not an elimination of nuances but rather an insistence vis-á-vis legal powers that psychological torture can be devastating and this should be appropriately evaluated.

The task is complex. Breaking with the notion held among both attorneys and the general population that torture is associated with physical pain, again, is as necessary as it is complex.

Where would the distinction lie?

The key is that what is being judged are the acts (what the perpetrator does intentionally to the victim and his/her purpose in doing so) not the consequences, especially in an immediate/short-term view (level of suffering). Undoubtedly, for there to be torture, there must be intentionality and purpose, with the nuances that must be included in those cases where the perpetrator is the State. This is the groundwork.

Doubt arises in those cases when the purpose is clear. Considering the severity of immediate suffering or severity of sequelae (criterion 1) does not seem to be the best approach.

In any event, it is impossible to use only one criterion, because as we saw, it is precisely in the *interaction* between torturer and victim, between the act of torturing and the way in which it is designed to break a person, where torture takes shape. Elements such as age, the personal vulnerability of the detainee, defencelessness and so forth, are relevant here.

TABLE 17.3 Elements to distinguish torture from inhuman or degrading treatment

Elements to be taken into account:
1. **Purpose of the acts**, i.e. of perpetrator or the institution that s/he represents (i.e. the State)
   a. Explicit purposes cited, for instance by the Convention (interrogation, confession, punishment, humiliation)
   b. More general and teleological purposes as appearing in the jurisprudence, and particularly the Inter-American Convention criterion of obliterating personality, the criterion of breaking one's identity and other elements reflecting the purpose of the torture from a more comprehensive standpoint rather than just a specific purpose
2. **Gravity of the acts** committed against the person particularly bearing in mind the intentionality indicators (see the Intentionality Assessment Checklist). Particularly pertinent are:
   a. Measures in the torturing environment
   b. Foreseeable potential damage
   c. Reiteration. Prolongation over time
   d. Cruelty. Defencelessness or particular vulnerability.
3. **Severity of the suffering** at the time of the events and/or subsequent evaluations, including physical and psychological suffering evaluated independently.

It therefore seems that a distinction should be made between torture and ill-treatment and that this distinction should reside in a set of criteria qualifying an act as torture and not something else. To a large extent, they have been included in the *Torturing Environment Scale* (see Appendix 5), which we feel is in an excellent position to help. *Severe physical and/ or psychological suffering* is yet another criteria among the rest of the legal and environmental criteria.

The work of an expert is imperative for this set of criteria to be evaluated. The expert is the one who can take all of these elements into consideration and facilitate for the judge access to the description of the torturing environment, to the victim's subjectivity and to the analysis of the specific interaction between the victim and the perpetrator.

Table 17.3 therefore includes elements that are pertinent and must be weighed on a case by case basis in considering something to be torture or cruel, inhuman and degrading treatment.

An abolition of the distinction between torture and ill-treatment would avoid using mis-classification as a common loophole for authorities and politicians in bad faith, but could paradoxically trivialise torture. We propose multiple criteria be used to both allow for finer definitions and prevent the notion of torture from being distorted by sui generis interpretations based on a sole criterion.

This is not a parsimonious approach in that the distinction between torture and cruel, inhuman and degrading treatment can be established as a response to a simple question. It requires expert intervention and a combination of more than one criterion. Parsimonious solutions, however, have run the risk of being oversimplified and easily manipulated. They are entirely inappropriate for such a delicate issue.

Who can perpetrate torture?

The Convention is clear. Torture is perpetrated by States. In the words of the Convention: *'when such pain or suffering is inflicted by or at the instigation of or with the consent or acquiescence of a public official or other person acting in an official capacity.'*

As discussed in Chapter 6, a series of circles demarcating torture can potentially ripple out from here. The initial circle, clear in nearly all legal systems, encompasses torture committed by agents representing the State or, although they are not the State themselves, agents performing functions that the State has delegated in them (though there are discrepancies as to exactly where to draw the line). The second blurrier circle includes torture committed by armed non-State actors or organised criminal structures acting as the State in areas under their control. Even blurrier and more controversial is the circle encompassing torture committed by private individuals working in institutions that must be monitored and supervised by the State, which therefore takes on subsidiary responsibility (i.e. physicians in a hospital who bind patients and force them to withstand their abstinence syndrome from alcohol or opiates untreated). Finally, the blurriest circle of all, which in all likelihood cannot be taken on board, includes torture committed by private individuals.

The relevance of the perpetrator's motivation and intention

Intentionality as a necessary criterion for determining perpetrator responsibility

The United Nations definition of torture requires perpetrator *intentionality* on the part of the perpetrator in order for the crime to be considered torture. This leads one to believe that the crime would always be *wilful*. Generally speaking, it has been established that it is precisely intentionality that separates torture from ill-treatment and degrading treatment (see Chapters 1 and 3).

As we analysed in Chapter 6, in the clearest situations, a person has to *know* that what s/he is doing amounts to ill-treatment or torture and must have that *aim*. Jurisprudence terms this *wilful misconduct*. Also covered by the definition, however, are situations where there is a basic, overall notion of the norms and none of the measures that should be been taken to avoid the damage and harm were, or else ill-treatment was accepted as either a minor or inevitable consequence (the former is known as *indirect wilful misconduct* and the latter *potential wilful misconduct*). Some jurists consider that if a State is responsible it makes no sense for intentionality of the specific perpetrating agent, for instance, to be legally debated because it is the system that acts through that person (i.e. in the Caso Algodonero – CIDH sentence). Alleging that a specific civil servant considers keeping a detainee naked and without food is 'standard procedure' – as some Uruguayan torturers did in Chapter 3, or justified by the United States Government under George Bush, should not be a cause to rule out torture.

When asserting that isolating out the State's responsibility is enough of a criterion for intentionality, what one is saying is that from a broader standpoint, intentionality can be inferred with no need to resort to dubious arguments regarding what the perpetrator thought or believed as the events were occurring, but instead from the torture environment indicators and interaction between the person exercising control and the person controlled. The Intentionality Assessment Checklist (Appendix 7) includes ten criteria for perpetrator intentionality and aims to be helpful in establishing this. Rather than a scale to quantify intentionality, it is a checklist of elements to bear in mind that come into play when evaluating intentionality.

Determination of purpose and alternatives

Determining purpose takes this one step further. Intention and purpose go hand and hand, and therefore when a purpose can be accredited, intentionality also is. And vice versa, it is hard to infer purpose if there is no proof of intentionality.

The Convention explicitly recognises four purposes, although it does leave the door open to others ('*such as . . .*'). Those that it recognises are closely tied to the State's role falling in line with safeguarding human rights: confession, intimidation, humiliation and punishment.[7] Ascertaining the perpetrator's intention is no simple matter, and it is one of the aspects that is left to the judge's discretion, which often means that s/he typically decides based on, for instance, his/her personal ideological position when weighing the individual's right to not be tortured against society's right to national security.

Here again, just as it makes no sense to aim to compile comprehensive lists of all methods of torture because the facts will always tend to supersede the list, and the underlying rationale for each must be sought instead, likewise, it makes no sense to establish a list of *purposes* and examine which additional purposes should be added to the four that are explicit in the definition. Other criteria, such as defencelessness put forward by Manfred Nowak (Nowak and McArthur, 2006) or 'obliterating personality' used by the Inter-American Convention seem to fall much more in line with the teleological principle, that is, they pursue substance as opposed to form. We have used this idea when putting forward the items in the Torturing Environment Scale, described in Chapter 18 and Appendix 5.

Delving into the perpetrator's mind: motivation

Lastly, the most complex step, beyond intentionality and purpose, is to ascertain motivation, i.e. the sociological and intra-psychic reasons that a person would torture someone else. This is doubtlessly the field that psychologists are most passionate about and with which philosophy and ethics have dealt amidst a host of experimental and theoretical models, which, generally speaking, concur (Bandura, 1999; Miller, 2004; Staub, 2003). *Grosso modo*, these theories can be divided into two paradigms. One is ecological and considers that anybody can become a perpetrator (Zimbardo, 2007, 2008) while the other paradigm considers that there are cognitive and personality traits providing an understanding of why certain persons are perpetrators and others not (perhaps Adorno can be cited as an emblematic figure). What is true is that it takes a certain combination of ecological *and* dispositional elements to generate a perpetrator (Haslam and Reicher, 2006; Miller, 2004). To a large extent because they have been detailed when describing torture training in Chapter 15, we have very briefly gone over some of the moral decision-making processes and have not gone into more global theories on perpetrating evil. This brief outline was more than enough to understand that this is complex and subjective and that a great deal of time may be spent on therapeutic work and personal thought to be able to demarcate individual processes and group influences whereby a specific person perpetrated evil. This holds true even more considering that exculpatory rational emotional and detachment can veil these aspects (Bandura, 1999).

This explains why these elements are not very pertinent legally speaking.[8] Yet these are precisely the decisive elements for developing pedagogical material to educate youth in values and design training programmes for State police forces and armies. Analysing individuals' motivations and group influence sets the groundwork for preventing torture in the future.

'Searching for the limits' as a solution in interrogation procedures

The definition of torture that emerged from the voice of torturers emphasised the art of searching for the limits of tolerance of the detainee, and finding the limit of physical and mental suffering that a particular detainee is capable of withstanding. According to that definition, there is no need to define the line between coercive interrogation and torture, because that limit is specific to each detainee (physical condition, age, tolerance, etc.) and the expert (torturer, psychologist, interrogator, etc.) is in the best position to 'sense' when the detainee is close to it.

This implies that there is a 'safety zone' that can be identified by the interrogator between what we called the Breaking Point of Resistance to Cooperation and the Breaking Point of Physical or Psychological Damage. What we saw in Chapter 3 was that such a safety zone does not in fact exist; it is a fantasy, like thinking that a trained landmines expert can prepare a minefield for the enemy and no civilians will be injured. Due to the nature of psychological damage (Chapter 8), when crossing certain limits that we know put the person in severe disequilibrium, it is impossible to be sure that the interrogator is not causing permanent damage.

In addition, the 'searching for the limit' solution assumes that a true professional can play with this imaginary line because he or she has the ability to *read* the suffering of others. But we have shown that suffering is a subjective experience, and social psychology shows how difficult it is to estimate the pain of others. Additionally, we learned that a person tends to justify his or her actions. People trained in the use of the Reid Technique tended to see juvenile delinquents as more mature and capable of enduring an 'adult' deceptive interrogation than interrogators trained in non-coercive interrogation. Like many other authors, Keller (2012), a former US soldier and author of *Torture Central*, exposed the slow but unavoidable process of getting involved in violence, normalising the abnormal and justifying the expansion of the 'limits' of what is acceptable. As time passes, the interrogator crosses one line of admissible conduct after another. Even if the interrogator wants to adhere to 'legal' procedures, he or she can easily slip into unauthorised territory if strict controls and regulations are not enforced.

Are behavioural psychologists the solution? Unfortunately, health professionals also believe in the fantasy of a safety zone. It is not a problem of possessing special skills or tools. The kind of damage we are evaluating does not appear mere hours or days following torture. He or she can assess how to press the detainee to extract information, but cannot assess how to protect the person in their 'care'. Pretending that psychologists who collaborate with interrogators are there to help protect detainees is simply untrue.

Is the answer to try to convert the *art* of searching for the limit into a *science* by developing a pre-planned log for each session (as seen in interrogations assisted by psychologists in Guantanamo)? Is it having a list of authorised procedures to control the interrogator? The 2014 Senate Intelligence Committee report clearly shows that these are not solutions. If we attempt these solutions, then the old (and false) idea that enough pressure will eventually produce results will prevail, and interrogators will resort to 'extraordinary measures' as soon as they need results.

Finally, we saw that there is a correlation between supporting torture as a necessary evil, and prejudice or desire for revenge or retaliation against the victim. Thus, in most cases the idea expressed by interrogators in Chapter 3 that they 'know' what is and isn't torture, that they know how to do the job without crossing the line into unprofessional behaviour, can be considered, at best, wishful thinking.

Alternative criteria: learning from a multidisciplinary view

The definitions raised earlier in this chapter open up the possibility of considering criteria other than those included in the UN's definition when determining the presence or absence of acts of torture from a legal or medical point of view. This possibility implies taking into account elements from other disciplines that are central to the concept of torture. Of particular importance are elements that involve (1) breaking the will of the subject, (2) a psychological break defined in terms of breakdown of the self and damage to identity and worldviews and (3) elements linked to the social and political context that suggest the existence of a *system* of torture. This will also help to resolve the gradient between torture and CIDT and allow for epidemiological research on torture.

In the next chapter we develop the necessary corollary: the formulation of an instrument that measures torturing environments.

Notes

1 There is, in fact, an additional view: that of society at large and the need for a shared truth.
2 An excellent example is the book *Torture: A Collection*, where Sanford Levinson (2004), the editor, asked for contributions from 18 prominent scholars who were for or against the legalisation of torture methods in certain circumstances. Levinson's conclusion (which ultimately only serves to disappoint the reader) is that society and legislators need to engage in further debate. The book shows how each contributor had a fixed opinion guided by his or her personal and political convictions, and that each of them tried to justify and convince others. The editor did not succeed in proposing a consensus among the contributors.
3 A principal components analysis of 46 captivity stressors revealed seven underlying factors: (1)*sexual torture* (e.g. rape, genital manipulation); (2) *physical torture* (beating, burning); (3) *psychological manipulation* (threats of torture, witnessing torture); (4) *humiliating treatment* (forced nudity, feces in food); (5) *forced stress positions* (forced standing for long periods, binding the body to restrict movement); (6) *sensory discomfort* (extreme cold, blindfolding); and (7) *deprivation of basic needs* (sleep, food) (Başoğlu, 2009).
4 To date, no one has tried to conduct a systematic Cochrane review of interrogation practices found (across studies) to produce serious damage to human health – practices which should, therefore, be banned. This is a challenge that remains to be resolved, probably when we have shared standardised tools.
5 The results of the experiment are not known and cannot be contrasted, although they were used to give legal support for using different techniques simultaneously. As explained in a memo from Steven G. Bradbury to John A. Rizzo: 'No apparent increase in susceptibility to severe pain has been observed either when techniques are used sequentially or when they are used simultaneously – for example, when an insult slap is simultaneously combined with water dousing or a kneeling stress position, or when wall-standing is simultaneously combined with an abdominal slap and water dousing. Nor does experience show that, even apart from changes in susceptibility to pain, combinations of these techniques cause the techniques to operate differently so as to cause severe pain. OMS doctors and psychologists, moreover, confirm that they expect that the techniques, when combined as described in the Background Paper and in the April 22 [redacted] Fax, would not operate in a different manner from the way they do individually, so as to cause severe pain' (Memorandum from Steven G. Bradbury, Principal Deputy Assistant Attorney General, for John A. Rizzo, Senior Deputy General Counsel, Central Intelligence Agency (10 May 2005): 12. Web. 11 Mar. 2010 http://i.cdn.turner.com/cnn/2009/images/05/22/bradbury3.pdf).
6 To a large extent, this book is based on the conventional definition of torture whose purpose is control although many of the situations described (such as sects or domestic violence) in Chapter 15 take place between private individuals.
7 In extreme cases, psychology can be used to construe the perpetrator as being actually a victim, and this was attempted by an expert advisor in a trial against one of the United States torturers in Iraq (Zimbardo, 2007). The torturer could be exonerated in the very rare event that s/he acted due to *force majeur*. (One example is the context of violence within paramilitary groups where certain members who were or are tortured must torture others or die.) But in this case, neither the intentionality or purpose criteria would be fulfilled and it does not seem that it would be necessary to resort to the more subjective criteria of motivation to exonerate the person.

18

A NEW OUTLOOK FOR DEFINING AND MEASURING TORTURING ENVIRONMENTS

Torturing environments instead of torture methods

Torture methods are always used in combination, never alone. We define a *torturing environment* as a milieu that creates the conditions for torture. It is made up of a group of contextual elements, conditions and practices that obliterate the will and control of the victim, compromising the self. This environment will amount to CIDT or torture when it has been generated for any of the purposes stated in the UNCAT: obtaining information or a confession, punishment, intimidation or coercion.[1]

In epidemiological terms, any element can be considered part of a torturing environment if it has been identified as likely to increase the relative risk of severe physical or psychological suffering, if it is used within the context of torture or if it is employed with the purpose of inflicting torture.

The idea of a torturing environment resolves many of the disputes and controversies surrounding the concept of torture. Politicians employ medical and psychological professionals to define the limits of acceptable suffering and to establish ethically 'acceptable' procedures. It is evident that this is an impossible endeavour. It is very difficult to determine the limits of human resilience. Moreover, conducting meaningful experimental research on torture is impossible for technical reasons,[2] and hardly acceptable because of obvious ethical concerns.

For this reason, research suggests *approximate* data in most cases. The rules at Guantanamo stated that the prisoners should sleep for *at least four continuous hours*, the Special Rapporteur on Torture suggested that solitary confinement should be limited to no more than 15 days and the World Health Organization suggested that prisoners must have at least six square meters of space in the cell. These are useful estimates, though they do not shed much light on the impact on prisoners or the sequelae they face following detention in such conditions. Four hours of sleep can be enough for someone used to sleeping little, or it can be the worst torture for a person with cluster migraines. And four hours of sleep do not have the same impact when used alone as when they are combined with dehydration, food restrictions, cold temperatures or continuous interrogation. Laboratory studies aimed to determine the tolerance of a human being to complete sensory isolation have found that while some people may begin hallucinating in less than ten minutes, others can resist for hours. But what is the effect of complete sensory isolation when the person is also hooded, handcuffed and terrified, fearing beatings or death at any moment?

This is exactly why the Behavioral Science Consultation Teams were incorporated into the process of interrogation at Guantanamo Bay. Knowing the limits of a person was (and is) considered an 'art': the army asks psychologists to use their expertise to determine if it is possible to continue an interrogation, if the person can endure more torture, and to identify the best ways to break him or her without provoking permanent damage.

We must abandon the idea of determining the limits of tolerance for individual torture methods, and shift our focus from the lab to real life by basing our understanding of torture on the complex combined effects of real scenarios and the way they act upon a detainee. This should be the focus of scientific research, epidemiological studies and informed political decisions. A necessary step in this direction is to establish measures that help determine the likelihood that torture will occur under this comprehensive and integrative view. That is why we have developed the Torturing Environment Scale (TES): a legal, medical and psychological measure of experiences and environments related to CIDT and torture.

The Torturing Environment Scale as a measurement tool

The idea of torturing environments and the possibility of measuring them is a major shift in the contemporary conceptualisation of torture. It provides a multifaceted and comprehensive way to face the problem of determining the existence of torture in general (and psychological torture in particular) and the conditions that promote it, based on a conceptual model that supports the construction and development of the TES.

Currently there is no tool to help visualise the combined effects of torturing methods. The TES meets this need (see the full scale with instructions for application in Appendix 5). The TES is based on a new paradigm by defining which human function is under attack, and grouping torture methods accordingly using a teleological approach (that is, organising methods according to a finite number of purposes – the intended impact they have on the person).

The scale can measure both torture *environments* and *experiences*. The TES is not a scale to assess psychological torture, as torture and psychological torture are two sides of the same coin and should not be considered as separate phenomena. Rather, it is a comprehensive scale the two, part and parcel of the same process.

The TES is not intended to quantify torture – or to measure the severity of suffering. Neither can be measured, because, as we have shown, each victim's experience is unique. Its aim is to serve as a guide for independent observers (e.g. decision-makers, judges, forensic experts, mental health professionals, researchers) by providing a comprehensive checklist of the main indicators of torture experiences or environments. Based on this list, the likelihood of a person's suffering torture can be determined. Furthermore, torturing scenario profiles can be defined. The TES does not distinguish between the legal concepts of CIDT and torture, although it provides strong arguments to qualify and define the facts. This is a legal distinction that is not medically or psychiatrically supported (see Chapter 17). It does, however, provide strong arguments for judicial officials.

Rationale

The TES provides an overview of risk factors for torture. The analysis focuses on conditions in the ethical, legal, medical, psychological and sociological contexts which offer a comprehensive view of a situation that is liable to constitute torture. Some indicators require the evaluator to acquire an emphatic and thorough understanding of the victim's experience. Other indicators can be evaluated based only on the narrative and testimony. The TES cannot be filled out as a simple questionnaire in the same way that a self-reported questionnaire would be, and no questions are posed directly to the survivor. The TES is best filled out after establishing trust with the survivor and getting to know each other, or after a visit to monitor detention conditions. Though ideally the TES would complement an evaluation based on the Istanbul Protocol, its structure allows a preliminary analysis pending further information.

The TES can also be applied as a collective measurement tool. In this sense its purpose would not be to assess the situation of a given person, but to provide an analysis of the conditions of a certain environment where people are held in custody. The TES can be a useful adjunctive tool for monitoring detention centres and reinforcing the work of National Prevention Mechanisms and NGOs.

Description

The TES does not need to be completed in a single interview. It is an open tool: information can be added in successive meetings as the evaluator gains knowledge of the person, the environment and the events.

It has 54 indicators of torture, 6 legal indicators and 12 medical and psychological corroborating elements.

Environment assessment: actions targeting the survivor's body and psyche

The scale looks at eight different blocks or groups of indicators (see Appendix 5) that follow the theoretical model represented in Figures 17.1 and 17.2. **Contextual manipulations** are attacks on basic physiological functions and environmental changes that would – in Jacobs' (2008) expression – disrupt the person's homeostasis: inhuman conditions of detention, sensory deprivation, restricting basic physiological functions, the use of time for generating confusion and anguish, and manipulation of environmental conditions. These types of manipulations relate to Biderman's (1961) 'monopolization of attention' concept and the KUBARK Manual's concept of 'forced absorption.'" **Fear-producing actions** target the need for security and preservation of life (threats of torture, threats to relatives, witnessing the torture of others, phobias and terror); **pain-producing actions** are attacks on the physical integrity of the person. These are distinguished from **extreme pain – mutilation – death** as suggested by most of the factorial analysis reviewed in Chapter 7 (Başoğlu, 2009; Phillips, 2011). **Actions against sexual integrity**, considered a specific, separate category, as shown in both the experience of survivors (see the testimonies of Jacqueline Gurruchaga and Beatriz Brenzano in Chapter 2) and factorial analysis of torture methods (Cunningham and Cunningham, 1997; Hooberman et al., 2007; Başoğlu, 2009; Phillips, 2011), **actions targeting the need for belonging, acceptance and care** include indicators related to isolation and breaking of ties (e.g. prolonged solitary confinement, incommunicado detention, cultural confinement [Koenig, 2013]). **Actions targeting needs of control, meaning and purpose** are elements that target the need for respect and dignity, question the inner sense of self, and provoke humiliation or shame, and attacks to cognitive, emotional and affective integrity, mostly linked to coercive interrogation techniques. For each block there are groups of torture methods organised teleologically (based on their function) within the overall torturing environment.

All of the blocks are open ended; the TES does not seek to define a limited or comprehensive set of torture methods, but rather classifies these methods according to their aims, or *targets*. We have seen that torture techniques are as infinite as the imagination of torturers. However, the number of targets *is* limited and can be properly defined.

There are six indicators related to **legal aspects**. Three indicators are criteria in the UNCAT definition of torture; the other two (the existence of a torturing system, and the demand for application of the exclusionary rule) are additional elements that signal the possible presence of torture from a legal point of view. Sometimes, even if a case does not fully fit the UNCAT definition, a court will rule that the case amounted to torture based on legal precedents. This is collected in the sixth indicator.

Medical and psychological indicators

The TES also has a list of additional corroborating items organised under **medical and psychological indicators**. These would likely fall outside the area of expertise of an assessor who is not a mental health professional. We refer to them as corroborating items because their presence supports the idea of torture, but their absence does not exclude torture – indeed, such absence may simply mean one is working with a resilient survivor. The medical and psychological indicators relate to the key elements of torture shown in Figures 17.1 and 17.2. Some involve clinical diagnoses (PTSD/Complex PTSD) that require the evaluation of a trained clinician.

We suggest that the TES be complemented with the Standardised Evaluation Form for Credibility Assessment (SEC) based on the Istanbul Protocol (see Appendix 6). This is a tool that should be used by a trained interviewer. It provides guidelines and criteria for the credibility analysis that a psychiatric forensic expert conducts based on the Istanbul Protocol.[3]

Instructions

Assessing the items

For each item on the scale, the person doing the assessment selects the most appropriate of three options: *No*, *Circumstantial or Limited* (C-L), or *Yes*:

Column 1. NO. Mark *No* when it is possible to reasonably ascertain that the indicator has not happened to the person (individual measure) or has never been documented in that location (collective measure). Leave it blank if there is *No Information Available* (NIA) and needs further clarification.

Column 2. C-L. *Present, but Circumstantial or Limited.* Mark *CC-LM* if the indicator has eventually appeared but it was not part of a systematic attack or one of the core techniques applied to the survivor. This is not a measure of the intensity of suffering, but a modulated assessment of the intensity and systematicity of the aggression.[4] For instance, a person may recall that he or she was treated in a humiliating way by a specific guard, but he or she felt that in general he or she was treated with respect during most of his detention; or a person may recall that while being detained during a demonstration, he or she was violently handcuffed and was repeatedly slapped by the police while being forced into a car. He or she recalls this, but does not attribute much importance to it and it has no physical or psychological consequences.

Column 3. YES. Mark *Yes* to signal the clear and consistent presence of the indicator according to the survivor's account. This is the core column of the TES. The allegations must be credible, and it is best to adopt a conservative approach to inconsistent statements (see Chapter 19 for more on credibility analysis in allegations of torture).

Sometimes there is a strong suspicion that the indicator happened. A survivor often needs time to open up and talk.[5] Decisive elements of the experience of torture may appear a long time after disclosure or after therapy was initiated.[6] It is not uncommon that the survivor has difficulty putting words to suffering. Feelings of shame or guilt, cultural factors, fragmented memories or dissociative states may prevent the person from describing the events clearly and thoroughly.

In exceptional cases, the person doing the assessment can mark *Yes* to signal the presence of the indicator if he or she:

- has *very* strong grounds to believe that the indicator of torture is present; and
- has marked at least 2 of the 12 corroborating medical or psychological indicators (in Part 2 of the TES) which he or she thinks relate to the torture indicator suspected to be present.

For example, one might strongly suspect the presence of Actions Targeting Sexual Integrity in a case involving a woman with mutism, severe depressive symptoms (corroborating elements 1, 2 and 9), and marks on her body, who was held in a detention camp where most women in her barracks were raped.

Note that the criteria to choose one indicator or another is the role of a certain action within the overall process of torture. For instance, *denying medical attention* when needed can be considered part of *inhuman conditions of detention* if denied regular attention (indicator 1), as a *pain-producing action*, if denied analgesia or treatment of a severe addiction in a drug addict (indicator 20), or even as *mutilation* if denial of medical attention results in the loss of a body part (indicator 27). *Forced feeding* of a prisoner can be a humiliating and debasing treatment (indicator 37), a pain-producing action (indicator 20), or an expression of absolute deprivation of will (indicator 45).

Many indicators include an additional bullet point for techniques or methods not included in the scale, and all subscales also have an additional point for actions not included in the available list of options. The TES is, in this sense, a living scale that can be adjusted to any context involving torture.

Measuring impact

Column 4. Impact. Additionally, the TES includes a column to measure *impact*. It should be marked when the indicator has great importance in the narrative of the survivor and is remembered as especially devastating. *Impact* is a key element for understanding the experience of the survivor. This column can be used to include a subjective evaluation of the contribution of a given indicator to the understanding of the sequelae in the survivor. *Impact* is related to the subjective perception of the survivor's experience, not to objective measurements of the severity of the situation (e.g. the number of days of continuous interrogation). For instance, a person might explain in his or her account that being naked in public was the most heinous and painful element of the experience, even more than being mistreated or beaten. For others, the indicator with maximum impact may have been the threat of rape against relatives or loved ones. Highlighting *impact* allows the evaluator to quickly detect the key elements of a torturing environment in a given population and helps to understand the deeper experience of survivors. In many cases we may not have access to such intimate information; in such cases the column is left blank.

Excerpts from a survivor's narrative are included at the end of this chapter. We invite the reader to practice filling out the TES based on this narrative (use copies from Appendix 5). You will likely discover that the survivor underwent many situations that are part of a torturing environment, but the experience she recognises as having affected her the most is probably not the one that the evaluator would have selected without taking *impact* into consideration.[7] Thus, the 'Impact' column in the TES highlights the importance of a particular indicator within the overall effect of the torturing environment from the point of view of the observer after working with the survivor.[8]

Sometimes it will be possible to connect the indicators that were more damaging in the victim's *subjective experience* with certain aspects of torture that were pre-planned and tailored to attack central aspects of the victim's identity. This would strongly support the motivational criteria that distinguishes CIDT from torture. Follow the scoring of the Torturing Environment Scale in Appendix 5.

Example of its application

Excerpts from an interview with Nagore X based on the Istanbul Protocol

The survivor was held for five days in incommunicado detention. We invite the reader to review her testimony, complete the TES based on her experience and compare the results with Table 18.1.

'They put me in a cell and started not allowing me to sleep. It was nighttime. I was exhausted from so much stress and from the ride there. I tried to sleep on a concrete bed, with no mattress or foam, and they began to beat me and turned on the light. I was told to stay standing in front of the peephole in order to be seen when they knocked on the door, and that's how it went every two or five minutes (. . .) I was scared, really scared, because I knew what was going to happen.'

Detention: Day 2

'It's humiliating, they are constantly humiliating you: they tell you that you're fat . . . I remember one detail, they said, "Yuck! She even has hairs on her nipples!" and other things like that; they stripped me and touched my breasts constantly. I was a little afraid that such things could go further and reach the point of rape. On one hand, they kept saying: "Yuck! I'm not fucking this one, because she has her period!" I thought, "Well . . . in the end, this is going to save me." But on the other hand, you don't know . . . You think: "Look: I'm an adult, I'm 32 years old." The nakedness you try to take in stride, but it brings about loads of impotence. You can't do anything, you're in their hands and you can't say, "You pig, take your hands off me!" Because you know it will be worse for you, so you just take it (. . .). And then from then on, they began the interrogation sessions. Well, in fact they had already started in the car, but there they asked questions again, about little things: "Where do you work? Where do you live?" And once you start to say something, they jump into questioning and bam! "Who recruited you?" If you keep quiet, they beat you, and then they start over again. (. . .) They used different techniques. They started with roles of the good and the bad cops. There was one, who was called "the coffee guy," who kept saying "Let's see, calm down . . . Let's have a coffee and talk." He was one of

TABLE 18.1 Torturing Environment Scale – Nagore X: summary sheet

TES – Summary Sheet

PART 1. Assessment of Environment Name: Nagore XXX

S: Score (0 = No, 1: CC–LMN, 2: Yes); I: Intensity Date: XX/XX/20XX

Contextual manipulations	S	I
1 a. Inhuman conditions of detention	0	
2 b. Environment conditions	1	
3 c. Basic physiological functions	0	
4 d. Sleep dysregulation	0	
5 e. Handling of time	1	
6 f. Sensory deprivation	1	
7 g. Mind-altering methods	0	
8 h. Other contextual manipulations		
Raw Score	3	

Fear-producing actions	S	I
9 a. Hopes and expectations	2	
10 b. Threats to the person	2	
11 c. Threats against family/ detainees	0	
12 d. Lack of information	0	
13 e. Experiences of near death	2	✓
14 f. Witnessing others' torture	0	
15 g. Phobias	0	
16 h. Other situations		
Raw Score	6	

Pain-producing actions	S	I
17 a. Beatings	1	
18 b. Battles against oneself	0	
19 c. Exhaustion exercises, forced work	2	
20 d. Other pain producing actions		
Raw Score	3	

Extreme pain – mutilation – death	S	I
21 a. Extreme pain	0	
22 b. Mutilation	0	
23 c. Brain damage	0	
24 d. Other (specify)		
Raw Score	0	

Actions targeting reproduction/ sexual integrity	S	I
25 a. Humiliation	2	
26 b. Sexual assault	2	✓
27 c. Rape	0	
28 d. Other (targeting sexual integrity)		
Raw Score	5	

Actions targeting the need to belong	S	I
29 a. Prolonged solitary confinement Incommunicado detention Cultural isolation	0	
30 b. Breaking social bonds	2	
31 c. Manipulation of affect	1	
32 d. Other (targeting need to belong)		
Raw Score	3	

Actions targeting identity [breaking/instilling new one]	S	I
33 a. Beliefs and worldviews Attacks on sense of self	0	
34 b. Helplessness induced	1	
35 c. Instilling guilt	0	
36 d. Induced shame	2	
37 e. Induced humiliation	2	✓
38 f. Violation of moral principles	0	

39	g. Installing goals and identity	0	
40	h. Other (targeting identity)		
	Raw Score	5	

Coercive interrogation techniques	S	I
41 a. Conditions during interrogation	2	
42 b. Style of interrogation	2	
43 c. Deception/cognitive manipulation	1	✓
44 d. Other (extreme coercive actions)		
Raw Score	5	

PART 2. Manner of Interaction

Relational indicators	S	I
45 a. Will	2	
46 b. Violation of autonomy	2	✓
47 c. Fostering unpredictability	1	
48 d. Systematic violation of dignity	1	✓
49 e. Personalised process	1	
50 f. Extreme signs of evil or cruelty	1	
51 g. Vulnerability factors	2	
52 h. Active role in own suffering	0	
53 i. Prolonged harm (physical/mental)	0	
54 j. Other (relational factors)		
Raw Score	10	

PART 3. Legal Criteria

Legal criteria	YES
1. Institutional agents	✓
2. Torturing system criteria	✓
3. Clear purpose or motivation – confession	✓
4. Clear purpose of punishment, humiliation or revenge	
5. Exclusionary rule	✓
6. Legal precedents	✓

PART 4. Medico-Psychological Criteria

Medical and psychological indicators Due to one or more of the above techniques, and within the cultural and social context of the examinee:	YES
1. Confusion or disorientation	
2. Anguish, fear or terror	✓
3. Emotional or cognitive exhaustion	✓
4. Signs of emotional manipulation	
5. Signs of damage to identity	
6. Brain damage	
7. Other acute medical disorders	✓
8. Chronic medical sequelae	
9. Acute or chronic PTSD	✓
10. Complex – PTSD/EPCACE	
11. Dissociative states	
12. Other relevant conditions	✓

(continued)

TABLE 18.1 Torturing Environment Scale (*continued*)

Part 1 TORTURING ENVIRONMENT	C-L (x1)	Yes (x2)	CF	Score	1	2	3	4	5	6	7	8	9	10	11	12	13	14	15	16	I
Block 1. Contextual manipulations	3	0		3																	
Block 2. Fear-producing actions	0	3		6																	✓
Block 3. Pain-producing actions	1	1	X2	6																	
Block 4. Extreme pain – mutilation – death	0	0	X2	0																	
Block 5. Sexual integrity	0	2	X2	8																	✓
Block 6. Attachment and need to belong	1	1	X2	6																	
Block 7. Actions targeting identity	1	2		5																	✓
Block 8. Coercive interrogation	1	2	X2	10																	✓
Overall Score (Sum of totals for each Block)				**44**	Mark YES if there is either [a] at least one FULL criteria in any of the 8 Blocks, or [b] an overall score or 5 or more.										YES ✓				NO

Part 2 RELATIONAL INDICATORS	CC-LM	Yes	*Overall Score*	Mark YES if there are at least 2 FULL relational criteria or an overall score of 5 or more.	YES ✓	NO
	4	3	**10**			

Part 3 LEGAL INDICATORS	1	2	3	4	5	6	Mark YES if legal criteria 1 and legal criteria 3 or 4 (or both) are fulfilled. Exceptionally consider criteria 6.	YES ✓	NO
	✓	✓	✓		✓				

Part 4 MEDICO-PSYCHOLOGICAL INDICATORS	NUMBER 5	Mark YES if there is at least 1 medico-psychological criterion	YES ✓	NO

ENVIRONMENTAL CONDITIONS AMOUNT TO TORTURE	NO	PARTIALLY	(YES)

Conditions amount to torture if
• Criteria of Part 1, 2 and 4 are fulfilled
Allegations additionally supported if
• Criteria of Part 3 are fulfilled
• There is an overall consistency of allegations according to the SEC

Psychological versus Physical Torture Methods

TORTURE	Blocks + Items	Weight	Method Score
Manipulation of Environment	[Block 1] + [items 29, 41]	Divide by 2	5/2: **2.5**
Mostly based on **Physical Pain**	[Block 3]+[Block 4]+ [items 3, 13, 27, 50]	Divide by 4	9/4: **2.2**
Mostly based on **Psychological Pain**	[Block 2]+[Block 6]+[Block 7]+ [Block 8] + [items 25, 26, 47]	Divide by 7	32/7: **4.5**

Sum as indicated and weight.

the good cops, and this was a constant throughout the five days . . . [Laughing] *In the end I don't remember if I ever got to drink that coffee . . . And then there were more interrogation sessions, and when he didn't like my answers, it got harder. (. . .) They take pieces of information from this guy, and from that guy, and they compile it. Then there are things you say when you have no answers, not even within yourself, and you say, "What can I do?" They told me they needed names, because they don't believe that you really don't know; "Come on, give us some answers" . . . And then they pull the bag over your head until you suffocate, until you give them a name. And again, and again . . . And you end up end up telling them about friends, giving names of people you don't know . . . Keeping silent is a victory over them, and the more you talk, the more you lose; besides, you say things that you don't even know are true.'*

'I was shocked, and I kept quiet, and they started hitting me on the head with something rolled up, like a magazine or something like that. (. . .) They beat me, and went on asking me. (. . .) I have no bruises, no marks, so I can't prove anything, either with the forensic doctor or with anyone else.'

'At that time I did not think, I just tried to sleep. I was obsessed with relaxing from the stress. I curled up in a fetal position, thinking about all that I had said and not said.'

Days 3–5

'They took me down the hall, head bowed, as usual, and eyes closed; and when I was to get in the interrogation room, they made me raise my head, and they stood behind me, so I couldn't see them. (. . .) I didn't know where I was or what I was doing there; they took me into a room and started asking me questions again. I don't know if they wanted to involve me in some other story . . . They rolled me into a blanket with only underwear on and tied me to a table leaving my head hanging off the table (. . .). They pulled the bag on my head. (. . .) The blanket is what broke me down completely, because I did not expect it. And besides, I peed on myself when I lost consciousness, another reason for humiliation. (. . .) [From that moment onwards] I was broken, that is the truth.'

'When they put "la bolsa" [the bag] on me, what I did was to try to push down my chin to stop them from tightening the bag so much, so that later when it loosened a bit, some air could flow in from below. But with my head [hanging off the back of the table], I couldn't do that. The body, in that situation, tends to escape because you are strong, [but] there were four people holding my body down.'

'I am half naked and they are putting things between my legs, sticks at crotch height, and then they tell you to "Get down!" so that the stick rubs against your genitals. These guys are obsessed with sex (. . .). It's a constant pattern.'

'I had to do "squats" to the point of exhaustion with my head covered by a woolen garment which hindered my breathing while my trousers and underwear had been pulled down. And more questions . . . And if they do not like what you answered, they force you to do squats, and up and down, and if you get tired you have to stretch your arms out, until you can't take any more, and then . . . a blow. And then the bag again, and again with the bag until you suffocated . . . And they got you undressed. . . and they tied you to a chair . . . . And squats and more squats . . . And then back to the cell, again.'

'They filled out [the police statement] as if they knew about you, and made you repeat the answers they wanted. Some of the things were things I had said in the interrogation and others weren't. They made you memorize the police statement: "When they ask you this, you say . . ." just like that, until I was ready. And they take you to a man who introduces himself to you as a lawyer, at a computer, and he asks you the same questions, and makes you sign; but I didn't sign it because even though I'd made those declarations, I disagreed. "You're not going to sign?! Come on . . . You are going to sign blank papers!" So once again they undressed me, [made me do] squats, until I signed.'

The TES shows that:

- It can be ascertained beyond reasonable doubt that Nagore was subjected to torture, according to [a] methods which were used on her (Part 1), [b] relational indicators (Part 2) and [c] legal aspects. The medical and psychological indicators also support the conclusion that she was tortured.
- Her torture was a short-term (five days) incommunicado detention (Block 6), in which interrogators used fear (Block 2), moderate but constant Pain (Block 3), attacks on identity (Block 7), and especially actions targeting sexual integrity (Block 5) in the context of an extremely coercive interrogation (Block 8).
- Globally she was submitted to environmental manipulations (2.5/10), physical pain (2.2/10) and psychological pain (4.5/10). Her torture was, thus, mainly psychological, although environmental manipulation and physical methods for torture were also used.
- She showed long-lasting psychological impact from her days of detention.
- The three elements that help better understand the long term impact of her experience were:
  [13] Experiences of near death (dry asphyxia)
  [37] Induced shame/humiliation (debasement based on physical appearance, forced to perform humiliating acts; being exposed in public; personal hygiene prevented; debasement based on cultural and socio–political background)
  [43] Conditions of interrogation that foster false confessions: lies; cognitive manipulation – cognitive exhaustion

Examples of torturing environment profiles

The following are examples of the application of the TES. They show different profiles of torturing environments based on two cases of survivors from Chapter 2, and three additional cases that could be especially difficult to elucidate for various reasons.

Vann Nath: survivor of the Khmer Rouge

In his memoir, Vann Nath describes hunger as an extremely painful torture method, and the slow death of the body as a method for breaking the psyche. His text also describes the environment of terror and the permanent state of fear and panic while waiting for the final moment of torture and killing, watching trucks arriving with new detainees and hearing how the newcomers were also tortured and disappeared. Time periods without limits, the total absence of hope and constant signs of evil and cruelty all caused irreversible damage to his worldviews. The TES gives a profile of a devastating system of destruction.

The TES final summary indicates that:

- Mr. Van Nath was subjected to torture, according to: [a] methods which were used on him (Part 1), [b] relational indicators (Part 2), and [c] legal aspects (Part 3). There are strong grounds to suspect, based on his memoir, strong medical and psychological consequences (Part 4).
- The torture methods used ranked the highest possible scores in almost all possible categories of physical and psychological attacks. In the TES, torture can be identified if scores are higher than 5 and fulfil one full criteria in Part 1. Mr. Van Nath scores 92 and fulfils criteria in all categories (contextual manipulations, fear-producing actions, pain-producing actions, extreme pain and mutilation, actions targeting attachment and need to belong, actions targeting identity and coercive interrogation techniques).
- His torture was prolonged (more than two years). During that time he was starved nearly to death and continuously interrogated in a context of extreme fear and pain, with the purpose of changing his identity to match the Khmer Rouge's vision of the new society. Hunger is remembered not as a manipulation of environment (Block 1) but as extremely painful and unbearable situation, a method to slowly kill the victim (Block 4).
- Treatment constitutes torture when there are at least two relational indicators. Mr. Van Nath fulfils seven out of ten (deprived of will, violation of autonomy, fostering unpredictability, systematic violation of dignity, extreme signs of evil or cruelty, active role in own suffering, and harm prolonged over time).
- He showed long-standing psychological impacts from his days of detention. The three elements that help better understand the deep impact of his experience are:
    [14] Cruelty/seeing others die
    [24] Hunger
    [41] [43] Conditions and style of interrogation

Carlos Liscano: The Truck of Fools

We learned from Liscano's experience in Chapter 2. In his testimony he gives a detailed account of nine months of daily torture suffered in Uruguay, with a unique description of the psychological mechanisms of destruction of identity, and the complexities of the relationships between the victim and the torturer and the victim and his own body. He rightly affirms that torture is unique for each person. The process of being alone with the pain, of trying to stay

TABLE 18.2 TES – Examples of application: Vann Nath

Part 1 TORTURING ENVIRONMENT	C-L (x1)	Yes (x2)	CF	Score	1	2	3	4	5	6	7	8	9	10	11	12	13	14	15	16	I
Block 1. Contextual manipulations	0	6		12																	
Block 2. Fear-producing actions	0	7		14																	
Block 3. Pain-producing actions	0	4	X2	16																	
Block 4. Extreme pain – mutilation – death	0	3	X2	12																	✓
Block 5. Sexual integrity	0	0	X2	0																	
Block 6. Attachment and need to belong	0	2	X2	8																	
Block 7. Actions targeting identity	0	7		14																	
Block 8. Coercive interrogation	0	4	X2	16																	✓
Overall Score (Sum of totals for each Block)				**92**	Mark YES if there is either [a] at least one FULL criteria in any of the 8 Blocks, or [b] an overall score or 5 or more.														YES ✓		NO

Part 2 RELATIONAL INDICATORS	CC-LM	Yes	Overall Score								
	0	7	14	Mark YES if there are at least 2 FULL relational criteria or an overall score of 5 or more.				YES ✓		NO

Part 3 LEGAL INDICATORS	1	2	3	4	5	6				
	✓	✓	✓	✓			Mark YES if legal criteria 1 and legal criteria 3 or 4 (or both) are fulfilled. Exceptionally consider criteria 6.	YES ✓	NO

Part 4 MEDICO-PSYCHOLOGICAL INDICATORS	NUMBER 7	Mark YES if there is at least 1 medico-psychological criterion	YES ✓	NO

ENVIRONMENTAL CONDITIONS AMOUNT TO TORTURE	Conditions amount to torture if • Criteria of Part 1, 2 and 3 are fulfilled Allegations additionally supported if • Criteria of Part 4 are fulfilled • There is an overall consistency of allegations according to the SEC	NO	PARTIALLY	(YES)

oriented despite manipulation and deceit, and the unbearable anguish of suffocation in the *tacho* (waterboarding), are all unique. So too is the ambivalence and the feeling of dependency and hatred towards the torturer.

According to his memoir, the TES final summary indicates that:

- Mr. Liscano was subjected to torture, according to: [a] methods which were used on him (Part 1), [b] relational indicators (Part 2) and [c] legal aspects (Part 3). The medical and psychological indicators (Part 4) also support the overall conclusion.
- Torture methods fell into the highest possible range of scores, especially in actions producing fear and pain, actions targeting identity and actions targeting attachment and need to belong. He was also subject to constant coercive interrogations.
- It can be said that torture has occurred when there are at least two relational indicators. Mr. Liscano fulfills eight out of ten (deprived of will, violation of autonomy, fostering unpredictability, systematic violation of dignity, torture as a personalised process, extreme signs of evil or cruelty, active role in own suffering and harm prolonged over time). The combined effect of these elements, more than any specific torture method, offers a portrait of a torturing system, including a full torturing environment and a torturing relationship.
- His torture was prolonged (more than nine months). Although he showed long-standing psychological impact from his days of detention, The two elements that help better understand the deep impact of his experience are:
  [18] Forced self-produced pain/Battle against oneself
  [41] Conditions of coercive interrogation
- He can be comparatively considered, with the passing of years, as a resilient survivor who managed to give meaning to his experience and slowly gain control over the consequences.

Ana: aggression and arbitrary detention during a mass protest

Country: Italy

Events: Ana is detained during an antiglobalisation protest. She is part of a group that is staying in a school that also serves as a media centre. The police break into the school in an extremely violent way and indiscriminately beat everyone present. There is widespread panic and many people are seriously injured. Ana is beaten on the head and arms, and (together with others) taken to the police station in a police van. At the station she is frisked, inappropriately touched and insulted; they take her photo, and she is fingerprinted. Then she is transferred to an old military barracks that has been refurbished as a detention centre. At the entrance, she is frisked again, and a police officer draws a red cross on the foreheads of several detainees and laughs. There she is forced to remain standing for hours, facing the wall, without eating, drinking or going to the bathroom. Once in a while a police officer comes in and insults them. Some of the detainees are kicked and slapped, but she isn't. After eighteen hours she is frisked again and, finally, released. When she gets home she goes to the nearest hospital, and is examined because of the pain she is in; they certify that she has a fractured rib and hematomas all over her body from the beatings.

TABLE 18.3 TES – Examples of application: Carlos Liscano

Part 1 TORTURING ENVIRONMENT	C-L (x1)	Yes (x2)	CF	Score	1	2	3	4	5	6	7	8	9	10	11	12	13	14	15	16	I
Block 1. Contextual manipulations	0	6		12																	
Block 2. Fear-producing actions	0	8		16																	
Block 3. Pain-producing actions	0	3	X2	12																	✓
Block 4. Extreme pain – mutilation – death	0	1	X2	4																	
Block 5. Sexual integrity	0	2	X2	8																	
Block 6. Attachment and need to belong	0	3	X2	12																	
Block 7. Actions targeting identity	0	6		12																	✓
Block 8. Coercive interrogation	0	3	X2	12																	

| Overall Score (Sum of totals for each Block) | | | | 88 | Mark YES if there is either [a] at least one FULL criteria in any of the 8 Blocks, or [b] an overall score of 5 or more. | | | | | | | | | | | | | | YES ✓ | | NO |

| Part 2 RELATIONAL INDICATORS | CC-LM 0 | Yes 8 | | Overall Score 16 | Mark YES if there are at least 2 FULL relational criteria or an overall score of 5 or more. | | | | | | | | | | | | | | YES ✓ | | NO |

| Part 3 LEGAL INDICATORS | 1 ✓ | 2 ✓ | 3 ✓ | 4 | 5 ✓ | 6 ✓ | Mark YES if legal criteria 1 and legal criteria 3 or 4 (or both) are fulfilled. Exceptionally consider criteria 6. | | | | | | | | | | | | YES ✓ | | NO |

| Part 4 MEDICO-PSYCHOLOGICAL INDICATORS | NUMBER 4 | | | | Mark YES if there is at least 1 medico-psychological criterion | | | | | | | | | | | | | | YES ✓ | | NO |

| ENVIRONMENTAL CONDITIONS AMOUNT TO TORTURE | Conditions amount to torture if • Criteria of Part 1, 2 and 3 are fulfilled Allegations additionally supported if • Criteria of Part 4 are fulfilled • There is an overall consistency of allegations according to the SEC | | | | | | | | | | NO | | | | PARTIALLY | | | | (YES) |

According to the Istanbul Protocol interview the TES final summary indicates that:

- Ana was subjected to torture, according to: [a] methods which were used on her (Part 1), [b] relational indicators (Part 2) and [c] legal aspects (Part 3). The medical and psychological indicators (Part 4) also support the overall conclusion.
- She was subjected to pain-producing actions, and during certain moments during her detention, she was subjected to conditions of environmental manipulation and fear-producing actions.
- She was subjected to a relationship with the detention officers that can be considered as torture-prone through violation of autonomy. She was also held in a context of violation of dignity, and was forced to play an active role in her own suffering (through prolonged stress positions).
- She had acute medical disorders attributable to the alleged events: a broken rib and hematomas documented in a subsequent hospital report. There were no psychological consequences at the time of the interview.

Khadim: racial profiling

Country: Spain

Events: Khadim is detained at a local police checkpoint at 7:00 PM for vending goods in a street market without a license. After asking for his papers, he's taken into a doorway and verbally attacked. Bystanders stop and protest the police's actions and someone begins to record what happens on a cell phone, causing the police to release Khadim. Two hours later, after nightfall, when Khadim is walking down a quiet street to a homeless shelter, two police cars appear and block his path – one in front of him and one behind. Several plainclothes officers get out and walk towards him, mentioning what happened a few hours earlier and saying that he's not going to make a fool of the police. They beat him violently for approximately three minutes. They punch and kick him. They throw him to the ground, causing him to hit the back of his head, and they continue kicking him. Then they handcuff him and take him to the hospital where he is attended to and detained. The police charge him with disobeying authority and accuse him of calling them racist, spitting on them and attacking them.

According to the Istanbul Protocol interview the TES final summary for Khadim indicates that:

- He was subjected to torture methods (fear and pain production and actions targeting identity) although in a limited or circumstantial way. Although there are indicators of being submitted to elements of a torturing environment, the overall score does not suggest it could amount to torture.
- He was subjected to a relationship with the acting officers that can be considered torture-prone (factors associated with increased vulnerability and, partially, torture as a personalised process), although overall it does not appear sufficient to qualify it as a relationship involving torture.
- He was in custody and there are clear elements of racial punishment in the beatings.
- At the time (and since then), he has shown steady signs of anguish, fear and terror.

Overall: The case fulfils the legal requirements for torture. Khadim was PARTIALLY SUBJECTED to torturing conditions and the case requires a careful evaluation of the context and personal circumstances. The fact that he suffers long-standing psychological consequences

TABLE 18.4 TES – Examples of application: Ana

Part 1 TORTURING ENVIRONMENT	C-L (x1)	Yes (x2)	CF	Score	1	2	3	4	5	6	7	8	9	10	11	12	13	14	15	16	I
Block 1. Contextual manipulations	3	0		3																	
Block 2. Fear-producing actions	2	0		2																	
Block 3. Pain-producing actions	1	1	X2	6																	
Block 4. Extreme pain – mutilation – death	0	0	X2	0																	
Block 5. Sexual integrity	0	0	X2	0																	
Block 6. Attachment and need to belong	0	0	X2	0																	
Block 7. Actions targeting identity	0	0		0																	
Block 8. Coercive interrogation	0	0	X2	0																	
Overall Score (Sum of totals for each Block)				11	Mark YES if there is either [a] at least one FULL criteria in any of the 8 Blocks, or [b] an overall score or 5 or more.														YES ✓		NO

| Part 2 RELATIONAL INDICATORS | CC-LM 3 | YES 1 | | Overall Score 5 | Mark YES if there are at least 2 FULL relational criteria or an overall score of 5 or more. | | | | | | | | | | | | | | YES ✓ | | NO |
| | 1 ✓ | 2 | 3 | 4 ✓ | 5 | 6 ✓ | | | | | | | | | | | | | | | |

| Part 3 LEGAL INDICATORS | | | | | Mark YES if legal criteria 1 and legal criteria 3 or 4 (or both) are fulfilled. Exceptionally consider Criteria 6. | | | | | | | | | | | | | | YES ✓ | | NO |

| Part 4 MEDICO-PSYCHOLOGICAL INDICATORS | NUMBER 1 | | | | Mark YES if there is at least 1 medico-psychological criterion | | | | | | | | | | | | | | YES ✓ | | NO |

| ENVIRONMENTAL CONDITIONS AMOUNT TO TORTURE | Conditions amount to Torture if
 • Criteria of Part 1, 2 and 3 are fulfilled
 Allegations additionally supported if
 • Criteria of Part 4 are fulfilled
 • There is an overall consistency of allegations according to the SEC | | | | | | | | NO | | | | PARTIALLY | | | (YES) | | |

TABLE 18.5 TES – Examples of application: Khadim

Part 1 TORTURING ENVIRONMENT	C-L (x1)	Yes (x2)	CF	Score	1	2	3	4	5	6	7	8	9	10	11	12	13	14	15	16	I
Block 1. Contextual manipulations	0	0		0																	
Block 2. Fear-producing actions	1	0		1																	
Block 3. Pain-producing actions	1	0	X2	1																	
Block 4. Extreme pain – mutilation – death	0	0	X2	0																	
Block 5. Sexual integrity	0	0	X2	0																	
Block 6. Attachment and need to belong	0	0	X2	0																	
Block 7. Actions targeting identity	0	1		2																	
Block 8. Coercive interrogation	0	0	X2	0																	
Overall Score (Sum of totals for each Block)				**4**	Mark YES if there is either [a] at least one FULL criteria in any of the 8 Blocks, or [b] an overall score or 5 or more.														YES ✓		NO

Part 2 RELATIONAL INDICATORS	CC-LM 1	Yes 1	*Overall Score* 3	Mark YES if there are at least 2 FULL relational criteria or an overall score of 5 or more.	YES	NO ✓

Part 3 LEGAL INDICATORS	1 ✓	2	3	4 ✓	5	6	Mark YES if legal criteria 1 and legal criteria 3 or 4 (or both) are fulfilled. Exceptionally consider criteria 6.	YES ✓	NO

Part 4 MEDICO-PSYCHOLOGICAL INDICATORS	NUMBER 1	Mark YES if there is at least 1 medico-psychological criterion	YES ✓	NO

ENVIRONMENTAL CONDITIONS AMOUNT TO TORTURE	Conditions amount to torture if • Criteria of Part 1, 2 and 3 are fulfilled Allegations additionally supported if • Criteria of Part 4 are fulfilled • There is an overall consistency of allegations according to the SEC	NO	(PARTIALLY)	YES

from the events, as certified by a forensic expert, supports the idea that his treatment could amount to torture.

Pedro: torture at the hands of drug dealers

Country: Honduras

Events: Pedro is 16 years old and belongs to a church group that does work in his neighbourhood. His cousin pressured him to join a gang that works for local drug dealers. After receiving death threats against himself and his mother, he agrees to do some 'deliveries' in the neighbourhood. During one of these deliveries he is captured by a rival gang who demands that he tell them which safe house his cousin is staying in. They hang him from a tree, and they proceed to beat him and threaten him with a gun (including several mock executions) for over 10 hours. They use a knife to cut him all over his body, including his genitals. They intended to decapitate him, but the police rescued him after an anonymous call.

According to the Istanbul Protocol interview the TES final summary of Pedro indicates that:

- He was subjected, beyond a doubt, to physical and psychological torture methods, some of them extreme.
- He was subjected to a relationship with the persons who detained him that can be considered to be a torture process. It fulfils five out of seven criteria of a relationship involving torture.
- He was not held under the control of a public institution (or anyone acting in an official capacity or with the knowledge or acquiescence of a public authority). There are no similar cases in Honduras' domestic jurisprudence in which it has been determined that torture has occurred.
- At the time, and since then, he showed steady signs of anguish, fear and terror.

Overall: Pedro was subjected to torture according to environmental and relational criteria; this is further supported by medico–psychological criteria. But the case does not fulfil the legal requirements for torture. This does not mean that a judge, taking the context and circumstances into consideration, wouldn't consider this treatment to be torture by arguing that the state is ultimately responsible for the events or by making a specific interpretation of national laws.

Inma: victim of sex trafficking

Country: Brazil

Events: Inma is 26 years old and lives in Asunción, Paraguay. She has two daughters, and both she and her husband are unemployed. An agency offers her work as a caretaker for elderly people in Brazil. When she arrives at the appointed location she is given lodging, and an older woman meets her and keeps her passport. She soon realises that she can't leave the building, and that she's trapped in a prostitution ring. The next day, several men enter her room and explain that she has to work in a club to pay her debt for the travel expenses to Brazil, which is several thousand dollars. When she tries to leave she is repeatedly raped and beaten by three men. The beatings and rapes continue for over a week, even though she no longer puts up any resistance. They tell her they have people in Paraguay,

TABLE 18.6 TES – Examples of application: Pedro

Part 1 TORTURING ENVIRONMENT	C-L (x1)	Yes (x2)	CF	Score	1	2	3	4	5	6	7	8	9	10	11	12	13	14	15	16	I
Block 1. Contextual manipulations	0	0		0																	
Block 2. Fear-producing actions	1	4		8																	
Block 3. Pain-producing actions	0	2	X2	8																	
Block 4. Extreme pain – mutilation – death	0	2	X2	0																	✓
Block 5. Sexual integrity	1	0	X2	2																	
Block 6. Attachment and need to belong	0	0	X2	0																	
Block 7. Actions targeting identity	0	0		0																	
Block 8. Coercive interrogation	0	2	X2	8																	

Overall Score (Sum of totals for each Block)	**26**	Mark YES if there is either [a] at least one FULL criteria in any of the 8 Blocks, or [b] an overall score or 5 or more.	YES ✓	NO

Part 2 RELATIONAL INDICATORS	CC-LM 1	Yes 5	Overall Score **11**	Mark YES if there are at least 2 FULL relational criteria or an overall score of 5 or more.	YES ✓	NO

Part 3 LEGAL INDICATORS	CC-LM 1	1	2	3 ✓	4	5	6	Mark YES if legal criteria 1 and legal criteria 3 or 4 (or both) are fulfilled. Exceptionally consider criteria 6.	YES	NO ✓

Part 4 MEDICO-PSYCHOLOGICAL INDICATORS	NUMBER 1	Mark YES if there is at least 1 medico-psychological criterion	YES ✓	NO

ENVIRONMENTAL CONDITIONS AMOUNT TO TORTURE	Conditions amount to torture if • Criteria of Part 1, 2 and 3 are fulfilled. Allegations additionally supported if • Criteria of Part 4 are fulfilled • There is an overall consistency of allegations according to the SEC	NO	*PARTIALLY*	YES

and that if she tries to escape they will go look for her family and burn them alive. For four years, she remains kidnapped in the club, forced to work nonstop shifts. She suffers regular humiliation and abuse and does not earn any money for her work. She is freed by the police during a raid; they discovered the operation after one of the other women succeeded in escaping the house.

According to the Istanbul Protocol interview the TES final summary for Inma indicates that:

- She was subjected, beyond a doubt, to physical and psychological torture methods: in addition to attacks on sexual integrity (including forced prostitution), she was also subjected to contextual manipulations (time, space, environment, etc.), extreme fear-producing actions and actions attacking identity and attachment.
- According to the TES, she had a relationship with her captors involving torture (deprived of will, violation of autonomy, situation fosters unpredictability, systematic violation of dignity, signs of evilness or cruelty, vulnerability factors, forced to play an active role in her own suffering and prolonged physical and mental harm).
- She showed permanent psychological consequences (chronic and complex PTSD and dissociative states related to the events).

Although the case does not fulfil the legal criteria for torture, there are many precedents of similar cases that were found to constitute torture which take into consideration the responsibility of the state to dismantle trafficking networks and protect immigrants from human trafficking.

Although the TES indicates that the case would not strictly be considered torture, the evaluator concludes that in the context in which he works there are sufficient legal precedents of trafficking which have been found to constitute torture by a court.

Further steps: from torturing environments to psychological torture

The definition and study of *torturing environments* brings us closer to a definition of psychological torture. The TES shows that some actions or attacks are considered torture in and of themselves; their mere existence points to torture. Rape is the best example. There is ample legal support for the idea that rape must be considered a form of torture in itself (Littleton, 2007; McGlynn, 2009; McHenry, 2002; Schwartz, 1994; Zawati, 2007). Other examples include prolonged sensory deprivation and mutilations. If the other requirements for identifying torture are met (motivation, acting in an official capacity), there is little doubt that the acts amount to torture.

Further research is needed to determine if it is possible to establish rough criteria that can help in other situations, and if there are certain combinations or patterns of *torturing environments* that can be also considered torture in themselves.

Torturing environments and documenting torture

The TES provides an overview of the experience of torture, but it should not substitute other methodologies that are closer to the direct experience of torture survivors. In the future, the TES will help compare patterns of torture across different countries, contexts and historical moments, map torture's evolution and work accordingly. However, the best way to create a map of a torturing environment is to work directly with the testimonies of survivors. A trans-theoretical tool like the TES helps to pool knowledge, but it risks neglecting idiosyncratic elements and specific experiences.

TABLE 18.7 TES – Examples of application: Inma

Part 1 TORTURING ENVIRONMENT	C-L (x1)	Yes (x2)	CF	Score	1–16	I
Block 1. Contextual manipulations	0	3		6		
Block 2. Fear-producing actions	0	6		12		
Block 3. Pain-producing actions	1	1	X2	6		
Block 4. Extreme pain – mutilation – death	0	2	X2	0		
Block 5. Sexual integrity	0	4	X2	16		✓
Block 6. Attachment and need to belong	0	2	X2	8		
Block 7. Actions targeting identity	0	4		8		
Block 8. Coercive interrogation	0	0	X2	0		
Overall Score (Sum of totals for each Block)				**53**		

Mark YES if there is either [a] at least one FULL criteria in any of the 8 Blocks, or [b] an overall score or 5 or more. — **YES ✓** **NO**

Part 2 RELATIONAL INDICATORS	CC-LM	Yes		Overall Score
	1	8		**17**

Mark YES if there are at least 2 FULL relational criteria or an overall score of 5 or more. — **YES ✓** **NO**

Part 3 LEGAL INDICATORS	1	2	3	4	5	6
	1	2	3	4	5	6 ✓

Mark YES if legal criteria 1 and legal criteria 3 or 4 (or both) are fulfilled. Exceptionally consider criteria 6. — **YES** **NO ✓**

Part 4 MEDICO-PSYCHOLOGICAL INDICATORS	NUMBER
	6

Mark YES if there is at least 1 medico-psychological criterion — **YES ✓** **NO**

ENVIRONMENTAL CONDITIONS AMOUNT TO TORTURE if

Conditions amount to torture if
- Criteria of Part 1, 2 and 3 and fulfilled

Allegations additionally supported if
- Criteria of Part 4 are fulfilled
- There is an overall consistency of allegations according to the SEC

NO | PARTIALLY | (YES)

Collecting testimonies, transcribing them, analysing them through software-aided qualitative methodology, elaborating a thesaurus of methods from the experience of survivors, and trying to derive frequencies of each method so as to create a portrait of the elements of a torturing environment are all important parts of the work that lies ahead in deepening our understanding of torture. Ideally, this would be done through a Participatory Action Research (PAR) process with survivors to gain a perspective from the survivor's own point of view. A qualitative and PAR approach to mapping torturing environments takes time and effort, but produces unique insights that no scale can offer. Both the TES and qualitative research are important tools and that bring us closer to a better definition and understanding of torturing environments (see Appendix 8: A Step-by-step guide for documenting torture).

Notes

1 This idea clearly connects with the Inter-American Convention against Torture: '[torture] shall also be understood to be the use of methods upon a person intended to obliterate the personality of the victim or to diminish his physical or mental capacities, even if they do not cause physical pain or mental anguish.'

2 Even if one could find volunteers willing to be 'tortured' in an experiment, the resistance of a human being clearly changes with context and motivation. It is impossible to experimentally re-create the fear and the pain of being at the mercy of others who exhibit cruelty. An experiment is always a 'safe' situation.

3 Istanbul Protocol, paras 141–3.

4 In fieldwork with preliminary versions of the TES, the main source of doubt was the intensity of the indicator necessary to consider that it was present. This led to the inclusion of this column.

5 Often the best forensic expert is the survivor's own therapist, because it can take months, and sometimes years, to remember, organise and be able to express everything that happened.

6 There are many explanations in therapy for this. Survivors may say, for example: 'I never found the right time to bring it up', or 'you asked, but I felt it was unimportant', or, 'it was too painful at the time', or even have confusing memories ('I was not sure that my memories were true because everything was so confusing, but now I've recalled images and became a bit more sure of what happened to me.').

7 It was not the extremely harsh conditions, the beatings, the stress positions and exhausting exercises, the nakedness, humiliation, sexual harassment, threats of rape, or even the guilt associated with giving false information that incriminated others in order to escape torture. The experience she identifies as having affected her the most was a seemingly endless moment when she was subjected – as she had been previously – to dry asphyxia with 'la bolsa' (the bag); but one day she was wrapped in a blanket and put on a table with her head hanging in a position from which she could not defend herself. She had been able to rationalise aspects related to shame and guilt, but this experience of *absolute lack of control* and being completely at the mercy of the interrogators was her breaking point. It will remain in her memory forever. Neither a checklist, nor an assessment of the 'severity' of a technique (for example, as part of an objective assessment of the threat to life or supposed pain) would have detected this.

8 The idea of impact is connected to one of the indicators proposed by Crampton and Rodley (2013): the significance of the technique of psychological maltreatment for the victim. They studied the *Estrella v. Uruguay* case, in which the Inter-American Court ruled that psychological torture had occurred when Mr. Estrella, a famous Argentine pianist, was threatened with having his hands irreversibly injured. They also included the example of rape in the context of ethnic cleansing and the unique, severe psychological significance it has for the victim. When Crampton and Rodley proposed 'significance' as a criterion for identifying torture, they focused on how torture targets elements that are key to the identity of the person. This is what the fifth column of the TES reveals.

19

THE NEED TO FURTHER DEVELOP THE ISTANBUL PROTOCOL

This book begins with a need: to document and analyse contemporary forms of state violence. One key milestone was the creation of the Istanbul Protocol in 1999, which became the tool of international consensus for the documentation of torture and ill-treatment. Endorsed by the United Nations, it has been adapted to different contexts: there are local versions; guidelines for doctors, psychologists and lawyers; and a broad range of training materials available in different languages and for different audiences (Baykal, Schlar and Kapkin, 2004; Den Otter, 2013; International Rehabilitation Council for Torture Victims, 2009; Redress, 2004; United Nations High Commissioner for Human Rights, 2004).

The Istanbul Protocol reflects a modern conception of torture that draws heavily from the experience of military dictatorships and totalitarian governments of the 1960s–1980s, and it incorporates many elements related to psychological torture. However, torture at the moment of the protocol's initial drafting was almost exclusively physical and focused on the production of pain, and the IP provides categories and detailed descriptions congruent with that fact (see Chapter 7 and Appendix 1). Torturers at that time learned more from France and the film *The Battle of Algiers* than from the sophistication of experimental research in the United States. The general idea was to produce the greatest physical pain that detainees could endure in order to ensure that they revealed any information they might have. The testimony of Hugo Rivas in Chapter 3 describes this type of scenario. In most cases, torture was subsequently followed by the forced disappearance of the detainee: no witnesses survived torture. Though contemporary torture no longer resembles these kinds of practices, they remain at the centre of how society imagines torture.

This type of torture is still prevalent in many areas of Africa and Asia, but it has little in common with contemporary torture as taught and practiced by democratic states and the countries they train. Interrogators from intelligence services of low and middle-income countries learn more over time and generally apply combinations of physical and psychological techniques. Slowly but steadily, contemporary torture is increasingly transitioning to a focus on producing psychological pain, creating confusion and attacking the self and identity.

The Istanbul Protocol provides excellent recommendations and guidelines for the exploration and documentation of the psychiatric consequences of torture (although some of the suggested diagnoses have become obsolete as classifications have changed over time).

But it offers only rough guidance on how to evaluate the impact of, for example, several days of varying forms of psychological attacks combined with coercive interrogations when such treatment is not combined with prominent physical violence. And yet psychological torture often causes greater destruction to the person. At some point in the future an international task group will have to take on the challenge of updating the IP, because it is the best and most highly-valued tool in the fight against torture.

To this end, we would like to suggest some preliminary ideas.

A reconsideration of psychological torture in the Istanbul Protocol

The Istanbul Protocol explicitly states in paragraph 145 that: '*The distinction between physical and psychological methods is artificial. For example, sexual torture generally causes both physical and psychological symptoms, even when there has been no physical assault.*' Perhaps it's time to refine this idea. The fact that the distinction is artificial (i.e. made for epistemological purposes) does not mean that we shouldn't keep in mind that the ultimate target of torture is the conscious self, and that we should reflect on contemporary torture and the complex ways in which this conscious self is attacked and controlled.

The IP considers 21 categories of torture methods[1] (Appendix 1), that we have classified here as either Physical, Psychological or Mixed (Table 19.1). We have used numbers (the IP uses letters). Methods *a* through *l* are more physical and *o* through *u* are more psychological. Methods (m) and (n) can be considered mixed.

These 21 categories are not accompanied by definitions in the Protocol, so we do not know the precise definition of IP18 *Psychological techniques to break down the individual*, the main category dealing with psychological torture, or how it differs conceptually from the category *Behavioral coercion / forced betrayal*.

The protocol cannot provide an exhaustive catalogue of techniques. Again, the number of techniques is as infinite as the human imagination. We need broad categories, but in the case of psychological torture they are not easy to apply. In Table 19.2, we have organised the 8 classical

TABLE 19.1 Physical versus psychological torture techniques in the Istanbul protocol

Physical Torture: Pain	*Psychological Torture*
[1] (a) Blunt trauma	[15] (o) Humiliation
[2] (b) Positional torture	[16] (p) Threats, mock executions
[3] (c) Burns	[17] (q) Threats of attack
[4] (d) Electric shocks	[18] (r) Psychological techniques to break
[5] (e) Asphyxiation	down the individual, forced betrayal,
[6] (f) Crush injuries	inducing helplessness
[7] (g) Penetrating injuries	[19] (s) Violation of taboos
[8] (h) Chemical exposure	[20] (t) Behavioral coercion
[9] (i) Sexual violence	[21] (u) Forcing the victim to witness torture
[10] (j) Traumatic removal of digits and limbs	
[11] (k) Medical amputation	
[12] (l) Pharmacological torture	

Mixed Conditions

[13] (m) Conditions of detention	[14] (n) Deprivation of normal sensory stimulation

TABLE 19.2 Psychological torture: selected categories and difficulties in applying IP categories

Biderman (1964)	Corresponding IP category
Isolation	IP 13. Conditions of detention?
Monopolisation of attention	NO EQUIVALENT
Induced debilitation and exhaustion	NO EQUIVALENT (IP 2. Positional torture?)
Cultivation of anxiety and despair Alternating punishment and rewards 'Omniscience' and 'omnipotence'	IP 18. Psychological techniques to break down the individual?
Enforcing trivial and absurd demands	IP 20. Behavioral coercion, forced betrayal
Degradation	IP 15. Humiliation
Ojeda (2008)	
Isolation Spatial disorientation Temporal disorientation Sensory disorientation Sensory deprivation	IP 13. Conditions of detention? IP 14. Deprivation of normal sensory stimulation
Sensory assault (overstimulation)	NO EQUIVALENT
Psychological debilitation	NO EQUIVALENT (IP 2. Positional torture?)
Induced desperation	IP 18. Psychological techniques to break down the individual?
Threats	IP 16. Threats
Feral treatment	IP 15. Humiliation, IP 19. Violation of taboos
Sexual humiliation	IP 9. Sexual violence, IP 13. Forced nakedness, IP 15. Humiliation
Desecration	IP 15. Humiliation
Pharmacological manipulation	IP 12. Pharmacological torture

groups of psychological techniques (described by Biderman in 1964) and the 13 categories proposed by Ojeda (as part of his *extensional* definition of psychological torture) into the IP categories.

Overall, this represents a classification of *processes of breaking the conscious mind*, instead of (or in addition to) methods for producing pain or psychological suffering.

The following points also deserve more detailed consideration:

- **Solitary confinement** should be analysed independently from conditions of detention (more related to cell and living conditions) and examined as a relevant factor in itself.
- Concepts like **self-inflicted pain** or **forced absorption / monopolisation of attention** which are key in the understanding of the process of modern psychological torture should be considered important subjects of analysis.
- **Actions targeting identity** (attacks on the self, inducing guilt, inducing shame, manipulation of affect and use of relatives or loved ones) are not described or taken into account in the Istanbul Protocol; they should be included.[2]

• Interrogation techniques in general and coercive or deceptive techniques in particular often go unnoted; their impact should be studied further.

Promoting the use of the Istanbul Protocol is a priority worldwide. The Special Rapporteur against Torture, Juan Mendez, in a thematic report before the General Assembly of United Nations, insisted in 2015 on the need for all countries to implement the IP. Perhaps it is time to consider updating some sections of the IP. This may seem strange, given the fact that the IP's universal adoption is an ongoing battle. But updating the IP is also a way to preserve it as a living tool and to foster reflection on the new challenges presented by torture in the decades to come.

Moral suffering

If the distinction between CIDT and torture means anything, it is only insofar as it is capable of describing the victim's level of moral suffering. Beyond the sequelae, there is a subjective component of torture: it is what Koenig describes when she discusses the significance of sexual assault against Arab prisoners in Guantanamo; it is what the Inter-American Court of Human Rights alluded to when they ruled that the anguish suffered by family members of detained or disappeared persons reaches a level that deserves to be qualified as torture. Such conclusions are only possible when the judicial process is capable of accessing the victim's subjective experience.

The Istanbul Protocol exhaustively investigates the actions in question, the torture methods used and their psychological consequences. But it does not offer guidelines for analysing the subject's narrative in a way that permits an understanding of the elements of abuse that affect identity. Understanding the survivor's reality is a process that goes beyond listing actions and consequences to understand how they come together in the specific lived experience of the subject, and why they produce certain impacts.

Some of this information can be collected in the *interpretation and conclusions* section, where it is possible to take a closer look at the human victim and his or her needs and vulnerabilities, and explain the impact of torture on him or her by examining the interaction between torture method and the victim.

Credibility analysis in the Istanbul Protocol

Terminology

One of the IP's main objectives is to judge *credibility*, defined as the evaluator's impression of the accuracy of the survivor's statement, and whether or not it leads the evaluator to believe that the events occurred as the survivor claims. This is one of the most neglected aspects of the IP: its power and potential for credibility analysis. Because scars may be invisible and wounds are mostly psychological, and because torture is almost always committed without witnesses, quite often the survivors lose hope that any credit will be given to their claims.

To define credibility, experts employ three inter-related factors:

1. Consistency, defined as a lack of contradictory elements. For instance, we can consider an account to be consistent when there is a logical thread with no substantial contradictory elements.

2.   Congruence, defined as harmony between different sources of information. For instance, we consider there is congruence when the acts described are in accordance or compatible with the associated mood, feelings or emotions.
3.   Coherence, understood as logical and meaningful in terms of assumptions and implications, especially as related to the general context. For instance, the narrative is orderly and systematic.

Theoretical considerations

Credibility versus consistency

Certain forensic experts refuse to judge a victim's credibility because they understand that they are being asked to define his or her trustworthiness, which is subjective, ethical and would place the expert before an ethical dilemma. From this standpoint, a forensic expert could analyse consistency without defining credibility, which would be tantamount to judging the person. If we turn the question around, the expert would be asked to discern whether or not the person is lying, which for certain forensic experts is an ethically unacceptable question.

The Istanbul Protocol specifically asserts that one must 'establish the credibility of the person' (p. 36, paragraph 140) and that establishing consistency is a fundamental tool to do so. When the protocol speaks of 'credibility' it is not referring to evaluating the person's honesty but rather to *the credibility of past and present core facts* ('Objectively assessed, is all or part of the claimant's story of torture, which he or she presents as a factual background to their case, accepted as "credible"?'). The person's credibility is not being analysed, but rather the set of events that s/he refers to (Mackey and Barnes, 2013)

Objective and subjective elements in credibility analysis

The point of contention here is when the expert evaluates the credibility of the facts letting him or herself be affected by the overall impression generated by the person being examined and not by the technical elements of consistency, congruency and coherence. Cultural similarity to interviewer; being well dressed, friendly and/or smiling; appearing to be respectful, kind or shy; being self-confident and relaxed while answering, free from hesitation or doubts; being pleasant to the interviewer and agreeing with him/her without being too willing to please in responding to questions about changes in facts; and not attacking or pressing the expert for a positive evaluation are all factors included in psychological literature as contributing to an overall impression (Brodsky, Griffin and Cramer, 2010). All these elements help build subjective criteria on the degree of belief we attach to what we see and hear.

These elements are not to be completely dismissed by a forensic expert, as they are part of what a clinical psychologist or a psychiatrist calls 'first impression' or 'transference'. Here, the issue is not an *intuition* that a lay member of a jury may have for instance, but rather the automatic mental comparison of what the expert observes with his/her years of experiences in clinical work. It is an *intuition* that is *informed* by experience. In any event, this type of intangible criterion must be complementary and in general terms be avoided by forensic experts to the extent possible. Credibility assessment should be based as much as possible on objective facts (i.e. coherence, consistency and congruence of the narrative, having cross-checked information with other sources, and so on). A reasoned opinion should be provided based on proper analysis of all of these elements. Our scale refers to just this.

Types of consistency

When analysing torture allegations, it is important to analyse the consistency of the account. There are various manuals for legal officials who evaluate asylum seekers' applications and these manuals consider the key to be findings on consistencies or discrepancies within the statements and other evidence presented by claimants from their first meetings, applications and personal interviews and examination at all stages of processing their application/appeal until final disposal (Mackey and Barnes, 2013). A wealth of literature shows that administrative or legal processes require protracted amounts of time and that inconsistencies between different statements made at different times by those who have undergone traumatic experiences not only do not indicate of a lack of credibility, but that their grounding in trauma or relationships (see Table 19.3) in many cases actually supports the credibility of their allegations (Pérez-Sales, 2009).

TABLE 19.3 Reasons for inconsistency in a torture narrative over time

1. Lack of trust in the interviewer. Inappropriate setting. Time constraints. Poor translation.
2. By definition, the extreme trauma is unspeakable, undescribable. When a traumatic experience is easy to tell, its authenticity may be called into question.
3. Memory is a constructed account, a pact of sorts between the actual and tolerable truth, between one's own memories and the narratives of others. Over time, in repeating the account, the survivor subtly accommodates to the resonance that the facts generate in the listener as well as to what s/he can tolerate (Herlihy, Jobson and Turner, 2012).
4. Feelings of guilt (guilt cuts across the survivor's entire experience) and of shame (particularly in certain types of sexual torture).
5. Dissociation. Between 25 and 50 percent of the time, extreme traumas are associated with muddled, fragmented or partial memories. What is demanded from the survivor is a narrative whose consistency was often never there originally, partly because one's own mind, in order to protect itself, retains only certain aspects of the traumatic events. It is estimated that roughly 50 percent of traumas are associated with more or less severe dissociative symptoms.
6. In research on the accuracy of memory where external verification sources are available, up to 30 percent inconsistencies are observed in the substantive portions of the accounts of trauma between different accounts separated at times by merely a few hours when minor elements in the interview are changed, i.e. the person asking, whether or not the interview is guided or allows for silence, the time available and the degree of intimacy (Brewin and Holmes, 2003).
7. A good deal of experimental research has shown that when the interrogator asks about aspects that the person does not remember, there is a tendency to reply with what the person believes s/he should. The belief is that silence or the lack of response will generate a lack of credibility. Subsequently, this will lead to inconsistencies in the account, as it is difficult to remember exactly what was said at that time (Gudjonsson, 2003).
8. Many psychiatric pathologies such as depression, phobic disorders and post-contusion syndromes occurring after consciousness is lost due to beatings and so forth can interfere with memories (Mind, 2010).
9. Negative elements of projection onto the interviewer when s/he is perceived to be a punitive authority, or when s/he conveys a lack of trust or incredulity, or when the interview is experienced as yet another interrogation.
10. Fear of the consequences of there being a written record of the account and of the name of those responsible for the events recounted.

Issuing an opinion

A *victim deserves a credibility analysis because many times this is the only proof s/he has in legal proceedings.* Credibility assessment is not a matter of personally trusting the alleged victim, but of assessing a past and present account of events. In this process, it is always assumed that a forensic expert acts with the utmost integrity and professionalism to the best of his/her knowledge, and this is why s/he makes a sworn statement as the culmination of the Istanbul Protocol. We consider that the forensic expert must, to the best of his/her knowledge, attempt to make a statement *based on scientific evidence and facts and not subjective impressions* about the degree of the survivor's narrative's credibility, that is, assert whether there are sufficient scientific grounds to affirm that what the survivor declared as past and present fact is essentially true.

The Protocol is confusing when setting out the tools that a forensic expert has to do so and how s/he must issue his/her opinion. It states that:

> For each lesion and for the overall pattern of lesions, the physician should indicate the degree of consistency between it and the attribution given by the patient. The following terms are generally used:
>
> a.   *Not consistent: the lesion could not have been caused by the trauma described;*
> b.   *Consistent: the lesion could have been caused by the trauma described, but it is non-specific and there are many other possible causes;*
> c.   *Highly consistent: the lesion could have been caused by the trauma described, and there are few other possible causes;*
> d.   *Typical: this is an appearance that is usually found with this type of trauma, but there are other possible causes;*
> e.   *Diagnostic: this appearance could not have been caused in any way other than that described.* (p. 43, para. 187)

No guidelines are offered as to how to evaluate overall credibility. Instead, all that is stated is 'it is the overall evaluation of all lesions and not the consistency of each lesion with a particular form of torture that is important in assessing the torture story' (p. 44, para. 188).

Thus, the Istanbul Protocol avoids mentioning the expressions that must be used in issuing an opinion on credibility. Most forensic experts address this by using the same expression for analysing credibility and consistency, and this is the approach we have adopted here (see Table 19.5).

This is not the only approach. In some legal systems, the forensic expert is required to issue an opinion on his/her degree of conviction regarding the past and present facts (Gyulai et al., 2013). A normal credibility scale might be:

Degree 1. Highly unlikely
Degree 2. Likely
Degree 3. Beyond reasonable doubt
Degree 4. Beyond any doubt

Other expressions (used for instance by the European Court of Human Rights) are 'substantial grounds have been shown for believing that the person provides a credible account of past and present facts'.

TABLE 19.4 Credibility analysis in the Istanbul Protocol: epistemological basis

- Evaluator's knowledge of human rights and political context; external sources of verification
- Interview focused on personal biographical history, with data collation by third parties
- Empathy in an open and horizontal setting characterised by listening
- No time pressure on the interviewee
- Pre-post analysis of personality structure; plausibility of torture as a reason for changes (cause-effect relationship); rejection of other causes
- Evaluator's knowledge of coping patterns in adverse situations in general and the assessed situation in particular
- Consistency across verbal and nonverbal communication
- Coherence of the events described
- Consistency between the events described and the emotions with which they are expressed
- Consistency between the events described and the actions taken to confront them
- Complementary tests: psychometric measures, images and others

Issuing an opinion of consistency or credibility will depend not only on the expert's convictions, but also on the legal environment. Through a detailed account of sentences, Good (2004) shows reluctance (when not outright anger) on the part of UK judges when a senior forensic expert dares to use the word 'credibility' in his or her conclusions, given that, most of the time, these are speculative expressions that go beyond the expert's functions and that only the judge can rule on. Attorneys are thus advised to give proper counsel on the acceptable limits of expert comment.

SEC: a new tool to assess credibility based on the Istanbul Protocol

Aim

The SEC (known in previous versions as SEF-IP is a standardised evaluation form for credibility assessment (Pérez-Sales et al., 2015) (Table 19.5). The SEC aims to reinforce the idea of using the IP as legal proof in Court or as evidence for administrative purposes (i.e. asylum claims).

The SEC complements the IP to assess credibility in a consistent and reliable way. It helps the evaluator to search for potential sources of credibility and systematise information, to make his or her final decision more objective and to have comparable results among experts and studies. It is based on clinical data and analysis and triangulation of available sources. It does not include the result of technological devices (i.e. RNM, thermal cameras, P300 waves and others), as they fall beyond the average clinician's scope. Some call into question cognitive liberty principles and involve ethical challenges remaining to be solved (see Chapter 16). The SEC goes far beyond the IP criteria and adds others, defining levels of consistency / coherence for each criterion, for comprehensive credibility assessment.

Target Audience

It can be an extremely useful tool for judges, solicitors, attorneys or forensic experts to provide an evidence-based and informed decision on credibility and avoid intuitive or speculative decisions. It will help judges to gather all available information and attain a comprehensive view of the case. It will help solicitors and independent experts appointed by a court to provide objective grounds for a credibility analysis. And it will provide the party-appointed experts, whose role is surely among the most complex and challenging in the legal world, the opportunity to show their impartiality.

Rationale

The SEC has a set of criteria, some of them based on IP recommendations, with additional corroborating criteria. It encompasses hard and soft criteria for the expert to make a decision in one of the four categories recommended by the Istanbul Protocol. The exact wording of these four categories can be changed according to whether the expert feels comfortable using the word credibility (as we do) or might prefer using the word consistency.

The overall credibility assessment, based on the expert's knowledge and conclusions after carefully reviewing all of the criteria, is not a product of numerical totaling. The matrix is an aid to be used as part of a decision-making process.

Instructions

The SEC provides a range of elements to assess credibility based on a three C analysis (i.e. consistency, congruency and coherence) and an ensemble for triangulating sources of verification.

The SEC requires an atmosphere of cooperation and trust between the expert and the survivor, and again, the way the interview is conducted is essential.

Hard and soft criteria. Some of the SEC criteria can be considered *hard*, for instance when there are medium- and long-term sequels which are pathognomonic of torture. Others are *soft*. Consistency between verbal and non-verbal communication in the event statement depends on the interviewee (i.e. being accustomed to speaking coherently in public in similar cultural channels, shyness . . .), the interviewer (preconceptions, interview abilities), the setting (the purpose and the potential consequences of the interview) and the interaction (cultural gap, background knowledge of the interview . . .). Because they are subject to important inter-rater variability, they must be considered soft criteria.

SEC criteria 3 to 6 are usually considered *soft*, and the others *hard*. While each individual case varies, it is best for the overall SEC assessment to be based on hard criteria.

While presence supports there being torture, absence does not exclude it. During the interview there might be certain criteria, even soft ones, that clearly support credibility. But their absence does not indicate a lack of credibility. For instance, if a survivor presents a dissociative state in his or her torture testimony, this will strongly support credibility. Dissociative states are a clear indicator of psychological damage. But a torture victim could withstand an interview without showing ostensible signs of distress, and this does not exclude credibility. It might simply show, for instance, a high degree of self-control or psychological resilience which, when contextualised, can be a positive indicator of credibility.

The SEC helps experts properly assess this by drawing a distinction between elements that support consistency (column 1), elements that support inconsistency (column 2) and a lack of either one of these two elements (column 3).

Column 3 does not cast a negative light on the witness. Let's imagine a survivor that provides a statement of torture ten years after the events. S/he is accustomed to sharing his/her experience and can do so in a normal conversation relatively easily. The items regarding verbal and nonverbal consistency, emotional answers, clinical symptoms or others stemming from the interview might not provide particularly useful information, and we are to honestly reflect this in the clear understanding that it does not necessarily undermine credibility. It simply states that these criterion are not particularly pertinent to the overall assessment. Column 3 can also be used when the expert believes that he/she cannot make a proper assessment of a given criteria for medical or cultural reasons, in which case we recommend prudence be exercised in the assessment. Only the criteria that the expert is convinced of should be used. For instance, an evaluator may consider that given his or her cultural distance, s/he cannot determine whether or not an emotional expression in the account is congruous with the person's culture, and would thus prefer to mark column 3.

The devil in the details. As explained below, placing too much emphasis in minor details is a common error when assessing credibility. An alleged victim may have to provide testimony many times over the course of legal proceedings that might take years. In asylum claims, this may sometimes involve more than twenty instances of re-telling a story, from social workers to the police, from asylum officers to lawyers and forensic experts, from health service personnel to resettlement service staffers and so forth. Statements made at different times for different purposes regarding different moments are put together and compared, and minor inconsistencies between versions are considered proof of lack of credibility. But this is a big mistake. Proper coherence assessments must take the following into account:

- Whether or not the survivor can answer most questions on key events and, when asked, provide a reasonable number of specific details showing that the person *was there*.
- Whether the overall narrative is maintained from one version to the next.
- Whether or not there are substantial inconsistencies in the overall narration. Psychopathologies, cultural factors, and the time elapsed since the events could account for minor inconsistencies. For clinicians, minor inconsistencies actually *support* credibility. A survivor of a traumatic experience is not expected to produce a perfectly consistent narration of past events and an expert clinician can relate the emotional and clinical state of the witness to the accuracy of the narrative.

Reassessment. On occasion it may take time for the most painful experiences to appear and SEC could therefore potentially change over time.

Establishing a numerical threshold for the SEC would not make sense because: (1) some of the criteria depend on the availability of external sources, or obtaining information from proxies which might not always be available; (2) not fulfilling certain criteria does not discount credibility, for instance not having sequelae (criterion 10), persistent personality changes (criterion 11), a clinical diagnosis (criterion 11) and (3) the conceptual weight of each of the 16 criteria is too dissimilar for them to be combined in a numerical total.

The SEC, as a tool that complements the IP, can improve studies on the efficacy of the IP in the evaluation of credibility in allegations of ill-treatment and torture.

Examples of application

A.J. is a Palestinian refugee seeking asylum in Spain. A four-hour interview revealed that he was born in Amman (Jordania) where his family settled after fleeing the Palestinian Occupied Territory. When he was fourteen, his parents decided to return to their original

TABLE 19.5 Standard Evaluation Form for Credibility Assessment (SEC)

	Standard Evaluation Form for Credibility Assessment (SEC)				
Mark as appropriate.		**1. Highly consistent** **2. Consistent** **3. Inconsistent** **4. Not applicable**			
	Criterion	*1*	*2*	*3*	*4*
1	Plausible and logical description of alleged torture (circumstances, type, methodology, duration, etc.).				
2	Triangulation of information from witnesses / other potential victims – *[Highly consistent – Blind independent interviews with open questions; Consistent – Non independent – closed questions – Collective interviews]*				
3	Documentation supporting relevant dates and locations cited by the survivor. Triangulation of the events with external sources of information (i.e. newspapers, Internet).				
4	Positive outcome. The alleged victim has ostensible direct benefits (economic, legal or otherwise) of being considered credible *[Positive outcome supports inconsistency; Absence supports consistency]*				
5	Negative outcomes. There are ostensible negative outcomes of testyfying (public exposure, shame, danger or otherwise) that making illogical a false testimony *[Negative outcome supports consistency; Absence supports inconsistency]*				
6	Facts are described in accordance with reports produced by human rights organisations, international organisations, or entities associated with or recognised by United Nations agencies working on preventing or denouncing torture.				
7	*At the time of the alleged facts*, expected or typical physical or psychological reactions to extreme stress, within the cultural and social context of the examinee.				
8	*At the time of the expert assessment* consistency between the description of events and the emotions with which they are expressed.				
9	*At the time of the expert assessment*, consistency between verbal and nonverbal communication in the statement of events.				
10	Medical tests (including x-rays, blood tests, EMG) consistent with the alleged events.				
11	Psychometric assessment (PTSD, depression, impact on worldviews, neuropsychological tests) consistent with the alleged events.				

(continued)

TABLE 19.5 Standard Evaluation Form for Credibility Assessment (SEC) (*continued*)

Standard Evaluation Form for Credibility Assessment (SEC)

			1. **Highly consistent** 2. **Consistent** 3. **Inconsistent** 4. **Not applicable**		

Mark as appropriate.

	Criterion	1	2	3	4
12	Medium / long term physical sequelae consistent with the alleged events.				
13	Objective and verifiable personality changes that can be temporally associated with the alleged events.				
14	Functional changes (in work, studies, personal relationships, etc.) after the events described attributable to the events described.				
15	*At the time of the expert assessment*, the evaluee's principal clinical diagnosis related to the events is consistent with allegations. [ICD/ DSM Diagnosis:]				
16	Events, physical and psychological consequences, personality or functional changes *blindly contrasted* with one or more other first-hand sources (family, friends, co-detainees or others).				
17	Previous medical or forensic assessments indicating immediate physical or psychological consequences or medium or long term sequelae consistent with the events described.				
18	Concurrence of two forensic experts and/or an external evaluator.				
19	Court sentence or legal administrative procedure (i.e. refugee status, asylum claim) in favour of the examinee that recognises degrading treatment, ill-treatment, or torture.				
OVERALL LEVEL OF CREDIBILITY 1. Maximum consistency 2. Highly consistent 3. Consistent 4. Not consistent					

Alternatively: Overall level of credibility: 1. Beyond any doubt. 2. Beyond reasonable doubt. 3. Likely. 4. Highly unlikely.

place of residence in Palestine where their land had been confiscated. Since then, A.J. has been living in a refugee camp near Bethlehem. Like most teenagers in Palestine, he had had several confrontations with members of the Israeli Army and was detained, at the age of 15, during a demonstration where he was video-recorded throwing stones at a bus of Israeli settlers that were now living on what had been his grandparents' land. During his three-month detention he claims to have been submitted to hooding and beatings, to being forcedly kept on a small kindergarten chair for hours and hours, and to have been subjected to intensive, misleading interrogations by security officers. He is the only one of his group of friends who was released. One of them died in strange circumstances during detention. A.J. sought revenge and his family decided to send him abroad to prevent him from joining a radical Muslim group. He can document his residence in a refugee camp, but does not have any official document to attest to his time in detention. He has a medical report in Arabic, issued by an international NGO a few days after his alleged release date that mentions his being detained but provides no details of detention. It attests to his signs of anxiety, weight loss and headaches and includes a prescription for mild hypnotic treatment. During the interview, A.J. did not initially show symptoms of distress, although when talking about his parents and family in the Occupied Palestinian Territories he increasingly showed signs of anxiety and guilty feelings for 'being saved'. The refugee centre where he was assigned confirms that he is upset and alone most of the day, and has had flashbacks and a violent outburst on one occasion when the educator forced him to remain in his chair during lunch and wait until everybody else had finished. His psychometric tests show a pattern of damaged worldviews consistent with torture allegations (see Table 19.6).

TABLE 19.6 SEC – Example of application: A.J.

Standard Evaluation Form for Credibility Assessment (SEC)

Mark as appropriate.		1. **Highly consistent** 2. **Consistent** 3. **Inconsistent** 4. **Not applicable**			
	Criterion	*1*	*2*	*3*	*4*
1	Plausible and logical description of alleged torture (circumstances, type, methodology, duration, etc.).	X			
2	Triangulation of information from witnesses / other potential victims – *[Highly consistent – Blind independent interviews with open questions; Consistent – Non independent – closed questions – Collective interviews]*				X
3	Documentation supporting relevant dates and locations cited by the survivor. Triangulation of the events with external sources of information (i.e. newspapers, Internet).		X		
4	Positive outcome. The alleged victim has ostensible direct benefits (economic, legal or otherwise) of being considered credible *[Positive outcome supports inconsistency. Absence supports consistency]* *Claiming Asylum*			X	
5	Negative outcomes. There are ostensible negative outcomes of testifying (public exposure, shame, danger or otherwise) that making illogical a false testimony *[Negative outcome supports consistency. Absence supports inconsistency]* *The Embassy will know and he will not be allowed to enter the OpT again and see his relative even if asylum is rejected.*		X		
6	Facts are described in accordance with reports produced by human rights organisations, international organisations, or entities associated with or recognised by United Nations agencies working on preventing or denouncing torture.	X			

(continued)

TABLE 19.6 SEC – Example of application: A.J. (*continued*)

Standard Evaluation Form for Credibility Assessment (SEC)

Mark as appropriate.		**1. Highly consistent** **2. Consistent** **3. Inconsistent** **4. Not applicable**			
	Criterion	*1*	*2*	*3*	*4*
7	*At the time of the alleged facts*, expected or typical physical or psychological reactions to extreme stress, within the cultural and social context of the examinee.		X		
8	*At the time of the expert assessment* consistency between the description of events and the emotions with which they are expressed.		X		
9	*At the time of the expert assessment*, consistency between verbal and nonverbal communication in the statement of events.				X
10	Medical tests (including x-rays, blood tests, EMG) consistent with the alleged events.				X
11	Psychometric assessment (PTSD, depression, impact on worldviews, neuropsychological tests) consistent with the alleged events.		X		
12	Medium / long term physical sequelae consistent with the alleged events.				X
13	Objective and verifiable personality changes that can be temporally associated with the alleged events.				X
14	Functional changes (in work, studies, personal relationships, etc.) after the events described attributable to the events described.	X			
15	*At the time of the expert assessment*, the evaluee's principal clinical diagnosis related to the events is consistent with allegations. [ICD/ DSM Diagnosis:]		X		
16	Events, physical and psychological consequences, personality or functional changes *blindly contrasted* with one or more other first-hand sources (family, friends, co-detainees or others).		X		
17	Previous medical or forensic assessments indicating immediate physical or psychological consequences or medium or long term sequelae consistent with the events described.		X		
18	Concurrence of two forensic experts and/or an external evaluator.				X
19	Court sentence or legal administrative procedure (i.e. refugee status, asylum claim) in favour of the examinee that recognises degrading treatment, ill-treatment, or torture.				X

OVERALL LEVEL OF CREDIBILITY
1. Maximum consistency. 2. Highly consistent. 3. Consistent 4. Not consistent

J.S. is a migrant from Cameroon living in Spain. He arrived ten years ago and is fully integrated into the life of the country. He leads a small anti-racial organisation and writes a blog on discrimination. He is well-known in Madrid's old city and Sub-Saharian people, particularly homeless black people, seek informal legal advice from him. He explains that he saw the National Police asking Latinos and blacks in the street for their IDs and mediated on behalf of someone who did not understand what the police were demanding of him. The two were detained together. The person was soon released. However, the police had beaten J.S. severely inside their van, threatening him for not minding his own business. J.S. was hit in the head, fainted, and was brought to hospital where a doctor filled out a medical report documenting some minor bruises, not including either J.S.'s description of the facts or a clinical opinion on the compatibility between the alleged facts and observed injuries. Two of the policemen also asked for medical reports alleging having being hit by J.S during his detention. After leaving the hospital, in the middle of the night, the police took J.S. to the Casa de Campo, a solitary park in Madrid where, for approximately an hour and a half he was allegedly severely beaten, pulled very painfully by his dreadlocks, repeatedly suffocated with a plastic bag while handcuffed, subjected to a mock execution with a gun and repeatedly threatened with the detaining and deportation of his wife to Cameroon. Finally, he was driven to the police station. The time recorded in the official police station custody log is fifteen minutes after leaving the hospital. He was kept for 48 hours after the last of his bruises disappeared and released with charges of attacking an authority. After his release, he stayed home for a full week, terrified, until friends came to see him and contacted a human rights organisation which subsequently accompanied him to a health centre. A further medical report documented no physical marks but severe posttraumatic symptoms (acute stress disorder) and recommended psychiatric treatment. After three weeks of hesitation, he denounced having been tortured by the police. His lawyer demanded an Istanbul Protocol procedure, including a credibility assessment from an independent forensic expert from a public hospital (see Table 19.7).

TABLE 19.7 SEC – Example of application: J.S.

Standard Evaluation Form for Credibility Assessment (SEC)				
Mark as appropriate.	1. **Highly consistent** 2. **Consistent** 3. **Inconsistent** 4. **Not applicable**			
	Criterion	*1*	*2*	*3*	*4*
1	Plausible and logical description of alleged torture (circumstances, type, methodology, duration, etc.).	X			
2	Triangulation of information from witnesses / other potential victims – *[Highly consistent – Blind independent interviews with open questions; Consistent – Non independent – closed questions – Collective interviews]*		X		
3	Documentation supporting relevant dates and locations cited by the survivor. Triangulation of the events with external sources of information (i.e. newspapers, Internet).				X

(continued)

TABLE 19.7 SEC – Example of application: J.S. (*continued*)

Standard Evaluation Form for Credibility Assessment (SEC)

Mark as appropriate.		**1. Highly consistent** **2. Consistent** **3. Inconsistent** **4. Not applicable**			
	Criterion	*1*	*2*	*3*	*4*
4	Positive outcome. The alleged victim has ostensible direct benefits (economic, legal or otherwise) of being considered credible *[Positive outcome supports inconsistency. Absence supports consistency]*				X
5	Negative outcomes. There are ostensible negative outcomes of testifying (public exposure, shame, danger or otherwise) that make a false testimony illogical *[Negative outcome supports consistency. Absence supports inconsistency]* He has been counter-denounced by the Police. His lawyer is offered an agreement if he withdraws the complaint.		X		
6	Facts are described in accordance with reports produced by human rights organisations, international organisations, or entities associated with or recognised by United Nations agencies working on preventing or denouncing torture.				X
7	*At the time of the alleged facts*, expected or typical physical or psychological reactions to extreme stress, within the cultural and social context of the examinee.	X			
8	*At the time of the expert assessment* consistency between the description of events and the emotions with which they are expressed.	X			
9	*At the time of the expert assessment*, consistency between verbal and nonverbal communication in the statement of events.	X			
10	Medical tests (including x-rays, blood tests, EMG) consistent with the alleged events.				X
11	Psychometric assessment (PTSD, depression, impact on worldviews, neuropsychological tests) consistent with the alleged events.				X
12	Medium / long term physical sequelae consistent with the alleged events.				X
13	Objective and verifiable personality changes that can be temporally associated with the alleged events.				X
14	Functional changes (in work, studies, personal relationships, etc.) after the events described attributable to the events described.	X			
15	*At the time of the expert assessment*, the evaluee's principal clinical diagnosis related to the events is consistent with allegations. [ICD/ DSM Diagnosis:]	X			
16	Events, physical and psychological consequences, personality or functional changes *blindly contrasted* with one or more other first-hand sources (family, friends, co-detainees or others).		X		

Standard Evaluation Form for Credibility Assessment (SEC)

Mark as appropriate.	1. **Highly consistent**
	2. **Consistent**
	3. **Inconsistent**
	4. **Not applicable**

	Criterion	*1*	*2*	*3*	*4*
17	Previous medical or forensic assessments indicating immediate physical or psychological consequences or medium or long term sequelae consistent with the events described.	X			
18	Concurrence of two forensic experts and/or an external evaluator.				X
19	Court sentence or legal administrative procedure (i.e. refugee status, asylum claim) in favour of the examinee that recognises degrading treatment, ill-treatment, or torture.				X

OVERALL LEVEL OF CREDIBILITY
1. Maximum consistency. 2. Highly consistent. 3. (Consistent) 4. Not consistent

Other aspects

Legal environment

The Istanbul Protocol lacks clear legal guidelines for collecting specific information about the type of violation, including the historical context, the aggressor's characteristics, specific details regarding the perpetrators and the physical detention space. And this information is of value as evidence for identifying the perpetrator or perpetrators in subsequent legal claims. These elements could eventually be used in cases where the documentation of torture is linked to criminal proceedings against alleged perpetrators.

Gender perspective

The IP lacks a clear gender LGTB perspective. While it does take into account the gender of interviewer and interviewee, it fails to include in-depth analysis of what the victim's gender or sexual orientation determines regarding torture methods and impacts. The entire protocol should be analysed from a gender perspective.

Transcultural issues

The IP pays scarce attention to transcultural issues. The protocol demands the presence of an interpreter when needed, but does not include a cultural formulation or attach any importance to emic perspectives in the assessment of torture methods, impacts and sequelae

Collective cases

Finally, forensic experts often need to document collective cases. Ill-treatment of demonstrators, forced displacement or scorched earth policies are examples of collective punishment.

Although the Convention does not consider collective torture to be an entity, on certain occasions, although there has indeed been torture, the cases cannot be individualised.

Conclusions

The Istanbul Protocol is the most widely used instrument for evaluating torture victims. Its implementation is currently slow, but steady. It is a powerful tool that on many occasions is the only element presented and considered as evidence in cases of alleged ill-treatment or torture.

However, the IP is lengthy to complete and could be improved through brief forms to be used when time is limited or when the conditions for conducting an exhaustive, confidential evaluation are lacking. At the same time, there is a need to update some elements of the IP based on the experiences gained since its approval in 1999. These changes should include a more systematic exploration of the elements of psychological torture and of harm to identity, guidelines for analysing, from the victim's viewpoint, key elements in the experience of harm, which we could call moral harm, improved gender and transcultural perspectives, and guidelines for collective cases. Stronger guidelines for producing legal documentation that can serve as evidence, including enhanced instructions regarding credibility analysis, are also necessary.

All of these elements, and others that may emerge in the future, could pave the way for the IP to serve as a living tool adapted to new realities, and certainly significantly enhance it.

Notes

1 Although the protocol advises wisely that '*The following list of torture methods is given to show some of the categories of possible abuse. It is not meant to be used by investigators as a checklist or as a model for listing torture methods in a report*', in fact it is regularly used as a checklist in forensic assessment.
2 Category [18] (r) is described as: 'Psychological techniques to break down the individual, including forced betrayals, accentuating feelings of helplessness, exposure to ambiguous situations or contradictory messages and [20] (t) Behavioral coercion, such as forced engagement in practices against the religion of the victim (e.g. forcing Muslims to eat pork), forced harm to others through torture or other abuses, forced destruction of property, forced betrayal of someone placing them at risk of harm.'

20

FINAL THOUGHTS AND AN AGENDA FOR FUTURE RESEARCH

In recent decades there has been a gradual shift from methods of torture based on physical pain and the breaking of the will through the claudication caused by that pain, to much more subtle and complex techniques based on directly attacking the conscious self. Decades of shared knowledge and training have been exchanged through the torture and interrogation schools of each of the international geopolitical powers. This has produced a corpus that, despite local idiosyncrasies, is essentially the same across countries. Over time, a more or less fixed set of techniques has been established and is recognisable in the history of recent decades.

When the objective of torture is intimidation, humiliation or punishment (in other words, when torture is used as a form of social control), physical pain still remains the fundamental element at work. Occasionally, in environments in which impunity is the norm, torturers leave ostensible marks; such marks are intended as a reminder of the humiliation and of who holds the power. But when torture is meant to obtain information or self-incrimination, or in cases in which intimidation or punishment work in more subtle ways, these visible physical techniques end up being too crude, and often outright damaging to the torturers.

Both psychological and biomedical research linked to armies or intelligence services in high-income countries, and decades of trial and error, imitation, training workshops and local innovations in the low- and middle-income countries, have produced a shared methodology in which the main objective of torture is increasingly the self and the conscious mind.

A leader in various protests against her national government was arrested in her home and then held incommunicado in a clandestine detention centre. In therapy, she later recounted the endless days of isolation and loneliness in an environment with no other sound than the locks opening and closing. She distinctly remembers the anguish of not knowing why she was detained or who might have given her name, the fear that her family might also be detained and maybe even tortured, and the anxiety of waiting for excruciating pain to be inflicted. That pain never arrived, nor was she interrogated. There was only silence and absolute loneliness. When she was released, four months later, without formal charges, she didn't know what hurt more: the stress of anticipation and imagining what would happen to her, or the reality of what she actually experienced. During her therapy, she was unable to understand why she had been fleeing from herself for years, and in fact never truly stopped.

In this book we have presented some of the elements that cause the understanding of psychological torture to be especially complex, and we have proposed practical solutions.

Psychological torture, or simply torture

We began this book by recognising the challenge of developing an operational definition of torture – especially one that applies to Western democracies. The definition in the United Nations Convention Against Torture has ambiguous elements that are subject to interpretation. What is to be understood by 'severe' suffering? How is to possible to know the 'motives' of the person inflicting harm?

Jurisprudence has tried to address these problems by coming up with more advanced definitions (like that of the Inter-American Convention Against Torture, which is, without a doubt, the most forward-thinking definition from the medical and psychological point of view that exists in international law), or through the litigation of paradigmatic cases. In this way, certain elements have taken shape: the distinction between torture, cruel and inhuman treatment, and degrading treatment becomes diluted and no longer makes sense in juridical or medical terms. Additional elements have come to be recognised in jurisprudence as forms of torture, including elements that don't lead to direct physical suffering (such as fear and threats), as well as the anguish that comes from denying information to family members of the detained/disappeared. Rape is unanimously recognised as a form of torture due to its unique psychological impacts on the self and identity. Psychological torture – we could even say torture (without qualification) – understood as *an attack on the will of the conscious self* is slowly gaining recognition as a defined entity.

Even though many victims describe the 'worst' forms of torture as humiliation and attacks against their dignity (as we saw in Chapter 5), most people underestimate the impact of methods that do not involve pain or physical injury. Many influential policy makers' idea of torture is based on images from medieval times, or the mostly physical, pain-based torture of the 1970s and 1980s. When evaluating whether or not torture has occurred, many people have strong misconceptions about what factors are most relevant to the victim. On one end, humiliation can be an end in itself and be considered degrading treatment, but on the other, humiliation can also be used as a means to break the will (in the sense of the word *torcere*, or *to twist* in Latin), and should be qualified as torture. Any use of physical or mental force with the purpose of humiliation can, in certain circumstances, amount to torture: society has yet to fully recognise this in the same way that it has already recognised fear's role in torture.

It is time for an integrative perspective on torture: society must learn from survivors' definitions of torture; the legal and juridical world must incorporate the findings of psychometric, neuropsychological and neurobiological data.

Meanwhile, the prevailing understanding of torture is that of torturers themselves: interrogation is seen as the art of finding the detainee's limits and becomes torture only when the interrogator goes too far in this pursuit, has unethical motives or uses methods that risk causing potentially lethal damage. But how can the interrogator know when he or she has gone too far? Is there a scientific basis upon which clear rules about what is permissible and what is not can be established? Only explicit regulations and firmly established principles can keep an interrogator from giving in to the fantasy of his or her omnipotence or succumbing to the temptation of crossing the line in the pursuit of a supposedly greater good.

We must abandon the focus on torture 'methods' and move towards understanding torturing environments. To grasp the central elements of torture, and to build classifications that will endure over time and allow new forms of mistreatment to be taken into account, it is necessary to first comprehend the objective that lies behind every torture method, and the combination of processes employed to break the individual's identity. Second, it is necessary to abandon the idea of single torture methods and focus on the idea of cumulative mistreatment, cumulative effects of torture methods or, as proposed here, torturing environments.

Over the decades, knowledge of torture has converged to form a shared corpus of techniques. Methods such as isolation, sleep deprivation, inhuman conditions of detention, manipulation of environment (light, heat, time), pain (harsh beatings and stress positions), nakedness and other forms of humiliation, threats and fear are universal and central to contemporary torture in situations of short-term detention. What varies from country to country is the way in which these universal elements are combined with local variations, which are often derived simply from the tools or resources that torturers have at hand. In the long term, more sophisticated techniques point to strategies of breaking the person and changing the victim's identity, and substituting it for an identity that serves the torturer. Strategies used in the long term are also recurrent: isolation, power imbalances, questioning basic values, normalising the abnormal, interpersonal manipulation, fear, group pressure, breaking assumptions and beliefs, guilt and shame, and finally the installation of a new ideology (see Figure 15.1).

When interrogation is the main purpose of torture, the torturing environment becomes inextricably intertwined with coercive interrogation techniques. They are one and the same. The interrogation becomes part of the torturing environment, and the purpose of torture becomes to interrogate the detainee. To affirm, as Kelly et al. (2013) do, that coercive interrogation and torture 'are simply different things' ignores the fact that it is the environment and the motives, not the techniques, that determine what torture is. All of the elements that comprise the detainee's treatment are part of what we call the torturing environment. Just as it does not make sense to debate whether sleep deprivation is or is not a torture method (it may or may not be depending on the duration, the rest of the environment and the intentions of the torturer), coercive interrogation may or may not be torture depending on the way in which it is conducted, the duration, the environment and the intentionality of the torturer.

For this reason, coercive interrogation requires clear, explicit limits, especially when – contrary to the belief that such interrogation is a necessary evil – the data reviewed in this book shows that coercive interrogation works only slightly better than cognitive interviewing in getting confessions. Such results come at the expense of an unacceptable increase in false confessions, in particular when certain techniques are used, such as false-evidence ploys or having to choose between two incriminating alternatives in a state of exhaustion. False confessions are not only a serious ethical and legal problem, they are also a practical problem that causes confusion and additional work for those seeking the truth. Experimental studies show that coercive interrogation is even less effective than cognitive interviewing for gathering information from a source.

A review of the interrogation techniques collected in Appendix 3 shows that the great majority of these techniques could easily form part of a harsh torturing environment. Moreover, according to the definition in the UN Convention, interrogation *per se* (without any other elements) could be considered psychological torture if it induces severe psychological suffering for the purpose of obtaining a confession, or for the purpose of debasing, humiliating or punishing a person. Interrogation techniques can amount to torture: as such they should be integrated into a general schema on how torture works, and included in the Istanbul Protocol. This is a neglected aspect in the research on psychological torture.

It has been debated whether it is possible to select a group of techniques that produce an 'uncomfortable' situation, but do not amount to torture (such as the five techniques proposed by Guiora (2008), discussed in Chapter 14). It is difficult to know why some techniques and not others would qualify as 'uncomfortable'; the distinction between 'torture' and 'discomfort' seems to be merely semantic.

Music – one of the five techniques considered by Guiora as 'uncomfortable', but not torture – is a good example. Music has been used for decades as a re-education tool. One ethnographic study (Papaeti, 2013) describes how left-wing political prisoners in Greek prison camps on the island of Makronisos (1947–1955), and at the prison camp on the island of Giaros during the military junta (1967–1974), remember music from loudspeakers as one of the worst torture methods. Music, as a disturbing experience and 'brainwashing' instrument, was instrumentalised as a way of breaking political prisoners and as part of an attempt to make detainees sign declarations of loyalty, renouncing their values and their comrades. Former detainees from both historical periods stress the damaging effects of the use of music, highlighting the need to understand music's capacity to degrade and torture individuals. Continuous loud sounds prevent people from thinking and structuring their minds. Music induces an automatic state, where messages permeate a mind that easily becomes blocked and, over time, broken. Music is a constant reminder of who has the power, and is described as a 'mental jail' that acts within the 'physical jail' of the concentration camp. The content of the music, which may have both nationalist and traditional messages and emotional resonance (such as songs from the prisoner's childhood), is debasing and humiliating. Similar reports refer to the constant use of rock music with Arab prisoners in Guantanamo. There are descriptions of its use in Chile, in Soviet gulags and by the Gestapo in Nazi camps. Research shows that music by itself does not produce 'brainwashing' (i.e., compliance with the new ideology being imposed) but can produce a state of cognitive exhaustion and irritability as it humiliates and pushes the detainee to question their own identity. Different authors have discussed the idea of *coercive music*, and proposed that music should be banned in detention centres when it is used for coercion (Cusick, 2006; Grant, 2013; Klause, 2013).

In any case, if 'discomfort' is used to twist the wills of detainees and make them act against themselves, what difference does it make if it is called by another name? The 'uncomfortable' method clearly violates the rights of detainees according to national and international laws, which should be non-negotiable, as Guiora himself says. In effect, a democracy should never doubt that all of its citizens' constitutional rights remain intact: the right to remain silent and not incriminate oneself, the right to be informed of the law and of one's legal situation, the right to choose a lawyer, the right to not be subjected to inhuman or degrading treatment or to torture.

The future of torture

We do not know how torture methods will evolve in the future. There are numerous biometric techniques that are often used in the marketing world (fMRIs, wireless electroencephalography, eye tracking, biometric sensors, skin galvanic conductance, facial recognition systems, etc.) to see what types of emotions specific commercials or brands generate. These types of devices are often used when interrogating suspects. Some airports in the United States use biometric sensor systems to detect anomalous responses to routine questions to filter people likely to be interrogated by immigration agents. It is highly probable that diverse military scientific research projects are underway, and that they involve developing sophisticated decision-making algorithms for optimising visualisation of real-time electric brain activity signals during interrogation. Though their use is not widespread, it is possible that in the near future, technology-assisted interrogations (coercive or not) will be routine; we can also foresee the increased use of hormones like oxytocin that stimulate empathy and the formation of emotional bonds with the interrogators. Situations that up until now have been unimaginable are becoming reality, such as forcing people to reveal traces of what they think or feel, twisting their conscious will. The idea of cognitive liberty undoubtedly deserves further attention. From one point of view, this could make torture unnecessary. From another, the final frontiers of human privacy are being breached: the right to think freely. Just as we understand rape to be a crime against humanity, we should not underestimate the seriousness of violating a detainee's thoughts. If we condemn attacks against sexual identity, how can we accept attacks against identity as a whole? There is much left to reflect upon. Perhaps in the future, an international convention on involuntary information extraction will be needed. For now, it seems that in future decades the extraction of information will occur more often via the interception and the technological control of communications than via interrogation. It is possible that the changes brought on by the information age will make interrogation unnecessary, and that torture will only retain its punitive or degrading character.

Recent years have shown how the 'need' to torture has been justified for security reasons, kindling a debate that was unthinkable just a few years ago regarding the legitimacy of torture when applying raison d'état. The undeniable growth of terrorism as a form of combat should not justify renouncing the principles that separate civilisation from barbarism. When torture occurs, the very sense of what constitutes humanity is lost. It is not possible to pay such a price, nor is it necessary. As the 2014 US Senate intelligence committee report on the CIA's detention and interrogation program concluded, torture is not useful. It not only fails to solve a problem, it creates another: inhumanity begins to spiral out of control. For example, ISIS has recently become the focus of international attention for their brutal mass beheadings; such violence is not unrelated to the torture in Western detention centres. Swept up in the frenzy of what we could call *raison d'torture*, this extremist group has dressed innocent people in uniforms similar to those used by prisoners in Guantanamo, tortured them using methods that they consider to be equivalent to those used in Guantanamo, and then decapitated them. We are trying to fight fire with gasoline.

Many definitions, one concept

Meanwhile, we have proposed several solutions to some of these issues. It is clear that there are different ways of understanding torture, and the juridical definition is not the only one. It is possible to legitimately affirm that what happened to a given person is torture from a medical, psychological or ethical point of view, even if it is not considered torture from a juridical point of view. It is important to vindicate other visions of torture, even though the shared point of reference is always, at the end of the day, the legal one. On more than a few occasions an expert has found that, when classifying acts as 'torture' during trial, the judge insists that he or she stick to technical criteria and leave the penal judgments to the court. There are far too many arbitrary and unjust laws in the world to accept that the legal world always aligns perfectly with real life.

The lack of a clear and objective definition within the juridical conception of torture leaves space for uncertainty and discretional interpretations that makes scientists uncomfortable. In training courses instructors are often obligated to say – to the surprise of their students – that torture, ultimately, is whatever a judge decides is torture. This includes, but is not limited to, the particular judge's evaluation of the degree of severity of suffering and the motivation deemed to underscore the acts of coercion or violence that are on trial.

Even after taking into account the subjective and interpretative nature of the law, the enormous differences among judges in their sentences regarding torture represent a challenge. Such wild variation is difficult to understand from a scientific standpoint. The interpretation of legal criteria is relative: this is reflected, for example, in the disparate criteria employed by the European Court of Human Rights in the cases of *Ireland v. UK* and *Selmouni v. France*. We see the same phenomenon in the conflicting conclusions of different judges in the former Yugoslavian tribunal who, after reviewing similar detention conditions in concentration camps, found that such conditions should be considered torture in some cases, but not in others (see Chapter 4). We recognise that these are the laws with which the juridical world operates and that a certain amount of subjective discretion is necessary, but it is clear that the legal decision-making process regarding torture is in serious need of more scientific criteria.

The political sphere, like the legal world, faces the same challenge.

Evaluation of torturing environments

In this context, looking for tools that delve into the medical and psychological logic of torture is a necessary step towards supporting human rights investigations, as well as supporting the work of lawyers, judges and others responsible for decision-making within detention and interrogation processes.

The heart of torture lies not in suffering, but in the breaking of the will through a systematic attack on the victim's capacity to *be*, and to understand themselves – an attack on his or her identity. And that does not necessarily require physical or psychological suffering; it requires putting mechanisms into motion that, alone or in combination, undermine the person's capacity for control. The Torturing Environment Scale is a first step on the path to better understanding these conditions.

Any instrument of measure is, of necessity, unfair. We speak of the validity of an instrument as its ability to measure exactly what it proposes to measure, and nothing else. Time will tell if the TES serves as a valid instrument, or if its character is too general, and more specific instruments adapted to specific contexts are required. For example, in a given context the manipulation of environment may be highly sophisticated, or include elements that the TES fails to reflect.

The questionnaire reflects the fact that it only takes a single torture method for torture to exist. The overall score produced by the TES should not be misconstrued: it is not intended to compare intensities of torture. Human suffering can never be compared. What is compared in the TES is the *intensity of the aggression* and a profile is built to reveal the *objectives* of that aggression. Nothing could be further from our intentions than attempting to compare distinct experiences of torture. Each experience is unique and two experiences cannot be compared, much less ranked. A torturing environment with an overall score of 7 is not necessarily less devastating than one with an overall score of 40; to suggest as much would be to ignore the essence of torture and the reality of the experiences that victims share during therapy.

Designing a set of measurements to analyse torturing environments can help to create profiles of different torture styles and different kinds of attacks on the human mind. This opens up a field of research for human rights groups as well as scholars who are conducting studies that correlate profiles of torturing environments, areas of brain involvement and eventually impairments in brain functioning. The results currently available that track correlations between torture and measurements of electrical activity or images are not specific enough. Attempting to see the correlation by measuring specific types of aggressions to the conscious mind could open up new areas of forensic research.

To date, it has also been difficult to correlate torture with measurements of clinical impact, both in terms of PTSD and in changes in worldviews. Obtaining more advanced measurements of torturing environments can help understand the specific type of psychological damage that those environments provoke. Although we know that the long-term impact of torture experiences depends on the post-traumatic living conditions of the survivor, obtaining better measurements of psychological trauma would allow more specific rehabilitation programs adapted to the precise type of harm provoked by psychological torture to be designed.

There are many remaining challenges to future research. Unfortunately, after reviewing the history of torture, we found that clinical and academic research lags an average of 10 to 20 years behind research in military psychology. There is no funding for scientific work on subjects related to human rights; intelligence services, on the other hand, have vast resources with which to research ways to improve information collection, manipulation and coercion techniques, and methods of social control.

The Istanbul Protocol

We must strengthen and expand the use of the Istanbul Protocol. In the years since its approval in 1999, the IP has shown that it is one of the great contributions to the contemporary fight against torture. The heart of the Protocol is not just the identification of torture situations and the assessment of their consequences; it is the evaluation of the credibility of the allegations, assessing the veracity of the victim's testimony in the absence of witnesses and physical scars. It is important to consolidate this idea among all of the legal actors who intervene in the evaluation of situations of torture. This is why we propose more systematic exploration of the elements that permit objective and precise evaluations of the credibility of allegations. To achieve this, we propose the use of the Standard Evaluation Form based on the IP (SEC) as a tool that helps develop a common language and promotes research into credibility analysis based on the IP.

The Istanbul Protocol needs to be updated, if only because it alludes to classification systems for mental illnesses that are now obsolete and to diagnoses that are no longer used. It would be useful to open up this new area of work. Updating the IP is also a way to preserve it as a living tool and to foster reflection on the new challenges presented by torture in the decades to come.

Reversing the paradigm

We have developed a theoretical framework and a standardised method to determine when a situation could be considered torture. The question that follows is: is it possible to reverse this reasoning in order to help establish clear rules about what techniques should and should not be considered psychological torture and make a catalogue of allowed and forbidden techniques?

It is clear that the answer is no. Every single element in the torture process, even the most banal, can be used to torture. Seemingly ordinary elements like a chair, silence or using the toilet can be decisive pieces within the torturing environment when used in specific ways. Although it is necessary that clear, pre-facto rules be established to delineate the *minimum acceptable conditions* for detention and the conditions for lawful interrogation, only transparency and monitoring will ensure proper compliance. Such rules should not be limited to banning individual techniques. Further research on torturing environments will help define which parts of a torturing environment imply high, middle and low probability of sustained damage.

Monitoring must always imply full video and tape recording of places of detention and interrogation, full records of interrogations and the availability of recordings for judicial procedures. Monitoring should also involve regular visits and interviews with detainees, and the systematic measurement of torturing environments, like the TES or other similar scales adapted to specifics contexts or countries. Though an exhaustive list of allowed and forbidden techniques would undoubtedly help, banning procedures has not been sufficient to prevent abuses in the past. The only way to prevent cumulative mistreatment, and the cognitive and emotional manipulation of identity that forces a person to act against his or her will, is regular monitoring of interrogation environments, careful oversight and a system of legal guarantees established by the state. Only then can democracy and the rule of law prevail.

All nations, openly or covertly, resort to torture – especially, but not only, when faced with what they consider serious security threats. Ending torture is a complex task that requires a brave political attitude and a clear stance from civil society to reject any attempts to support torture in our name or with our taxes. Medical and psychological research and other branches of science can help. But in the end, each one of us must decide what kind of world we leave to the next generation. To work towards a world without torture we must begin by defending our very humanity, and to protect our humanity we must do everything in our power to stop torture.

Appendix 1

INTERNATIONAL CLASSIFICATION SYSTEMS

Classification of torture methods according to the Istanbul Protocol (1985)

TABLE A1.1 Classification of torture methods according to the Istanbul Protocol (1985)

a. Blunt trauma, such as a punch, kick, slap, whipping, beating with wires or truncheons, or falling down;

b. Positional torture, using suspension, stretching limbs apart, prolonged constraint of movement, forced positioning;

c. Burns with cigarettes, heated instruments, scalding liquid, or a caustic substance;

d. Electric shocks;

e. Asphyxiation, such as wet and dry methods, drowning, smothering, choking, or use of chemicals;

f. Crush injuries, such as smashing fingers or using a heavy roller to injure the thighs or back;

g. Penetrating injuries, such as stab or gunshot wounds, wires under nails;

h. Chemical exposure to salt, chilli pepper, gasoline, etc. (in wounds or body cavities);

i. Sexual violence to genitals, molestation, instrumentation, rape;

j. Crush injury or traumatic removal of digits and limbs;

k. Medical amputation of digits or limbs, surgical removal of organs;

l. Pharmacological torture using toxic doses of sedatives, neuroleptics, paralytics, etc.;

m. Conditions of detention, such as a small or overcrowded cell, solitary confinement, unhygienic conditions, no access to toilet facilities, irregular or contaminated food and water, exposure to extremes of temperature, denial of privacy, and forced nakedness;

n. Deprivation of normal sensory stimulation, such as sound, light, sense of time, isolation, manipulation of brightness of the cell, abuse of physiological needs, restriction of sleep, food, water, toilet facilities, bathing, motor activities, medical care, social contacts, isolation within prison, loss of contact with the outside world (victims are often kept in isolation in order to prevent bonding and mutual identification and to encourage traumatic bonding with the torturer);

o. Humiliation, such as verbal abuse, performance of humiliating acts;

p. Threats of death, harm to family, further torture, imprisonment, mock executions;

q. Threats of attack by animals, such as dogs, cats, rats or scorpions;

r. Psychological techniques to break down the individual, including forced betrayals, accentuating feelings of helplessness, exposure to ambiguous situations or contradictory messages;

(continued)

TABLE A1.1 Classification of torture methods according to the Istanbul Protocol (1985) (*continued*)

s. Violation of taboos;
t. Behavioral coercion, such as forced engagement in practices against the religion of the victim (e.g. forcing Muslims to eat pork), forced harm to others through torture or other abuses, forced destruction of property, forced betrayal of someone placing them at risk of harm;
u. Forcing the victim to witness torture or atrocities being inflicted on others.

HURIDOCS: thesaurus for the classification of torture methods

TABLE A1.2 HURIDOCS: thesaurus for the classification of torture methods

03	Methods of violence against a person (such as torture)	
03 01	Beating	05.21
03 01 01	Slapping, kicking or punching	05.211
03 01 02	Blows with rifle butts, whips, straps or heavy sticks	05.212
03 01 03	'Telefono' – clapping on ears with the mouth shut	05.2191
03 01 04	'Falanga' – beating of the soles of the feet	05.2192
03 02	Wounding	
03 03	Maiming or breaking bones	05.214
03 03 01	'Operating table' – the victim is forced to lie on a table with the upper half of the body unsupported while the abdomen is beaten Forced jumping or being thrown from heights	05.2193
03 04	Burns	05.24
03 04 01	Burns with boiling water	05.241
03 04 02	Burns with cigarettes	05.232
03 04 03	Burns with chemicals	05.243
03 04 04	Burns with burning sticks or live fire	05.244
03 05	Rape	
03 05 01	Rape with forced performance of particular sexual acts	05.252
03 05 02	Rape through introduction of inanimate objects into the genitalia	05.255
03 05 03	Rape through introduction of animate objects into the genitalia	05.256
03 06	Sexual harassment and molestation	
03 06 01	Sexual harassment and molestation, with forced performance of particular sexual acts	05.252
03 06 03	Sexual comments and other forms of sexual harassment	

03	Methods of violence against a person (such as torture)	
03 06 04	Touching as a form of sexual harassment and molestation	05.252
03 07	Exposure to extreme heat or cold	05.66
03 08	Application of electric shock	05.257
03 08 01	'Black slave' – an electric apparatus which inserts a heated metal skewer into the victim's anus	05.2571
03 08 02	'Picana' or 'parrilla' – use of heavy metal bed frame	05.321
03 09	Asphyxiation	05.26
03 09 01	'Submarino' – includes the use of water	
03 09 02	'Submarino seco' – putting the head in a plastic bag	05.262
03 09 03	'Submarino mojado' – immersion in filthy fluid such as water with urine and excrement	05.2631
03 10	Strangulation	05.261
03 11	Forced postures	05.27
03 11 02	'Pau de arara' (parrot's perch), or hanging the victim from a stick between the knees and arms bound tightly together	05.2711
03 11 03	'Planton' (forced standing), often exposed to the elements, for many hours	05.272
03 11 04	'Potro' – stretching of limbs and trunk	02.273
03 11 05	Forced sitting or kneeling	05.274
03 11 06	'Saw horse' – victim is forced to sit straddling a metal or wooden bar	05.2741
03 12	Nail removal	05.28
03 13	Use of animals (rats, spiders, etc.) as a method of violence	05.31
03 14	Amputation	05.34
03 15	Deprivation	05.4
03 15 01	Deprived of food and/or water	05.41
03 15 02	Deprived of sleep	05.43
03 15 03	Deprived of needed medical attention	05.44
03 15 04	Deprived of needed medication	05.45
03 16	Forced feeding	05.411

(continued)

TABLE A1.2 HURIDOCS: thesaurus for the classification of torture methods (*continued*)

03	Methods of violence against a person (such as torture)	
03 17	Immobilisation	
03 17 01	Being bound or tied up as a form of immobilisation	05.651
03 18	Isolation	03 18
03 19	Stress to the senses	05.6
03 19 01	Stress from loud/disagreeable noises	05.61
03 19 02	Stress from screams and voices	05.62
03 19 03	Stress from powerful lights	05.63
03 19 04	Blindfolding	05.64
03 19 05	Overcrowding	05.48
03 20	Psychological torture and ill-treatment	05.7
03 21	Degradation	05.76
03 21 01	Verbal abuse	05.71
03 21 02	Nakedness as a form of degradation	05.762
03 21 03	Being forced to act in a degrading way	05.764
03 22	Threats (not including death threats)	05.72
03 22 01	Threats against the victim	05.721
03 22 02	Threats against the victim's family	05.722
03 22 03	Threats against the victim's friends and colleagues	05.723
03 24	Torture as a witness	05.77
03 25	Pharmacological manipulation	05.8
03 90	Other methods of violence against a person	

Appendix 2
CIA AND ARMY MANUALS

The KUBARK Interrogation Manual: techniques[1]

[C1] **Monopolization of Attention:** The more completely the place of confinement eliminates sensory stimuli, the more rapidly and deeply will the interrogatee be affected [. . .] An early effect of such an environment is anxiety [. . .] The interrogator can benefit from the subject's anxiety [. . .] The deprivation of stimuli induces regression [of the interrogatee to his or her childhood] by depriving the subject's mind of contact with an outer world and thus forcing it upon itself (90).

[C2] **Induced Debilitation and Exhaustion:** An over-stuffed chair for the use of the interrogatee is sometimes preferable to a straight-backed, wooden chair because *if he is made to stand for a lengthy period or is otherwise deprived of physical comfort*, the contrast is intensified and increased disorientation results (45, emphasis supplied) | *When the individual is told to stand at attention for long periods* [. . .] the immediate source of pain is not the interrogator but the victim himself. The motivational strength of the individual is likely to exhaust itself in this internal encounter (94, *emphasis supplied*).

[C3] **Cultivation of Anxiety and Despair:** The interrogator can and does make the subject's world not only unlike the world to which he had been accustomed but also strange in itself – a world in which familiar patterns of time, space, and sensory perception are overthrown (52). | A pale face indicates fear and usually shows that the interrogator is hitting close to the mark (55). | What we aim to do is to ensure that the manner of arrest achieves, if possible, surprise, and *the maximum amount of mental discomfort* [. . .]. The ideal time at which to arrest a person is in the early hours of the morning because surprise is achieved then (85, emphasis in the original). | The circumstances of detention are arranged to enhance within the subject his feelings of being cut off from the known and the reassuring, and of being plunged into the strange. Usually his own clothes are immediately taken away, because familiar clothing reinforces identity and thus the capacity for resistance. [. . .] Detention permits the interrogator to cut through these links and throw the interrogatee back upon his own unaided internal resources. [. . .] Control of source's environment permits the interrogator to determine his diet, sleep pattern, and other fundamentals. Manipulating these into irregularities, so that the subject becomes disoriented, is very likely to create feelings of fear and helplessness [. . .]. In any event, it is advisable to keep the subject upset by constant disruptions of patterns (86f). | It is usually useful to intensify [the subject's feelings of guilt] (103). | See also *Monopolization of Attention.*

[C4] **Alternating Punishments and Rewards:** The commonest of the joint interrogator techniques is the Mutt-and-Jeff routine: the brutal, angry, domineering type contrasted with the friendly, quiet type. This routine works best with women, teenagers, and timid men [. . .] an interrogator working alone can also use the Mutt-and-Jeff technique [. . .] (72f). | Half-hearted efforts to cooperate can be ignored, and conversely he can be rewarded for non-cooperation (for example, a successfully resisting source may become distraught if given some reward for the 'valuable contribution' that he has made) (77). | Meals and sleep granted irregularly, in more than abundance or less than adequacy, the shifts occurring on no discernible time pattern, will normally disorient an interrogatee and sap his will to resist more effectively than a sustained deprivation leading to debility (93).

[C5] **Demonstrating 'Omniscience' of Captor:** [The interrogator] can create and amplify an effect of omniscience in a number of ways. For example, he can show the interrogatee a thick file bearing [the interogatee's] name. Even if the file contains little or nothing but blank paper, the air of familiarity with which the interrogator refers to the subject's background can convince some sources that all is known and that resistance is futile (52). | The interrogator [. . .] explains to the source that the purpose of the questioning is not to gain information; the interrogator knows everything already. His real purpose is to test the sincerity (reliability, honor, etc.) of the source. The interrogator then asks a few questions to which he knows the answers. If the subject lies, he is informed firmly and dispassionately that he has lied. By skilled manipulation of the known, the questioner can convince a naive subject that all his secrets are out (67).

[C6] **Demonstrating 'Omnipotence' of Captor:** [The interrogator] exercises the powers of an all-powerful parent, determining when the source will be sent to bed, when and what he will eat, [and] whether he will be rewarded for good behavior or punished for being bad (52).

[C7] **Temporal Disorientation:** The subject may be left alone for days; and he may be returned to his cell, allowed to sleep for five minutes, and brought back to an interrogation which is conducted as though eight hours had intervened. The principle is that sessions should be so planned as to disrupt the source's sense of chronological order (49f). | There are a number of non-coercive techniques for inducing regression [. . .]. Some interrogatees can be re[g]ressed by persistent manipulation of time, by retarding and advancing clocks, and serving meals at odd times – ten minutes or ten hours after the last food was given. Day and night are jumbled. Interrogation sessions are similarly unpatterned[;] the subject may be brought back for more questioning just a few minutes after being dismissed for the night (76f).

[C8] **Sensory Disorientation:** The Confusion [or *Alice-in-Wonderland*] technique is designed not only to obliterate the familiar, but to replace it with the weird [. . .]. When the subject enters the room, the first interrogator asks a double talk question – one which seems straightforward but is essentially nonsensical [. . .]. The second interrogator follows up [. . .] with a wholly unrelated and equally illogical query [. . .]. No pattern of questions and answers is permitted to develop [. . .]. As the process continues, day after day if necessary, the subject begins to try to make sense of the situation, which becomes mentally intolerable (76). | [One example of the *magic room* technique involves giving the prisoner] a hypnotic suggestion that his hand is growing warm. However, in this instance, the prisoner's hand actually does become warm, a problem easily resolved by the use of a concealed diathermy machine. Or it might be suggested . . . that . . . a cigarette will taste bitter. Here again, he could be given a cigarette prepared to have a slight but noticeably bitter taste (77f).

[C9] **Threats:** The threat of coercion usually weakens or destroys resistance more effectively than coercion itself. The threat to inflict pain, for example, can trigger fears more damaging than the immediate sensation of pain [. . .]. The same principle holds for other fears: sustained long enough, a strong fear of anything vague or unknown induces regression, whereas the materialization of the fear, the infliction of some form of punishment, is likely to come as a relief [. . .]. Threats delivered coldly are more effective than those shouted in rage (90f).

[C10] **Pharmacological Manipulation:** Persons burdened with feelings of shame or guilt are likely to unburden themselves when drugged, especially if these feelings have been reinforced by the interrogator [. . .]. Drugs (and the other aids discussed in this section) should not be used persistently to facilitate the interrogative debriefing that follows capitulation. Their function is to cause capitulation, to aid in the shift from resistance to cooperation (100).

FM 2–22.3 Human Intelligence Collector Operations (2006)

- **Direct approach.** Pertinent questions are asked directly 'as long as the source is answering the questions in a truthful manner'. In almost all HUMINT collection this is the first approach used, and an alternative approach is chosen once the source refuses to answer, avoids answering or answers falsely.
- **Incentive approach.** A real or emotional reward is given, or a real or perceived negative stimulus is removed, within the limits of what can be delivered and what is permissible by national and international law.
- **Emotional approaches** join an emotional response with some attached incentive. These are:
  - **Emotional love.** 'Sincerity and conviction are critical' for the questioner to be persuasive. 'For example, if the source cooperates, he can see his family sooner, end the war, protect his comrades, help his country, help his ethnic group.'
  - **Emotional hate.** The questioner persuades the source that cooperation will harm his enemies. The manual prohibits the questioner from promising that a unit will be denied a chance to surrender or that it will be mistreated.
  - **Emotional fear-up.** 'The HUMINT collector must be extremely careful that he does not threaten or coerce a source', but can rely on justifiable fears such as

[the fear] that the prisoner may be killed for cooperating unless he receives protection; and he can rely on non-specific fears, such as asking, 'You know what can happen to you here?'

- **Emotional fear-down.** A fearful subject is reassured 'through verbal and physical actions' to calm him and cause him to view the interrogator as a 'protector'.
- **Emotional pride and ego-up.** The subject is 'flattered into providing certain information in order to gain credit and build his ego' using a 'somewhat-in-awe tone of voice'. The subject might be complimented on a well-done operation or be persuaded to begin talking about an aspect of his job at which he is skilled.
- **Emotional pride and ego-down.** The questioner attacks the subject's 'loyalty, intelligence, abilities, leadership qualities, slovenly appearance, or any other perceived weakness'. If the subject tries to defend himself he may provide useful information. This must not 'cross the line into humiliating and degrading treatment of the detainee', and the manual advises that the 'experience level' and intended actions of subordinates be considered before an interrogation plan is approved using this method.
- **Emotional futility.** The questioner uses factual information to try to convince the source that resistance is futile. This approach generally must be combined with another, such as the emotional love approach, to be effective.
- **Cognitive manipulation and deceit.**
  - **We know all.** The interrogator 'subtly convinces the source that his questioning of the source is perfunctory because any information that the source has is already known' by providing detailed information and answering himself when the source hesitates. The approach requires the interrogator to have a large amount of information already, and have committed much of it to memory.
  - **File and dossier.** The interrogator prepares himself with a large dossier (padded with paper if necessary) indexed with tabs for 'education, employment, criminal record, military service, and others' and proceeds as in the 'We know all' approach.
  - **Establish your identity.** The subject is told that he has been 'identified as an infamous individual wanted by higher authorities on serious charges'. In a sincere effort to correct this mistake, against the interrogator's persistent denials, he may provide leads for further development.
  - **Repetition.** The interrogator 'listens carefully to a source's answer to a question, and then repeats the question and answer several times. He does this with each succeeding question until the source becomes so thoroughly bored with the procedure, he answers questions fully and candidly.'
  - **Rapid fire.** One, two or more interrogators 'ask a series of questions in such a manner that the source does not have time to answer a question completely before the next one is asked. This confuses the source, and he will tend to contradict himself as he has little time to formulate his answers.' The source may then be persuaded to explain the inconsistencies.
  - **Silence.** The interrogator 'says nothing to the source, but looks him squarely in the eye, preferably with a slight smile on his face . . . [he forces the source to] break eye contact first. The source may become nervous, begin to shift in his chair, cross

and re-cross his legs, and look away. He may ask questions . . .' After much delay, the interrogator asks questions such as 'You planned this operation for a long time, didn't you?'

- **Change of scenery.** When removed from the formal environment, 'the source may experience a feeling of leaving the interrogation behind'. The interrogator steers conversation toward the topic of interest, and 'the source may never realize he is still being questioned'.

- Two additional techniques require previous approval:

  - **Mutt and Jeff.** Two interrogators who are 'convincing actors' are chosen. The first may, for instance, "'be very strict and order the source to follow all military courtesies during questioning. Although he conveys an unfeeling attitude, the HUMINT collector is careful not to threaten or coerce the source.' The second scolds the first, may offer the source a beverage or a cigarette, and tries to persuade the source that they 'share a high degree of intelligence and sensitivity'. However, he is very busy and 'cannot afford to waste time on an uncooperative source. He can broadly imply that the first HUMINT collector might return . . .'

  - **False flag.** The goal is to 'convince the detainee that individuals from a country other than the United States are interrogating him, and trick the detainee into cooperating with US forces'. It may be 'effectively orchestrated with the Fear Down approach and the Pride and Ego Up'.

Separation is described at much greater length than the other methods in Appendix M of the manual, with the warning that it is forbidden under Geneva Conventions and requires approval. 'The purpose of separation is to deny the detainee the opportunity to communicate with other detainees in order to keep him from learning counter-resistance techniques.' The approach can be combined with the Futility, Incentive, or Fear Up approaches. The separation 'must not preclude the detainee getting four hours of continuous sleep every 24 hours'. The two forms of separation are:

- **Physical separation,** which prevents the detainee from communicating. Limited to 30 days of initial duration. Requires O-6 or above approval.
- **Field expedient separation.** 'Prolong the shock of capture' by using 'goggles or blindfolds and earmuffs' to prevent the detainee from communicating for up to 12 hours, plus the time these are used 'for security purposes during transit and evacuation'. 'Use of hoods (sacks) over the head, or of duct tape or adhesive tape over the eyes' is prohibited. The manual states that the technique shall not amount to **sensory deprivation**.

Note

1 Modified from Almerindo Ojeda (2008).

Appendix 3

CLASSIFICATION OF INTERROGATION TECHNIQUES (KELLY ET AL., 2013)

TABLE A3.1 Classification of interrogation techniques (Kelly et al., 2013)

DOMAIN 1 RAPPORT AND RELATIONSHIP BUILDING	DOMAIN 2 CONTEXT MANIPULATION	DOMAIN 3 EMOTION PROVOCATION	DOMAIN 4 CONFRONTATION AND COMPETITION	DOMAIN 5 COLLABORATION	DOMAIN 6 PRESENTATION OF EVIDENCE
1. Find common ground or shared experiences	1. Conduct the interrogation in a small room	1. Appeal to self-interest	1. Emphasise your authority and expertise over source	1. Offer rewards or reinforcement for desired information	1. Confront source with *actual* evidence of involvement
2. Show kindness and respect	2. Move the interrogation from a formal room to a more neutral setting	2. Appeal to conscience	2. Challenge the values held by the source	2. Make bargains with source	2. Confront source with fabricated or knowingly unsubstantiated evidence of involvement
3. Identify and meet basic needs	3. Move the interrogation from a neutral setting to a more formal room	3. Appeal to religion	3. Threaten source with consequences for non-cooperation	3. Appeal to sense of cooperation	3. Bluff or bait source about supposed evidence of involvement
4. Be patient	4. Isolate source before interrogation	4. Interrogate source while very stressed	4. Express impatience, frustration or anger	4. Present scenario so that source may regain or assert control	4. Identify contradictions within source's story
5. Allow source to play role of teacher	5. Disorganise source by manipulating the physical space	5. Offer moral rationalisations	5. Use deception	5. Offer special rewards (e.g. cigarettes, candy) for cooperation	5. Reveal evidence to source, demonstrating that s/he can offer no more useful information, until s/he eventually does
6. Build a bond	6. Consider the time of day	6. Capitalise on capture shock	6. Obscure source's fate	6. Offer intangible rewards (e.g. encouragement, respect)	6. Use polygraphs or other physiological tools
7. Present self as in a role/persona other than being an interrogator	7. Consider your physical appearance (clothing)	7. Appeal to negative feelings for individuals or organisations	7. Ask the same question over and over	7. Present a scenario where interrogator's job is to accurately represent the source as innocent or helpful to higher authorities	7. Show source photos or statements from witnesses or others
8. Touch source in a friendly manner	8. Prisoner's Dilemma	8. Identify and exaggerate fears	8. Ask a series of questions quickly without allowing source to answer		8. Use visual aids
9. Find identities in common	9. Consider where operator and detainees' chairs are in relation to one another	9. Reduce fears	9. Do not allow denials from source		
10. Attempt to become source's lifeline	10. Create setting that is culturally attractive	10. Flatter source	10. Do not speak to source, only stare at source		
11. Present oneself as similar to the source	11. Consider the effect of certain colors or sounds	11. Instill hopelessness in source	11. Confront source without insulting		
12. Show concern for source and his/her situation		12. Encourage source to take responsibility for the outcome	12. Adopt a non-friendly stance		
13. Use similar language as the source (e.g. slang)			13. Insult source		
14. Employ active listening skills (e.g. eye contact, nodding, summarise source's statements)			14. Get another interrogator and employ good cop/bad cop		
			15. Directly accuse source of being involved		
			16. Accuse source of being someone s/he is not		
			17. Disparage or dismiss information source provides		
			18. Misconstrue the source's own words		
			19. Ask unexpected / alternative questions		

Appendix 4
TOOLBOX

Semi-structured interview for torture survivors – Exposure to Torture Scale (Başoğlu & Paker, 1995)

The module is part of a broader interview, the Semi-structured Interview for Survivors of War (SISOW), which also includes demographic variables, personal history (infancy, psychosocial history, socio-political background), the Exposure to Trauma Scale (57 items of combat-related events), and the psychological preparedness to trauma and post-trauma measures (social support and post-trauma adaptation). The full SISOW protocol is available from the author (metin.basoglu@kcl.ac.uk).

SEMI-STRUCTURED INTERVIEW FOR SURVIVORS OF TORTURE
- (SIST) MODUL -

[**Definition of torture**: For the purposes of this study the following definition of torture provided by the 1986 United Nations Declaration of Human Rights has been adopted: "...any act by which severe pain or suffering, whether physical or mental, is intentionally inflicted on a person for such purposes as obtaining from him or a third person information or a confession, punishing him for an act he or a third person has committed or is suspected of having committed, or intimidating or coercing him or a third person, or for any reason based on discrimination of any kind, when such pain of suffering is inflicted by or at the instigation of or with the consent or acquiescence of a public official or other person acting in an official capacity."

According to this definition, indiscriminate violence or sporadic acts of sexual assault or rape are not regarded as torture, although they may share common elements with it. Multiple incidents of rape, however, occurring in a context of prolonged captivity or detention accompanied by other forms of ill treatment and/or torture can be defined as torture. Multiple rape of female victims over the course of several months to ensure pregnancy and delivery of a child is a case in point. Most incidents of systematic physical and/or mental ill treatment during captivity in a detention / concentration camp or a prison would be regarded as torture, provided they satisfy the definition given above. Such systematic torture incidents may also occur during the course of a war such as during house raids, hostage situations or kidnapping.

In this section the term **'torture experience'** refers to all torture events the person has experienced throughout the war. **'Torture incident'** refers to a single episode of systematic torture. A person might have had repeated 'incidents' of torture during captivity in a detention / concentration camp / prison or such incidents might have occurred sporadically outside the context of prolonged captivity (e.g. during a house raid).]

A. HISTORY OF TORTURE EXPERIENCE

Now I would like to ask about your torture experience. You told me earlier that you have been tortured on ..... occasions. [quote frequency figure for torture from Exposure to Trauma Scale] *Can you tell me more about each of these torture incidents, when and where it occurred* [location: concentration camp, prison etc.; specify where in the country and the surrounding events, e.g. during an enemy raid to the village], *who were involved* [soldiers, paramilitaries etc., names of persons not required], *and the reasons why they did that to you?* [e.g. was it used as a means of interrogation, punishment, vengeance, or was it carried out as part of indiscriminate action against the community?]

[Provide details of all torture incidents below. Use a separate sheet if necessary

	Date	Location	Carried out by	Reasons
1.	....			
2.	....			
3.	....			
4.	....			
5.	....			

A. EXPOSURE TO TORTURE SCALE

[The respondent may have had more than one incident of torture and had experienced different forms of torture during different torture incidents. In administering the scale, determine whether the person has ever experienced a particular form of torture, regardless of during which incident that form of torture may have taken place. Score "Present" as 0 if an event is absent and as 1 if an event is present.

Base the following ratings on the survivor's report and not on your own assessment. If a particular type of torture occurred more than once, base ratings on the most distressing / traumatic occurrence of the event.

Watch for any signs of distress in the respondent during the interview. If distress gets intolerable, allow the respondent some time to calm down or consider discontinuing the interview. Never continue the interview against the respondent's will.]

Now I would like to go through a list of common torture methods and ask you whether you have ever experienced them. I will also ask about various aspects of each torture event such as how much distress you felt during the event, what you did to cope with the situation, and how much control you had over the event. I will ask you to rate each of these events on these two scales. [Note: Detach the page with the scales and put it in front of the respondent]

1. *How distressed were you at the time you experienced the event?* [Base rating on how the survivor felt at the time of the event and not how s/he perceives it now.]

0= Not at all distressing	1= Mildly	2= Moderately	3= Fairly	4= Extremely distressing / intolerable

2. *How much control did you have over the situation? Were you able to do anything to avoid the event or lessen the distress it involved?* [Assess coping strategies and whether they were perceived to be effective in avoiding the event or lessening the pain or distress while the event was taking place. Take into account both behavioural and cognitive strategies used to cope with the event. The latter includes dissociation, distraction strategies, and beliefs, thoughts, or interpretations of event that reduce distress.]

0= **Completely in control**	1= **Fairly**	2= **Moderately**	3= **Slightly**	4= **Not at all in control / Entirely helpless**

		Present*	**Distress**	**Control**
1.	Beating	____	____	____
2.	Falaqa	____	____	____
3.	Electric torture	____	____	____
4.	Stretching of the body	____	____	____
5.	Burning	____	____	____
6.	Rope bondage	____	____	____
7.	Forced standing	____	____	____
8.	Throwing of urine / faeces at detainee	____	____	____
9.	Pulling / dragging / lifting by hair	____	____	____
10.	Needles under toenails or fingernails	____	____	____
11.	Forced extraction of teeth	____	____	____
12.	Hanging by hands or feet	____	____	____
13.	Palestinian hanging	____	____	____
14.	Sexual advances (by hand, etc)	____	____	____
15.	Fondling of genitals	____	____	____
16.	Threats of rape	____	____	____
17.	Rape	____	____	____
18.	Beating over the ears with cupped hands	____	____	____
19.	Forced standing with weight on	____	____	____
20.	Suffocation / asphyxiation (details: …………)	____	____	____
21.	Isolation	____	____	____
22.	Food deprivation	____	____	____
23.	Water deprivation	____	____	____
24.	Sleep deprivation	____	____	____
25.	Cold showers	____	____	____
26.	Exposure to extreme heat or cold	____	____	____
27.	Restriction of movement	____	____	____
28.	Blindfolding	____	____	____
29.	Exposure to bright light	____	____	____

30.	Exposure to loud music	____	____	____
31.	Threats of death	____	____	____
32.	Threats against family	____	____	____
33.	Threats of further torture	____	____	____
34.	Witnessing torture of close ones	____	____	____
35.	Witnessing torture of others	____	____	____
36.	Sham executions	____	____	____

* 0 = Absent 1 = Present

37.	Prevention of personal hygiene	____	____	____
38.	Denial of privacy	____	____	____
39.	Verbal abuse	____	____	____
40.	Mockery / humiliation	____	____	____
41.	Excrement in food	____	____	____
42.	Infested surroundings	____	____	____
43.	Stripping naked	____	____	____
44.	Fluctuation of interrogator's attitude	____	____	____
45.	Prevention of urination / defecation	____	____	____
46.	Deprivation of medical care	____	____	____
47.	Other:	____	____	____
48.	Other:	____	____	____
49.	Other:	____	____	____
50.	Other:	____	____	____
51.	Other:	____	____	____

* 0 = Absent 1 = Present

52. *Overall, how distressing was the torture experience for you?* ____

 0= Not at all distressing 1= Slightly 2= Moderately 3= Fairly 4= Extremely distressing

53. *How would you rate your overall control over everything you experienced?* ____

 0= Completely in control 1= Fairly 2= Moderately 3= Slightly 4= Not at all in control / entirely helpless

Torture Checklist (Jaranson et al., 2004)

Administered through semi-structured interview. Rated Yes/No

★	Experienced attempts at thought control	
★	Did you suffer any head injuries from torture?	
★	Beating soles of the feet	
★	Burned with boiling water	
★	Burned with cigarettes	
★	Use of animals or objects in a sexual manner	
★	Electric shock of genital areas	
★	Weights tied to testicles	
★	Immersion in water	
★	Immersion in dirty fluids	
★	Hanging the victim by thumbs, arms, or legs	
★	Rope bondage—tightening of ropes over a period of hours	
★	Forced to stand, sit, or kneel for many hours	
★	Stretching of limbs and body	
★	Removal of fingernails or toenails	
★	Needles under fingernails or toenails	
★	Electric shock	
★	Forced teeth extraction	
★	Forced ingestion/injection of harmful drugs	
★	Water slowly dripped onto head	
★	Subjected to powerful lights or forced to look directly into the sun	
★	Placed in total darkness for more than two days	
★	Abuse with excrement	
★	Mock execution	
★	Forced to watch or listen to the torture or murder of others	
★	Change of repressor role to that of ally in order to disorient the victim, fluctuation in torturer's attitude toward victim	
★	Forced choices (e.g. which person dies, which type of torture used next on self or others)	
★★	Slapping, kicking, or punching	
★★	Blows with rifle butts, whips, straps, heavy sticks, etc.	
★★	Flogging with rope, whip, or stick	
★★	Attacks with knives or other sharp instruments	

★★	Maiming or breaking bones	
★★	Blows to ears with mouth shut	
★★	Forced to jump or being thrown from heights	
★★	Burned with chemicals	
★★	Burned with live fire or burning sticks	
★★	Physical assault and touching sexual parts	
★★	Forced performance of particular sexual acts excluding actual rape	
★★	Rape by someone of the opposite sex	
★★	Rape by someone of the same sex	
★★	Lifting by hair	
★★	Prevention of urination or defecation	
★★	Deprived of food	
★★	Deprived of water	
★★	Immobilized, bound, or tied up	
★★	Isolated from others for more than three days	
★★	Deprived of regular sleep frequently or for extended periods	
★★	Subjected to constant loud noises (e.g. music, screams, voices)	
★★	Detonation of explosives nearby	
★★	Blindfolding	
★★	False accusations, recanting, or forced self-incrimination	
★★	Degradation through deprivation of personal hygiene (e.g. lack of access to toilets, showers, sanitary supplies)	
★★	Being forced to act in a degrading way (e.g. bark like a dog, dance, etc.)	
★★	Made to harm others	
★★	Made to tell on other people	
★★	Release and immediate rearrest	
★★	Other (10 techniques not in the questionnaire but identified by participants during interviews)	

★ 27 torture techniques used to classify participants as torture survivors even though they don't acknowledge torture.

★★ Trauma techniques which could occur during either torture or civil war.

Torture Screening Checklist, Revised (TSCL-R) (Rasmussen, 2011, 2016)

The following is a guide for clinicians to collect relevant information to help determine and document whether or not an interviewee qualifies as tortured under international statutes. It is based on United States Torture Victims Relief Act (TVRA; 18 USC 2340(1)) and the

United Nations Convention against Torture (UNCAT), and intended to become part of the record and justification for delivering services funded through either TVRA or the United Nations' Voluntary Fund. This guide may also be useful in developing legal cases in which torture is at issue.

Interviewee (i.e., client): _____

Interviewer: _____ Location of interview: _____

1. Was the interviewee in a situation in which someone in a government or other organized authority, acting under "color of law," intentionally hurt him/her in any way?
    ❑   Yes, act(s) by authorities/person(s) acting as authorities
    ❑   No
    1a. *IF "No"*: Did any authority know that someone might hurt interviewee and ignore this information?
    ❑   Yes, with the consent or acquiescence of a public official
    ❑   Yes, with the consent or acquiescence of a person acting in an official capacity
    ❑   No
    ❑   Don't know
2. Who perpetrated the acts? (specify; e.g. "police," not just "government"):
    _____
3. In what country did this happen? _____
4. Where did this take place? (Check all that apply)
    4a. ❑ Police station
    4b. ❑ Jail, prison or detention center
    4c. ❑ Military base or camp
    4d. ❑ Compound
    4e. ❑ Hospital
    4f. ❑ School
    4g. ❑ Home
    4h. ❑ Public space (e.g. street, public park, athletic arena)
    4i. ❑ Other: _____
5. Was the interviewee in the custody of or under the physical control of the actor(s) described in 1?
    ❑   Yes
    ❑   No
    IF "Yes": 5a. Explain answer:

    _____
6. Describe acts:

    _____
    _____
7. Were these acts deliberate or intentional? I.e., were they not accidentally perpetrated?
    ❑   Yes
    ❑   No

8. What was the purpose of the acts? (check all that apply)

    8a. ❑ Obtaining information

    8b. ❑ Confession of guilt (whether real or false)

    8c. ❑ Punishment for something he/she did

    8d. ❑ Punishment for something alleged but not done

    8e. ❑ Intimidation of self

    8f. ❑ Intimidation of someone else

    8g. ❑ Other reason based on discrimination:_____

    8h. ❑ Other reason:_____

    8i. ❑ Interviewee reports that he/she does not know

9. Did the acts result in severe pain or suffering?

    ❑ Yes

    ❑ No

    9a. Was the harm (physical or mental) prolonged, extending over a long period of time?

    ❑ Yes

    ❑ No

    IF *"Yes"*: 9a.1. Explain answer (include *length of time* and how harm was extended):

    9b. Did the harm have its source in:

        9b.1. The infliction of severe physical pain or suffering?

        ❑ Yes ❑ No

        9b.2. The threatened infliction of severe physical pain or suffering?

        ❑ Yes ❑ No

        9b.3. The forced administration or application of psychoactive drugs or other psychological procedures designed to disrupt profoundly the senses or the personality?

        ❑ Yes ❑ No

        9b.4. Death threats made against the person, where death is made to appear imminent?

        ❑ Yes ❑ No

        9b.5. Threats made against others of imminent death, severe physical pain or suffering, or forced administration or application of psychoactive drugs or psychologically disruptive procedures?

        ❑ Yes ❑ No

10. Were the acts intended by the perpetrator to cause severe pain or suffering?

    ❑ Yes

    ❑ No

    IF *"Yes"*: 10a. Explain answer (include how intention is inferred):

---

11. Did the perpetrator specifically target the interviewee? I.e., the interviewee was *not* only one of several persons randomly subjected to the act(s).

    ❑ Yes

    ❑ No

    IF *"Yes"*: 11a.1. Explain answer (include how targeting is inferred):

---

12. Did the acts occur as part of a legal punishment for something he/she did? (I.e., does what happened to him/her happen as part of *legally sanctioned* punishment for the alleged crime in that country? Answering this may involve knowledge of foreign legal codes.)

   ❑ Yes

   ❑ No

   ❑ Don't know

SCORING	
TVRA	**UNCAT**
Is 1 marked "Yes"? ❑ True	Is 1 *or* 1a marked "Yes"? ❑ True
Is *at least one* from 4a–4f "Yes"? ❑ True	Is 7 marked "Yes"? ❑ True
Is 5 marked "Yes"? ❑ True	Is *at least one* from 8a–8g "Yes"? ❑ True
Is 7 marked "Yes"? ❑ True	Is 9 marked "Yes"? ❑ True
Is 9a marked "Yes"? ❑ True	Is 12 marked "No"? ❑ True
Is *at least one* from 9b.1–5 "Yes"? ❑ True	
Is 11 marked "Yes"? ❑ True	If all of the above conditions are met, then individual meets criteria for **United Nations Convention Against Torture**.
Is 12 marked "No"? ❑ True	
If all of the above conditions are met, then individual meets criteria for **United States Torture Victims Relief Act**, 18 USC 2340(1).	

Other Information

This instrument is the result of development and research at the Bellevue/NYU Program for Survivors of Torture. For more information, please contact the Research Director, Andrew Rasmussen, at rasmua01@nyumc.org or (212) 562-8449.

Vital Impact Assessment Questionnaire – VIVO Questionnaire
(Pérez-Sales et al., 2012)

We kindly request that you respond to the following questions, not based on whether you agree with them or not, but based on whether **they truly describe you**, using the following scale:

1. Doesn't describe me or define me whatsoever
2. Describes me or defines me a little
3. In a certain way, it describes me or defines me
4. Describes me or defines me well
5. Describes me or defines me completely

		1	2	3	4	5
1.	Most days the world is full of beautiful things.					
2.	I am constantly thinking that I'd be happy if I could only fix the damage I've done.					
3.	I tend to trust people.					
4.	What isn't talked about ends up being forgotten and stops being painful.					
5.	Destiny doesn't exist.					
6.	It helps me to talk about the grave experiences of my life, like sicknesses, accidents, or losses, with those I care about.					
7.	I don't think life makes sense but I guess it has to be lived.					
8.	Suffering is useless pain.					
9.	There can only be happiness when there is no suffering.					
10.	I don't believe that one should ever give up on life.					
11.	Mistakes help change the way you are.					
12.	I believe that in this world, evil wins.					
13.	I've made mistakes in the past that I can't bear to remember.					
14.	I don't believe in ideologies, or if I do they haven't helped me in difficult times.					
15.	I'm incapable of enjoying life to the fullest.					
16.	I tend not to completely trust people.					
17.	I believe that when others assign me responsibilities, they are in good hands.					
18.	Life is about controlling uncertainty and ambiguity.					
19.	It calms me to think that things simply happen.					
20.	I have never considered suicide as an option.					

© 2017, *Psychological Torture*, Pérez-Sales, Routledge

21.	Some things are too horrible for words to describe.					
22.	You learn from suffering.					
23.	When something serious happens to me I tend to think calmly and coolly about how to solve it.					
24.	Most days the world is grey.					
25.	What isn't talked about gets stuck inside you.					
26.	I don't think it's helpful to talk about the grave experiences in my life like sicknesses or accidents, to others, even to those I care about.					
27.	I believe than even the worst feelings of guilt can be forgiven.					
28.	I don't have spiritual convictions, or if I have them they haven't helped me in difficult times.					
29.	I feel like I break everything I touch.					
30.	I believe that in this world, good wins.					
31.	Suicide is a dignified option that I have seriously considered.					
32.	Life is about accepting uncertainty and ambiguity.					
33.	I express my suffering through dreams.					
34.	Life makes sense and that's why it has to be lived.					
35.	I spend a lot of time thinking about things that have happened to me.					
36.	You never really learn from your mistakes.					
37.	Sometimes I have fears that I can't seem to identify.					
38.	I don't usually remember my dreams and if I remember them I don't usually find them important.					
39.	There are always words to describe even the most horrible things.					
40.	Even when there is suffering there can be moments of happiness.					
41.	I've learned from my mistakes in life.					
42.	Forgetting depends on yourself.					
43.	I feel that in order to get rid of my guilt, I need to be punished.					
44.	You don't choose to forget.					
45.	Our lives are predetermined by destiny.					
46.	My ideological convictions have been of great help to me in difficult times.					
47.	Suffering makes you sink, or break down.					
48.	It's impossible to feel safe and secure in this life.					
49.	All suffering is an opportunity for growth.					

© 2017, *Psychological Torture*, Pérez-Sales, Routledge

50.	I don't think that living through horrible experiences makes me stronger, like people say.					
51.	I believe that I've been through some tough experiences which have made me stronger.					
52.	People don't usually help those close to them.					
53.	When something serious happens to me, I tend to freeze up.					
54.	Talking about things relieves suffering.					
55.	I don't usually feel guilty for things that can't be fixed.					
56.	I can stop thinking about something that worries me when I know that there's nothing I can do about it.					
57.	What happened is in the past. Thinking about it doesn't help anything.					
58.	I always know what my fears are.					
59.	Even considering the mistakes I've made, I can accept my past without regret.					
60.	It is possible to live safely and securely and out of danger.					
61.	When I try not to think about something that worries me, I end up thinking about it more.					
62.	The mistakes I've made haven't caused me to lose my self-confidence.					
63.	I am more courageous than before when confronting situations.					
64.	It calms me to think about why things happen.					
65.	My spiritual convictions have helped me in difficult times.					
66.	People help those close to them whenever they can.					
67.	The way you are never really changes.					
68.	Fear stops me from doing things that I used to be able to do.					
69.	Suicide is a dignified option that I could come to consider.					
70.	Talking about things brings more suffering.					
71.	The mistakes I've made have made me lose confidence in myself.					
72.	I've learned to fully enjoy life.					
73.	What happened has not changed who I am.					
74.	Now I feel like the future is full of possibilities.					
75.	I ask myself, why me?					
76.	I've tried to communicate almost everything.					
77.	I haven't changed my priorities in life.					
78.	I feel like I'm unable to love anyone like I used to.					

© 2017, *Psychological Torture*, Pérez-Sales, Routledge

No.	Statement					
79.	Looking back, I'm left with a feeling of humiliation.					
80.	To bear witness or testify to what has happened or what is happening brings meaning to life.					
81.	I've never felt like I've lost control.					
82.	I always look towards the future with expectations that everything will turn out fine.					
83.	I feel more compassion towards others.					
84.	What happened has only changed small aspects of the way I see myself and the world.					
85.	I've changed my priorities about what is important in life.					
86.	I felt silence and a void. No one wanted to talk.					
87.	I don't feel like what happened affects my identity.					
88.	I don't care enough about things that happen around me.					
89.	Looking back, I feel proud of how I reacted.					
90.	Now the future feels like something I'll never reach.					
91.	I had a feeling of absolute loss of control that I couldn't get rid of.					
92.	My ability to love remains intact.					
93.	It's as if society holds you responsible for what happened to you.					
94.	I do not wonder "why me," things are the way they are.					
95.	There are some things I have preferred to keep to myself.					
96.	I saw myself as vulnerable, helpless.					
97.	I struggle against my feelings.					
98.	What happened became a point of reference from which I see myself and the world.					
99.	To bear witness or testify to what happens is irrelevant.					
100.	You always find someone who will listen to you.					
101.	I accept my feelings.					
102.	I feel like what happened broke me.					
103.	I didn't feel like anyone was making me feel guilty for what happened.					
104.	Even in the worst times I can feel moments of happiness.					
105.	Happiness stopped existing for me.					
106.	Looking back, I'm left with a profound feeling of dignity.					
107.	I feel involved in everything I do.					

© 2017, *Psychological Torture*, Pérez-Sales, Routledge

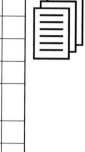

108.	When I think about the future I imagine it dark.					
109.	I feel like this has become part of my identity.					
110.	Everyone did what they could to help me/us.					
111.	I can only see reality from my point of view as a victim.					
112.	I have become tougher and the suffering of others seems now normal to me.					
113.	I saw myself as strong, resistant					
114.	Looking back, I'm embarrassed to think about how I reacted.					
115.	I do not see the world from a victim's point of view.					
116.	Most of society turned its back on me/ us.					

Items 1–72. General population. 73–116. Survivors' items.

© 2017, *Psychological Torture*, Pérez–Sales, Routledge

Appendix 5
THE TORTURING ENVIRONMENT SCALE

The Torturing Environment Scale (TES) measures the likelihood that a person has suffered torture, or whether an environment can be considered to be torture.[1] The analysis focuses on conditions in the ethical, legal, medical, psychological and sociological contexts that offer a comprehensive view of a situation that is liable to constitute torture.

The TES is best filled out after establishing trust and getting to know the survivor, or after a visit to monitor detention conditions. The TES does not need to be completed in a single interview.

Mark Column 1 (NO) when it is possible to reasonably ascertain that the indicator has not happened to the person (individual measure) or has never been documented in that location (collective measure). Leave it blank if there is *No Information Available* (NIA) and needs further clarification.

Mark Column 2 (C-L) *Present, but Circumstantial or Limited (CC-LM)* if the indicator has eventually appeared but it was not part of a systematic attack or one of the core techniques applied to the survivor. This is not a measure of the intensity of suffering, but a modulated assessment of the intensity and systematicity of the aggression.

Mark Column 3 (YES) to signal the clear and consistent presence of the indicator according to the survivor's account. The allegations must be credible. In exceptional cases, mark *Yes* if the evaluator: (1) has *very* strong grounds to believe that the indicator of torture is present; and (2) has marked at least 2 of the 12 corroborating medical or psychological indicators (in Part 2 of the TES) which the evaluator thinks relate to the torture indicator suspected to be present. The criteria for choosing one indicator or another should be based on the role of a certain action within the purpose of the overall torturing process.

Column 4 (Impact) is related to the subjective perception of the survivor's experience. It should be marked when the indicator has great importance in the narrative of the survivor and is remembered as especially devastating. In many cases we may not have access to such intimate information; in such cases the column is left blank.

TABLE A5.1 Torturing Environment Scale – TES

Choose the best option:
- No presence of indicator: Mark *0* under *NO*
- Present, but Circumstantial or Limited: Mark *1* under *Cc-Lm*
- Presence of indicator or Strongly Suspected: Mark *2* under *Yes*
- Additionally: Mark *X* under *I* (*Impact*) if indicator caused significant impact

PART 1. Assessment of Environment

	Torturing Environment Scale (TES)	NO	Cc-Lm	YES	I
	Contextual manipulations			Select	
1	a. Inhuman conditions of detention according to international standards (e.g. cell size and conditions, overcrowding, lack of hygiene)				
2	b. Manipulation of environmental conditions (specify) ❑ Temperature (heat/cold) ❑ Humidity ❑ Noise, white noise, music ❑ Permanent bright light ❑ Others:				
3	c. Altering basic physiological functions (specify) ❑ Starvation ❑ Thirst ❑ Restricting urination/defecation ❑ Others:				
4	d. Sleep dysregulation (e.g. deprivation, shifting hours)				
5	e. Manipulating sense of time				
6	f. Partial deprivation of senses/disorientation (e.g. blindfolds, earmuffs, hooding)				
7	g. Medical induction of altered states/ mind-altering methods ❑ Use of drugs/pharmacological torture ❑ White noise, visual or kinetic manipulations ❑ White or monochrome environments ❑ *Complete* sensory isolation ❑ Others:				
8	Other contextual manipulations. Specify:				

(continued)

TABLE A5.1 Torturing Environment Scale – TES (*continued*)

	Fear	NO	Cc-Lm	YES	I
9	a. Manipulation of hopes and expectations to produce extreme fear or terror (e.g. inducing helplessness; denying information; grotesque, absurd, illogical or terrorising environments; constructing scenarios; creating expectations of pain or death; prolonged waiting or silence)				
10	b. Threats against the person (e.g. endless isolation, endless interrogation, rape, pain, torture, death)				
11	c. Threats against family or relatives (next-of-kin) (e.g. rape, detention, punishment, retaliation), or threats against other detainees				
12	d. Anguish associated with lack of information (e.g. relatives of people detained/disappeared)				
13	e. Experiences of near death (e.g. mock executions, dry/wet asphyxia . . .)				
14	f. Forced witnessing of others' torture or death				
15	g. Use of situations evoking insurmountable fear (e.g. phobias, total darkness)				
16	h. Other situations provoking fear or terror. Specify:				
	Physical pain	NO	Cc-Lm	YES	I
17	a. Blunt trauma (specify) ❑ Punches, kicks, slaps; blows with sticks, falaqa ❑ 'Clean' whipping / flagellation, beating with wires or truncheons ❑ Beatings over the ears with closed hands, eyeball press ❑ Being thrown/dragged/shaken ❑ Other:				
18	b. Forced battles against oneself. Forced self-induced pain (specify) ❑ Positional torture: suspension, hanging ❑ Stretching body/limbs ❑ Prolonged constraint of movement, sweatboxes, coffins, blackholes, straitjackets, ties ❑ Forced to stand, sit or kneel for hours; chair tortures ❑ Forced to stand under heavy sun, ice, strong electric light ❑ Other:				

Torturing Environment Scale (TES)				
Physical pain	NO	Cc-Lm	YES	I

19   c. Exhaustion exercises
      ❑   Forced running, military training, drilling
      ❑   Step-ups, knee bends, push-ups, squats, crunches
      ❑ Other:				

20 d. Other pain-producing actions not included in the methods that produce mutilation or extreme pain. Specify:				
Extreme pain – mutilation – death	NO	Cc-Lm	YES	I

21   a. Devices that produce excruciating pain
      ❑   Burns with cigarettes, heated instruments, scalding liquid or caustic substances
      ❑   Cuts with knives, blades or other sharp objects
      ❑   Electric shocks (e.g. electric prod or 'picana', dinamos, electrical wires, electroshock weapons (batons, rifles and guns (tasers), stun belts)
      ❑   Dry and wet asphyxia, suffocation, strangulation
      ❑   Chemical exposure to salt, chili pepper, gasoline, etc. (in wounds or body cavities)
      ❑   Mechanical devices that produce extreme pain (e.g. wooden horse ('caballete'), parrot's perch, standing on sharp objects)
      ❑ Other:				

22   b. Mutilation
      ❑   Crush injury, smashing parts of the body
      ❑   Disfigurement
      ❑   Traumatic removal of skin, digits, nails, teeth, hair, ears
      ❑   Amputation, surgical removal of organs, dismemberment
      ❑   Permanent organ damage, ischemia
      ❑   Permanent penetrating injuries, such as sticks with nails or spikes, stab or gunshot wounds, hard whipping
      ❑   Mutilation by insects (e.g. worms, ants, bees) or animals (e.g. dogs, rats)
      ❑ Other:				

23   c. Brain damage
      ❑   Open head wounds
      ❑   Severe brain contusions, loss of consciousness due to repeated traumatic head injuries
      ❑   Non-medical electroconvulsive therapy, insulin therapy, or other physical or chemical direct attacks on the brain (excluding pharmacological torture)
      ❑ Other:				

(continued)

TABLE A5.1 Torturing Environment Scale – TES (*continued*)

	Extreme pain – mutilation – death	NO	Cc-Lm	YES	I
24	d. Other actions producing extreme pain, mutilation or death. Specify:				
	Reproduction/Sexual integrity	NO	Cc-Lm	YES	I
25	a. Humiliation related to sexual identity (e.g. forced nakedness, debasing treatment targeting sexual characteristics or sexual orientation)				
26	b. Sexual assault (including violent acts targeting genitals)				
27	c. Rape				
28	d. Other actions targeting sexual integrity. Specify:				
	Need to belong. Acceptance and care	NO	Cc-Lm	YES	I
29	a. Prolonged solitary confinement (more than 15 days). Incommunicado detention				
30	b. Breaking social bonds/isolation from family, social, cultural, political networks				
31	c. Manipulation of affect (e.g. actions encouraging traumatic bonding with the torturer, ambivalent feelings of love/hate and care/rejection, 'testing' loyalty, occasional discretional favors…)				
32	d. Other actions targeting the need to belong. Specify:				
	Identity, control, meaning and purpose	NO	Cc-Lm	YES	I
33	a. Beliefs and worldviews. Attacks on sense of self (e.g. forcing detainee to break with his or her past/identity, questioning basic values, breaking worldviews)				
34	b. Helplessness. Induced submission and compliance (e.g. changing rules, trivial orders, random punishment or rewards)				
35	c. Instilling guilt (e.g. detainee forced to harm others; forced choices such as deciding who's next to die; forcing betrayal)				
36	d. Induced shame (e.g. forced to perform humiliating acts in public, public debasement, preventing personal hygiene, debasement based on ethnic or cultural background)				
37	e. Induced humiliation (e.g. insults, deprecation, deprecation based on physical appearance, feral treatment, debasement based on ethnic or cultural background)				
38	f. Violation of taboos (i.e. coerced actions that go against the person's moral principles)				
39	g. Installing goals and identity (e.g. forced to adopt new values and a new sense of meaning, pushed into a grafted identity)				
40	h. Other actions targeting identity. Specify:				

Torturing Environment Scale (TES)				
Coercive interrogation techniques	NO	Cc-Lm	YES	I
41	a. Extreme conditions during interrogation (e.g. oppressive or intimidating setting, night interrogation, disruption of sleep, prolonged and exhausting interrogations or continuous interrogation for several days, interrogation combined with elements that produce confusion (e.g. beatings to the head, strenuous physical exercise, asphyxia)				
42	b. Conditions of interrogation that foster false confessions: provoking extreme emotions or emotional exhaustion, for example, omnipotence, omniscience (showing absolute power over the body and fate of the detainee during interrogation), maximisation (exaggerating evidence, data, responsibility or guilt), minimisation (alleviating responsibility, providing justifications or excuses), threats for not confessing, use of personal information to break the self				
43	c. Conditions of interrogation that foster false confessions: lies or deliberate deception (e.g. direct accusations with false, fabricated, or unsubstantiated evidence; false or deceptive information regarding family, detention site, or interrogators; use of false witnesses; offering leniency or rewards for cooperation); cognitive manipulation or cognitive exhaustion (e.g. forced choices between two incriminating options, contradictory and confusing messages, prisoner's dilemma, role–playing such as good cop/bad cop, manipulation of detainees' words)				
44	d. Other extreme coercive actions to intimidate, obtain information, or force self-incrimination. Specify:				

PART 2. Manner of Interaction – Indicators of a Torturing Environment

Relational indicators	NO	Cc-Lm	YES	I
45	a. Person completely deprived of will (the individual freedom that requires reflection and conscious choice)				
46	b. Violation of autonomy, expressed in the absolute power and imposing control of the perpetrator and the lack of control and helplessness of the victim				

(continued)

TABLE A5.1 Torturing Environment Scale – TES (*continued*)

	Relational indicators	NO	Cc-Lm	YES	I
47	c. The situation fosters unpredictability (e.g. no restraints on time or location, no one knows where the detainee is held, uncertain or vague accusations, abrupt changes in rules or scenarios)				
48	d. Systematic violation of dignity; lack of recognition and respect for the victim as a human being				
49	e. Torture designed and planned as a personalised process (torture tailored to the subject's characteristics and identity)				
50	f. Signs of evil or extreme cruelty in the torture process				
51	g. Increased vulnerability associated with age (e.g. victim is a child, elder), gender and sexuality (e.g. victim is a woman, LGBTI), ethnic group or other factors				
52	h. Forcing the victim to play an active role in his or her own suffering and fighting against his or her own body and self (e.g. prolonged stress positions, prolonged impediments to physiological functions)				
53	i. Physical and or mental harm is prolonged or repeated over a period of time				
54	j. Other relational factors. Specify:				

PART 3. Legal Criteria

Legal criteria	NO	YES
1. The interviewee was in the custody of or under the physical control of institutional agents.		
2. There are legal cases, testimonies, documentation or other contextual information that provides grounds to suspect that this treatment is part of a state policy (*torturing system* criteria).		
3. There is a clear purpose or motivation related to obtaining information or a confession.		
4. There are grounds to think that the main purpose of ill-treatment was punishment, humiliation or revenge against the detainee or the group he or she represents.		
5. The subject rejects the statements made during his or her detention and claims that he or she gave those statements because of ill-treatment (detainee demands *Exclusionary Rule*).		
6. There are legal precedents of similar cases considered to amount to torture.		

PART 4. Medico–Psychological Criteria[1]

The presence of one or more of the following indicators *supports the idea of a torturing environment or a torturing situation.* The absence of these indicators does not preclude the existence of a torturing environment, and may indicate physical or psychological resilience. Please check the appropriate box.

	NO	YES
Medical and psychological indicators *Due to one or more of the above techniques or situations, and within the cultural and social context of the examinee, the person shows:*		
1. Steady signs of confusion or disorientation during or after detention		
2. Steady signs of anguish, fear or terror during or after detention		
3. Steady signs of emotional exhaustion or cognitive impairment during or after detention		
4. Signs of emotional manipulation during or after detention (e.g. guilt/shame, emotional dependence, ambivalent emotions toward alleged perpetrator)		
5. Signs of damage to identity and self-questioning worldviews		
6. Indicators of brain damage (e.g. neurological examination, neuropsychological assessment, EEG and/or related tests or other measures of brain damage, CT-SCAN, MNR or other brain imaging evidence)		
7. Other acute medical disorders attributable to the alleged acts. Specify:		
8. Chronic medical sequelae attributable to the alleged acts. Specify:		
9. Acute or Chronic PTSD related to the alleged acts		
10. Complex PTSD/Enduring Personality Change after Catastrophic Experience (EPCACE) related to the alleged acts		
11. Dissociative states related to the alleged acts		
12. Other medical or psychiatric disorders attributable to the alleged acts. Specify:		

1. If the TES is used for forensic or legal purposes, complement this section with the SEF-IP (Standardised Evaluation Form for an Assessment of Credibility based on the Istanbul Protocol). See Chapter 19.
2. Pérez-Sales, Pau (2016). Intentionality Assessment Scale. In Pérez-Sales, Pau (2016). *Psychological Torture: Definition, Evaluation and Measurement.* Routledge. London.

TES – SUMMARY SHEET

PART 1. Assessment of Environment

S: Score (0 = No, 1= CC-LMN, 2= Yes); I: Intensity

Name:

Date:

	Contextual manipulations	S	I
1	a. Inhuman conditions of detention		
2	b. Environmental manipulation		
3	c. Basic physiological functions		

4	d. Sleep dysregulation
5	e. Handling of time
6	f. Sensory deprivation
7	g. Mind-altering methods
8	h. Other (contextual manipulations)

Raw Score

(continued)

TABLE A5.1 Torturing Environment Scale – TES (*continued*)

	Fear-producing actions	S	I
9	a. Hopes and expectations		
10	b. Threats to the person		
11	c. Threats against family/detainees		
12	d. Lack of information		
13	e. Experiences of near death		
14	f. Witnessing others' torture		
15	g. Phobias		
16	h. Other situations		
	Raw Score		

	Pain-producing actions	S	I
17	a. Beatings		
18	b. Battles against oneself		
19	c. Exhaustion exercises, forced work		
20	d. Other pain-producing actions		
	Raw Score		

	Extreme pain – mutilation – death	S	I
21	a. Extreme pain		
22	b. Mutilation		
23	c. Brain damage		
24	d. Other (specify)		
	Raw Score		

	Actions targeting reproduction/sexual integrity	S	I
25	a. Humiliation		
26	b. Sexual assault		
27	c. Rape		
28	d. Other (targeting sexual integrity)		
	Raw Score		

	Actions targeting the need to belong: acceptance and care	S	I
29	a. Prolonged solitary confinement. Incommunicado detention		
30	b. Breaking social bonds		
31	c. Manipulation of affect		
32	d. Other (targeting need to belong)		
	Raw Score		

	Actions targeting identity, control, meaning	S	I
33	a. Beliefs and worldviews. Attacks on sense of self		
34	b. Helplessness induced		
35	c. Instilling guilt		
36	d. Induced shame		
37	e. Induced humiliation		
38	f. Violation of moral principles		
39	g. Installing goals and identity		
40	h. Other (targeting identity)		
	Raw Score		

	Coercive interrogation techniques	S	I
41	a. Conditions during interrogation		
42	b. Style of interrogation		
43	c. Deception/cognitive manipulation		
44	d. Other (extreme coercive actions)		
	Raw Score		

PART 2. Manner of interaction

Relational indicators	S	I
45 a. Will		
46 b. Violation of autonomy		
47 c. Fostering unpredictability		
48 d. Systematic violation of dignity		
49 e. Personalised process		

Relational indicators	S	I
50 f. Extreme signs of evil or cruelty		
51 g. Vulnerability factors		
52 h. Active role in own suffering		
53 i. Prolonged harm (physical/mental)		
54 j. Other (relational factors)		
Raw Score		

PART 3. Legal Criteria

Legal criteria	YES
1. Institutional agents	
2. *Torturing system* criteria	
3. Clear motivation for obtaining confession	
4. Clear purpose of punishment, humiliation or revenge	
5. *Exclusionary rule*	
6. Legal precedents	

PART 4. Medico–Psychological Criteria

Medical and psychological indicators. *Due to one or more of the above techniques, and within the cultural and social context of the examinee:*	YES
1. Confusion or disorientation	
2. Anguish, fear or terror	
3. Emotional or cognitive exhaustion	
4. Signs of emotional manipulation	
5. Signs of damage to identity	
6. Brain damage	
7. Other acute medical disorders	
8. Chronic medical sequelae	
9. Acute or chronic PTSD	
10. Complex PTSD/EPCACE	
11. Dissociative states	
12. Other relevant condition	

TABLE A5.2 Torturing Environment Scale scoring form

Part 1 TORTURING ENVIRONMENT	C-L (x1)	Yes (x2)	CF	Score	1	2	3	4	5	6	7	8	9	10	11	12	13	14	15	16	I
Block 1. Contextual manipulations																					
Block 2. Fear-producing actions																					
Block 3. Pain-producing actions			X2																		
Block 4. Extreme pain – mutilation – death			X2																		
Block 5. Sexual integrity			X2																		
Block 6. Attachment and need to belong			X2																		
Block 7. Actions targeting identity																					
Block 8. Coercive interrogation techniques			X2																		
Overall Score (Sum of totals for each Block)					Mark YES if there is either [a] at least one FULL criteria in any of the 8 Blocks, or [b] an overall score or 5 or more.														YES		NO

Part 2 RELATIONAL INDICATORS	CC-LM	Yes		Overall Score	Mark YES if there are at least 2 FULL relational criteria or an overall score of 5 or more.														YES		NO
Part 3 LEGAL INDICATORS	1	2	3	4	5	6	Mark YES if legal criteria 1 and legal criteria 3 or 4 (or both) are fulfilled. Exceptionally consider criteria 6.												YES		NO
Part 4 MEDICO-PSYCHOLOGICAL INDICATORS	NUMBER				Mark YES if there is at least 1 medico-psychological criterion														YES		NO

ENVIRONMENTAL CONDITIONS AMOUNT TO TORTURE	Conditions amount to torture if • Criteria of Part 1, 2 and 4 are fulfilled Allegations additionally supported if • Criteria of Part 3 are fulfilled • There is an overall consistency of allegations according to the SEC		NO		PARTIALLY		YES

Scoring and interpretation of results

The Overall Score provides a combined view of techniques and relational, legal and medico-psychological criteria for **determining whether or not torture has occurred**. Thus, the TES is an aid for obtaining an objective definition of torturing environments or experiences for forensic, legal or research purposes. It is **not** intended to quantify the *experiences of torture*. Personal experiences of survivors are unique and cannot be quantified or compared. Any individual element considered in the Torturing Environment Scale can destroy a human being and amount to torture in itself.

Steps to score the TES

1. Sum up scores for each block (CC–LM = 1, Yes = 2) and multiply by the Correcting Factor (CF) to obtain the score for each block of torture methods. Values range from 0 to 16.
2. Obtain the Overall Score by summing up the scores of the 8 blocks. Values range from 0 to 128.
3. Mark YES if there is at least one full criteria ('YES') in any of the 8 blocks or an overall score of 5 or more.

TABLE A5.3 TES – Blocks scoring

Part 1	CC-LM (1)	Yes (2)	CF	Score [0–16]
Block 1. Contextual manipulations				
Block 2. Fear-producing actions				
Block 3. Pain-producing actions			X2	
Block 4. Extreme pain – mutilation – death			X2	
Block 5. Sexual integrity			X2	
Block 6. Attachment and need to belong			X2	
Block 7. Actions targeting identity				
Block 8. Coercive interrogation techniques			X2	
Overall Score [0–128] (Sum of totals for each Block)				

Torturing Environment – Assessment of Environment/Experience Mark YES if there is either [a] at least one FULL criteria in any of the 8 Blocks, or [b] an overall score or 5 or more.	YES	NO

4. Color in the cells at the right to obtain a visual portrait of the torturing environment, and mark the column (I) according to the methods which were deemed to have maximum destructive impact according to the survivor's experience.
5. Calculate the score for relational indicators. Values range from 0 to 20. Mark YES if there are at least 2 FULL relational criteria or an overall score of 5 or more.

TABLE A5.4 TES – Relational indicators

Part 2. Relational Indicators (Mark the number of indicators that are met)	Cc–Lm	YES (Full criteria)	Score TOTAL
		Overall Score [0–20]	
Torturing Environment – Relational Indicators Mark YES if there are at least 2 FULL relational criteria or an overall score of 5 or more.			YES	NO

6. Indicate the legal criteria. Mark YES if legal criteria 1 *and* legal criteria 3 or 4 (or both) are fulfilled Exceptionally consider, additionally, criteria 6.

TABLE A5.5 TES – Legal indicators

Part 4	1	2	3	4	5	6
Legal Indicators (Mark which indicators are met)						
Torturing Environment – Legal Criteria [Mark YES if Legal criteria 1 *and* Legal criteria 3 or 4 (or both) are fulfilled Exceptionally consider Criteria 6.	YES	NO

7. Calculate the score for medico-psychological indicators. Values range from 0 to 12. Mark YES if there is at least 1 full medico-psychological criterion.

TABLE A5.6 TES – Medico-psychological indicators

	YES
Part 3. Medico-Psychological Indicators (Mark the number of indicators that are met)	
Torturing Environment – Medico-Psychological Indicators Mark YES if there is at least 1 Medico-Psychological criterion	YES	NO

8. The combination of all the above will indicate whether conditions amount to torture.

TABLE A5.7 TES – Overall score

Torture has occurred if:
A. There is at least one FULL criteria in any of the 8 Blocks or a score or 5 or more summing up all indicators in Part 1 AND
B. There are at least 2 FULL relational criteria in Part 2
   AND
C. Legal criteria 1 and legal criteria 3 or 4 are fulfilled in Part 3. Exceptionally consider Criteria 6.
Additionally, results support the presence of torture if:
D. At least 1 medico-psychological indicator in Part 3 is present
E. There is an overall consistency of allegations according to the SEC

CONDITIONS AMOUNT TO TORTURE:	NO	PARTIALLY	YES

The structure in eight blocks and the graphic offer a portrait of torture methods at a glance. Additionally, it is possible to calculate comparative scores between environmental, physical and psychological methods. Sum as indicated in the table and weight. Final scores range from 0 to 10.

Psychological versus physical torture methods

TABLE A5.8 TES – Subscales: physical vs. psychological torture

TORTURE	Blocks + Items	Weight	Methods Score
MANIPULATION OF ENVIRONMENT	[Block 1] + [items 29, 41]	Divide by 2	
Mostly based on PHYSICAL PAIN	[Block 3]+[Block 4]+ [items 3, 13, 27, 50]	Divide by 4	
Mostly based on PSYCHOLOGICAL PAIN	[Block 2]+[Block 6]+ [Block 7]+[Block 8] + [items 25, 26, 47]	Divide by 7	

The values do not measure the intensity of each category of torture methods, but simply allows for comparison among methods. A final score of, for example, 1.3, 3.1 and 5.2 would mean that the torturing environment was heavily focused on producing psychological pain as compared to environmental manipulation and physical pain. It would not say anything about the *intensity* of that pain, and could not be used for that purpose.

Note

1 We suggest that the TES be complemented with the Standardized Evaluation Form for an Assessment of Credibility based on the Istanbul Protocol (SEF-IP). This is a tool that should be used by a trained interviewer. It provides guidelines and criteria for the credibility analysis that a psychiatric forensic expert conducts based on the Istanbul Protocol.

Appendix 6

STANDARD EVALUATION FORM FOR CREDIBILITY ASSESSMENT (SEC)

The SEC is an aid for an evidence-based assessment of credibility of allegations of ill-treatment or torture by legal professionals (judges, attorneys, medical and psychological examiners and forensic experts). It helps the evaluator to search for potential sources of credibility and systematise information, to make his or her final decision more objective, and to have comparable results among experts and studies. It is based on clinical data and analysis and triangulation of available sources.

The SEC has a set of criteria, some of them based on IP recommendations, with additional corroborating criteria. It encompasses hard and soft criteria for the expert to make a decision in one of the four categories recommended by the Istanbul Protocol.

The SEC helps experts properly assess this by drawing a distinction between elements that support consistency (column 1), elements that support inconsistency (column 2) and a lack of either one of these two elements (column 3). Column 3 can also be used when the expert believes that he/she cannot make a proper assessment of a given criteria for medical or cultural reasons.

The Overall Level of Credibility, based on the expert's knowledge and conclusions after carefully reviewing all of the criteria, is not a product of numerical totaling. The SEC is an aid to be used as part of a decision-making process. The Overall Level of Credibility is derived from a qualitative assessment of the applicable criteria. The exact wording of these four categories can be changed according to whether the expert feels comfortable using the word credibility (as we do) or might prefer using the word consistency.

There might be certain criteria, even soft ones, that clearly support credibility. But the evaluator must bear in mind that their absence does not indicate a lack of credibility.

See instructions in Chapter 19.

TABLE A6.1 Standard Evaluation Form for Credibility Assessment (SEC)

Standard Evaluation Form for Credibility Assessment (SEC)

Mark as appropriate.

1. **Highly consistent**
2. **Consistent**
3. **Inconsistent**
4. **Not applicable**

	Criterion	*1*	*2*	*3*	*4*
1	Plausible and logical description of alleged torture (circumstances, type, methodology, duration, etc.).				
2	Triangulation of information from witnesses / other potential victims – *[Highly consistent – Blind independent interviews with open questions; Consistent – Non independent – closed questions – Collective interviews]*				
3	Documentation supporting relevant dates and locations cited by the survivor. Triangulation of the events with external sources of information (i.e. newspapers, Internet).				
4	Positive outcome. The alleged victim has ostensible direct benefits (economic, legal or otherwise) of being considered credible *[Positive outcome support Inconsistency. Absence support consistency]*				
5	Negative outcomes. There are ostensible negative outcomes of testyfying (public exposure, shame, danger or otherwise) that making illogical a false testimony *[Negative outcome supports consistency. Absence supports inconsistency]*				
6	Facts are described in accordance with reports produced by human rights organisations, international organisations, or entities associated with or recognised by United Nations agencies working on preventing or denouncing torture.				
7	*At the time of the alleged facts,* expected or typical physical or psychological reactions to extreme stress, within the cultural and social context of the examinee.				
8	*At the time of the expert assessment* consistency between the description of events and the emotions with which they are expressed.				
9	*At the time of the expert assessment,* consistency between verbal and nonverbal communication in the statement of events.				
10	Medical tests (including x-rays, blood tests, EMG) consistent with the alleged events.				
11	Psychometric assessment (PTSD, depression, impact on worldviews, neuropsychological tests) consistent with the alleged events.				

(continued)

TABLE A6.1 Standard Evaluation Form for Credibility Assessment (SEC) (*continued*)

Standard Evaluation Form for Credibility Assessment (SEC)

Mark as appropriate.		1. **Highly consistent** 2. **Consistent** 3. **Inconsistent** 4. **Not applicable**			
	Criterion	*1*	*2*	*3*	*4*
12	Medium / long term physical sequelae consistent with the alleged events.				
13	Objective and verifiable personality changes that can be temporally associated with the alleged events.				
14	Functional changes (in work, studies, personal relationships, etc.) after the events described attributable to the events described.				
15	*At the time of the expert assessment*, the evaluee's principal clinical diagnosis related to the events is consistent with allegations. [ICD/ DSM Diagnosis:]				
16	Events, physical and psychological consequences, personality or functional changes *blindly contrasted* with one or more other first-hand sources (family, friends, co-detainees or others).				
17	Previous medical or forensic assessments indicating immediate physical or psychological consequences or medium or long term sequelae consistent with the events described.				
18	Concurrence of two forensic experts and/or an external evaluator.				
19	Court sentence or legal administrative procedure (i.e. refugee status, asylum claim) in favour of the examinee that recognises degrading treatment, ill-treatment, or torture.				
	OVERALL LEVEL OF CREDIBILITY 1. Maximum consistency 2. Highly consistent 3. Consistent 4. Not consistent				

Pérez-Sales, Pau (2017). Standard Evaluation Form for Credibility Assessment. In Pérez-Sales, Pau (2017). *Psychological Torture: Definition, Evaluation and Measurement*. Routledge. London.

Appendix 7
INTENTIONALITY ASSESSMENT CHECKLIST (IAC)

The IAC is an aid to assess the alleged torture perpetrator's intent. It helps to systematically assess all potentially pertinent elements, without aiming to provide a score.

TABLE A7.1 Intentionality Assessment Checklist (IAC)

		Intentionality Assessment Checklist (IAC)	1. Consistent	2. Not Present, Unknown or Irrelevant	3. Inconsistent
		OVERALL INDICATORS			
1	Torturing Environment	Situation and context analysis. The overall detention context constitutes a torturing environment.			
2	Plan – Malice	There is a plan, understood as a planned sequence of events designed to produce a specific result or consequence (malice aforethought).			
3	Pattern or strategy	There is a similar pattern of strategies, behaviours or procedures taken against different people.			
		SPECIFIC INDICATORS			
4	Social role	The social role of the people involved is compatible with an alleged intentionality.			
5	Interaction	Absolute suppression of the victim's will. The victim is maintained at the mercy of others.			
6	Intensity	The aggression is particularly intensive or the techniques used are particularly grave.			

(continued)

TABLE A7.1 Intentionality Assessment Checklist (IAC) (*continued*)

Intentionality Assessment Checklist (IAC)

			1. Consistent		
				2. Not Present, Unknown or Irrelevant	
					3. Inconsistent
		SPECIFIC INDICATORS			
7	Prolongation or Reiteration	The acts are prolonged or repeated over time, particularly when this occurs even when perceiving the consequences.			
8	Viciousness	Harm is sustained despite the victim's defencelessness.			
9	Attitude (the end justifies the means)	The person knows the adverse consequences but would have continued even in the knowledge that the final result would be the worst possible.			
10	Objective	A functionality or clear objective can be established.			

Pérez-Sales, Pau (2017). *Intentionality Assessment Scale.* In Pérez-Sales, Pau (2017). *Psychological Torture: Definition, Evaluation and Measurement.* Routledge. London.

Appendix 8

A STEP-BY-STEP GUIDE FOR DOCUMENTING TORTURE

Documenting torture requires a mixed-method approach that conjugates the unique perspective of individuals and the subjectivity of victims' narratives with the use of scales in order to compare data from different cultural environments and geographical and historical contexts. Here we aim to provide a very simple, useful guide for doing so.

Stage 1. Testimonies

In order to ascertain the victims' experience, providing them with a voice to give their own testimony stands as an irreplaceable imperative. Moreover, testimony may constitute a therapeutic tool when it is taken within a process and certain methodological safeguards are kept in place (Agger & Jensen, 1990; Cienfuegos & Monelli, 1983).

In order to document torture in a given social, geographical or political context, whenever possible, it is best to start by collecting testimonies using qualitative methodologies preferring open questions and doing content analysis of testimonies. The following steps are desirable (Figure A.8.1):

1. Gather previous reports, files of testimonies, clinical records (with informed consent to use them) as well as any other available documents.
2. Take testimonies from a representative sample of victims. These testimonies are better collected in writing, and whenever possible, also kept in sound or image recordings.
3. Make a separate text file of each interview.
4. Analyse the contents of the texts creating conceptual categories[1] ('nodes'). Whether using a software programme (like Atlas-ti), the preferable approach, or creating categories by hand, the process is similar: the team builds a thesaurus of terms referring to:
    4.1. Context (situations, places, periods, types of centre, perpetrating agent)
    4.2. Traits and specific characteristics of the testifier
    4.3. Methods of torture (as perceived by the survivor); assess whether to pool from TES categories (see Appendix 5)

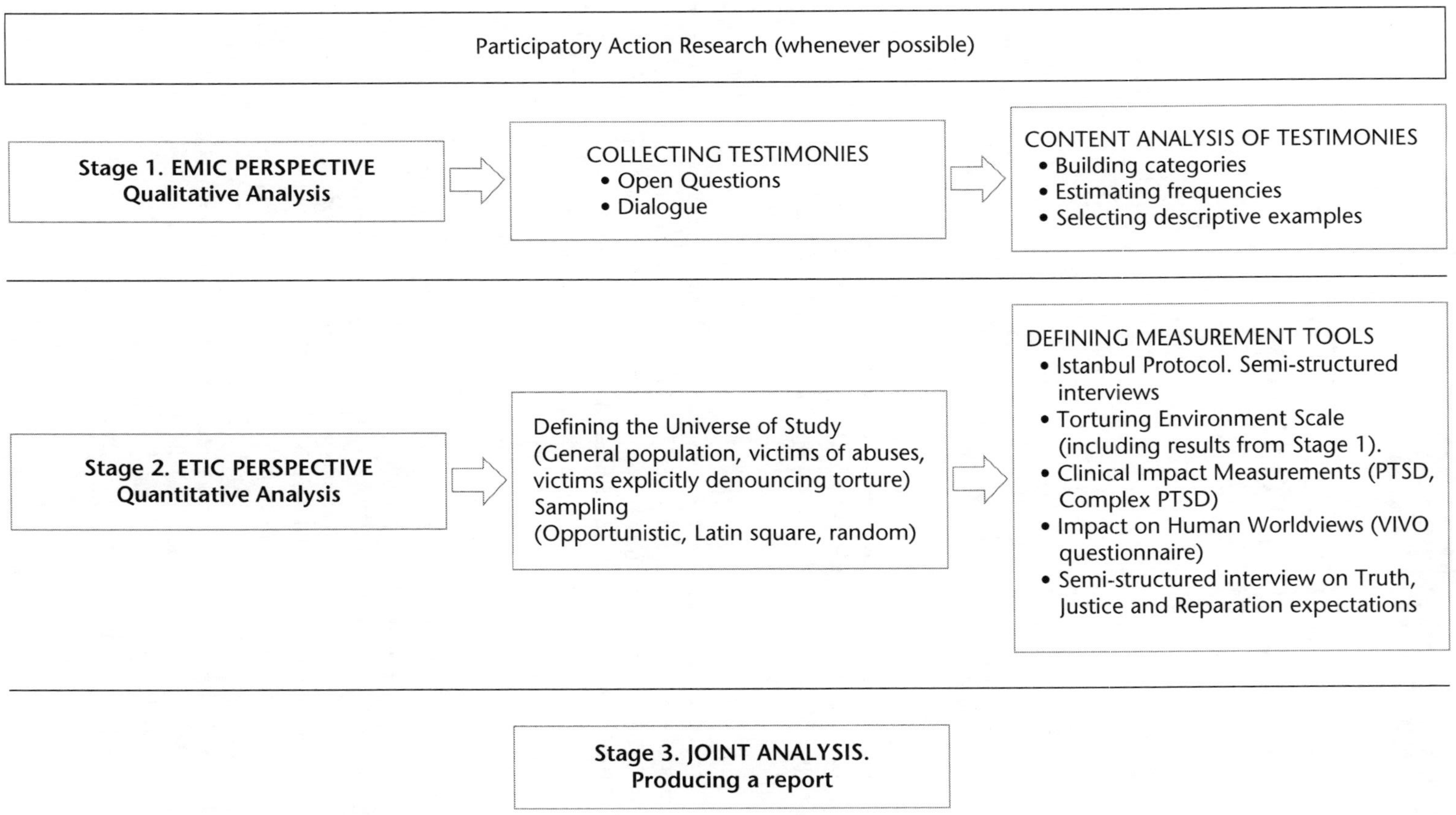

Participatory Action Research (whenever possible)

Stage 1. EMIC PERSPECTIVE
Qualitative Analysis

COLLECTING TESTIMONIES
• Open Questions
• Dialogue

CONTENT ANALYSIS OF TESTIMONIES
• Building categories
• Estimating frequencies
• Selecting descriptive examples

Stage 2. ETIC PERSPECTIVE
Quantitative Analysis

Defining the Universe of Study
(General population, victims of abuses,
victims explicitly denouncing torture)
Sampling
(Opportunistic, Latin square, random)

DEFINING MEASUREMENT TOOLS
• Istanbul Protocol. Semi-structured
  interviews
• Torturing Environment Scale
  (including results from Stage 1).
• Clinical Impact Measurements (PTSD,
  Complex PTSD)
• Impact on Human Worldviews (VIVO
  questionnaire)
• Semi-structured interview on Truth,
  Justice and Reparation expectations

Stage 3. JOINT ANALYSIS.
Producing a report

FIGURE A8.1 Documenting torture: mixed-method approach.

4.4.   Impacts
    4.4.1. Emotions
    4.4.2. Psychological 'symptoms' (in the victim's own terminology and cultural framework)
    4.4.3. Physical symptoms
    4.4.4. Impacts on the family, community and other cultural, social or political groups the victim may belong to
4.5.   Other pertinent elements to understand the torture narrative.

5.   Group the thesaurus terms into families of terms, when required, to simplify analysis.
6.   Obtain a list of all the terms (or families) with all the citations in which this word or expression was used. The software does this automatically.
7.   Elaborate by categories, analysing which elements appear in the narratives, emotions, coping mechanisms and context, and the meanings attributed to it. This should give rise to an early framework and an overall theory for understanding torture in a given historical and geographical context.
8.   Try generalisation and comparison with other ethnographies or similar reports, where applicable.

Participatory Action Research

The first option to be considered is always working with survivors using any of the many forms or variants of the Participatory Action Research (PAR) methodology (Fals-Borda & Rahman, 1991; Heron, 1997; Maiter et al., 2008; Tringer, 2007).

PAR has the survivors themselves, accompanied by the technical team, design and implement the process. This makes it a research tool itself while at the same time empowering them and enabling them to network in order to work together and support each other. It is those affected themselves who, in the final instance, define what should be asked, how, where, and by whom, and those affected who work on compiling and analysing the databases and give meaning to the results. This is particularly noteworthy in stage 1 where the questions are open and the testimony content must be analysed and validated.[2]

It is sometimes impossible to work with PAR methodologies and conventional top-down methods must be used. This holds true especially when safety and security are a problem and the victims are exposed to retaliation for merely going to a victim care facility or conversing with a researcher or therapist (for instance in visits to people hold in detention centres). In these cases, testimonies must be gathered with methodologies protecting anonymity and the security of the victims as much as possible.

In any event, it is always desirable for the interviewers to be as emotionally, culturally and politically close as possible to the victims as this facilitates building trust and ties.

The Istanbul Protocol offers an excellent guide to protection and safeguard measures that must be taken into account when gathering testimonies on torture (Section III, paras 74–119).

Building an information-gathering tool

When collecting testimonies, interviews can be purely open or a semi-open model can be used including certain guided questions. Here again, the Istanbul Protocol can serve as an excellent guide and should be the first reference. However, although certain brief versions are available, they may also require several hours of work and one may therefore choose to develop a more specific tool for gathering information.

For collecting testimonies, open or semi-structured interviews should cover at least three areas:

1. Facts, including circumstances during detention and pertinent legal issues to identify the perpetrators.
2. Experiences, thoughts and emotions during the torture or ill-treatment and their relationship with specific aspects of torture where culturally appropriate and where there is no risk of harming the survivor with exceedingly painful questions without having the opportunity to elaborate on it.
3. Subjective psychological and psychosocial consequences in the medium to long term.

Semi-structured interviews can be used in a pilot phase seeking pertinent elements to subsequently be developed into questions giving rise to both quantitative and qualitative replies. For instance, when questioning on torture, one can ask:

Should checklists of torture methods be used in interviews for collecting testimonies? There is debate as to whether checklists of torture methods should be used. Some argue that this technique leads to affirmative answers while others sustain it enhances the accuracy in memory. The debate remains open, however there are at least three reasons not to use these checklists in qualitative research: (1) when asking open questions, the interviewee refers to what s/he *subjectively remembers the most* or is *most relevant*, and this is precisely the subjectivity we want; (2) when using checklists we truncate or steer spontaneous narratives while open questions lead the person to say *what s/he believes s/he should share*, which is undoubtedly more respectful; (3) more credibility issues are posed.

Similarly, there are also arguments in favour of using checklists: (1) in an open account, the person may conceal methods of torture that s/he associates with guilt or shame, such as sexual violence. It is easier to give a 'yes' to a closed question; (2) the person may not remember all of the elements involved in the torture; (3) considering it 'normal', the person may not mention certain conduct that in fact corresponds to torture.

Choosing whether or not to use a checklist depends on the circumstances. Working in a climate of trust with open questions, in an interview free of time constraints, without a checklist would be ideal. In this scenario, information would flow due to the bond gradually built, and the checklist would be used later as a complement to complete the information.

Sample size

Individual testimonies. There are marvellous, deeply insightful individual testimonies that shed more light on the methods and impacts of torture than very costly research using great samples of aggregate data that sometimes offer confusing poorly interpretable results. Both the testimonies in Chapter 2 and the research on factors presented in Chapter 6 clearly illustrate this.

It may be useful to use manuals including autoethnography methodologies, which help those wishing to provide testimony of their experience to be systematic in collecting and analysing the information (Muncey, 2010).

Small samples. Good qualitative research can be done starting from ten in-depth interviews or even fewer under certain conditions: (1) the persons interviewed must be carefully selected in terms of their representativeness; (2) they must be highly capable of elaborating on their experience and the interviewer must do in-depth work with each one of the interviewees; (3) there must be an opportunity to share experiences through discussion groups in order to complement the individual interviews and foster a process where knowledge is built collectively by survivors; and (4) the results must subsequently be compared with other sources.

Nevertheless, it is hard to generalise the results or extrapolate them to fit other contexts or even other persons in the same context.

Stage 2. Using tools and scales

Sampling

Quantitative studies aim at attaining generalisable results, and selecting the sample size is key. Various methods can be used:

Opportunistic sampling. This type of research is done with a non-representative sample of survivors, for instance persons from a victim centre where it is impossible to ascertain whether or not they are representative of all survivors. Snowball selection is a special type of opportunistic sampling where an initial group of victims subsequently puts the interviewer in contact with other victims, and so forth.

Opportunistic sampling is the weakest method as it only enables results to be generalized within the researched sample.

Latin square. Here also one works with an opportunistic sampling of survivors, but attempts to control some of the key variables that may impact the participants' experience and steer participant selection as a result.

This methodology ensures the required minimum sample size for comparing different groups.

When the Latin square methodology is used, as the interviews are conducted, a checklist is filled out to indicate the number of persons fulfilling key characteristics to be analysed. For instance, if the aim is to have a representative sample by gender, age group and detention centre, a matrix with these variables would be used so that certain profiles would gradually be 'closed' while others whose representation had not yet been covered would be sought. An attempt should be made to cover a minimum of between 5 and 30 persons per Latin square cell.

The results of research using opportunistic sampling and a Latin square approach cannot be generalised to be applied to all victims, but certain key aspects that are otherwise usually lost, such as the differing impact on women, can be analysed further in depth.

Random sampling. This is the only way to achieve prevalence indicators and be able to generalise results. This can only be done based on an official census, which might be a census of inmates in a detention centre or an official Truth Commission victim census. The persons to be interviewed could be drawn at random for instance from the entire list, or after stratifying the sample using key variables.

These sampling methods can be combined to increase sample size and power of results, for instance conducting multi-centre research or paralleling different groups with comparable methodologies or working with on-line samples.

Selecting tools

Whichever scale is chosen, its transcultural validation is important. In other words, the faithfulness to the original of the translation into the local language must be verified. All necessary adaptations must be made to ensure that there is both linguistic correlation and also conceptual correlation to the original.

The wording must also be specifically tailored to the experience of torture in contexts where there may have been a host of types of violence (war, prison, forced displacement. . . .). This is to say that it is not merely the symptoms that should be asked about, but whether these symptoms are *related to* the victims' experience of torture. Alternatively, the survivor should be asked about symptoms related to torture or other symptoms separately through the questionnaire.

It is important for the time period covered by the question to be clearly and specifically determined. One helpful approach is to ask whether the person had the symptoms immediately after the facts, i.e. during the first six months, whether s/he experienced them any time subsequently (overall prevalence), and whether the person had them at the time of the research (point-prevalence). Asking these questions enables subsequent comparability of the results to be ensured.

The following should be used as a minimum:

1. A torture methods checklist (see Appendix 4), adapted to the local context, based on Stage 1 of testimony collection. Chapter 7 addressed this type of tool's shortcomings. The Torturing Environment Scale (TES) stands as an alternative to classical checklists and puts the accent not on the methods and the mechanics of torture, but on the objective that each method pursues in the overall torture process. This enables a torturing environment profile to be drawn up and each one of the dimensions it contains to be quantified. The TES affords a new, etiological, comprehensive approach.
2. One or several clinical impact measurements. At least a Post-Traumatic Stress Test (i.e. the PCL-C), and/or a measurement of Complex Post Traumatic Stress (DESNOS, EPCACE or similar) should be used with additional optional general measurements of anxiety or depression.
3. Psychosocial impact measurements. The way in which the torture impacted the survivor's life (work, studies, activism . . .) including family networks and types of social support (see box for a sample question).

'Do you believe that torture changed the way you perceive the world?'   Yes   No
'Can you explain your answer?'

'Can you give examples?'

Several additional measurements may be added, including:

4.   Impact on belief system of others and oneself. Impact on worldviews.
5.   Scale of emotions linked to the torture, particularly shame and guilt.
6.   Measurement of mechanisms to face torture and resilience indicators.
7.   Measurement of the perception of social climate, representations of violence, truth and justice. Needs for reparation and rehabilitation.

The VIVO scale encompasses aspects (4), (5) and (6) in a single questionnaire. Availability of a wealth of samples of its use with survivors enables data comparison (see Appendix 4).

Ethical aspects

Lastly, in an issue as sensitive as torture, it is particularly important:

1.   To maintain database confidentiality according to data protection laws, particularly considering the participants' safety and potential retaliation.
2.   To obtain a signature of informed consent regarding the information's use and custody. Should the data be gathered for documenting research, it cannot be used subsequently for legal purposes without express consent.
3.   To provide the survivor feedback regarding the results without generating the feeling of being 'a subject of an investigation' but rather 'part of the research team'.
4.   To plan for careful, attentive follow-up measures when significant damage is detected.

Notes

1 This process is extremely simple when using specific software for text analysis such as Atlas-ti or N6.
2 While it is important for it to be survivors who generate the conceptual categories, particularly in cultural environments that differ greatly from those doing the documentation, this may make the process more complex. Given that the categories may be fairly standard, it might be more useful for the survivors to perform the analysis of the results for the final report.

BIBLIOGRAPHY

Abootalebi, V., Moradi, M. H., & Khalilzadeh, M. A. (2009). A new approach for EEG feature extraction in P300-based lie detection. *Computer Methods and Programs in Biomedicine, 94*(1), 48–57. doi:10.1016/j.cmpb.2008.10.001.

Adcock, J. (2012). Is the Reid technique really the problem? *IIIRG Bulletin, 3*(1): 1–43.

Adenauer, H., Catani, C., Keil, J., Aichinger, H., & Neuner, F. (2010). Is freezing an adaptive reaction to threat? Evidence from heart rate reactivity to emotional pictures in victims of war and torture. *Psychophysiology, 47,* 315–22. doi:10.1111/j.1469-8986.2009.00940.x

Adorno, T. (1950). *The authoritarian personality.* New York: Harper.

Agger, I., & Jensen, S. B. (1990). Testimony as ritual and evidence in psychotherapy for political refugees. *Journal of Traumatic Stress, 3,* 115–30. doi:10.1007/BF00975139

Ahuja, N. (2011). Abu Zubaydah and the Caterpillar. *Social Text, 29*(1), 127–49. doi:10.1215/01642472-

Albarelli, H. (2009). *A terrible mistake: the murder of Frank Olson and the CIA's secret Cold War experiments.* Trine Day. Waltersville, USA.

Albu, R., & Grier, D. (2010). Quantum Orbital Resonance Spectroscopy (QORS). In *DARPA NEST FORUM, At San Diego, CA.* doi:10.13140/2.1.2555.2008.

Alleg, H. (1958). *The question.* Cambridge, MA: Plunkett Lake Press.

Allhoff, F. (2005). A defense of torture: separation of cases, ticking time-bombs, and moral justification. *International Journal of Applied Philosophy, 19*(2), 243–64.

Allodi, F. (1991). Assessment and tratment of torture victims: a critical review. *Journal of Nervous and Mental Disease, 179,* 4–11.

Allodi, F., & Cowgill, G. (1982). Ethical and psychiatric aspects of torture: a Canadian study. *Canadian Journal of Psychiatry. Revue Canadienne de Psychiatrie, 27,* 98–102.

Almond, I. (2013). British and Israeli assistance to U. S. Strategies of torture and counter-insurgency in Central and Latin America, 1967–96: an argument against complexification. *Journal of Critical Globalisation Studies,* (6), 57–77.

Alonso, J., Angermeyer, M. C., Bernert, S., Bruffaerts, R., Brugha, T. S., Bryson, H., . . . Almansa, J. (2004). Prevalence of mental disorders in Europe: results from the European Study of the Epidemiology of Mental Disorders (ESEMeD) project. *Acta Psychiatrica Scandinavica, 109,* 21–7.

Altemeyer, B. (2006). *The Authoritarians.* University of Manitoba. Manitoba, Canada.

American Bar Association. (2011). *Treatment of prisoners. ABA standards for criminal justice.* Washington DC.

American Civil Liberties Union. (2012). *Revising the standard minimum rules for the treatment of prisoners: statement on solitary confinement.* Expert Group Meeting. New York.

American Psychiatric Association. (1994). *Diagnostic and statistical manual of mental disorders (4th ed.).* Washington, DC.

American Psychiatric Association. (2005). *APA submits comments on solitary confinement policy to senate judiciary subcommittee.* APA News. Washington, DC.

American Psychiatric Association. (1980). *Diagnostic and statistical manual of mental disorders.* Washington, DC.

American Psychiatric Association. (2013). Post-Traumatic Stress Disorder – DSM V Fact Sheet. Retrieved from http://www.dsm5.org/Documents/PTSDFactSheet.pdf

Amery, J. (1980). *At the mind's limits: contemplations by a survivor of Auschwitz and its realities.* Indiana University Press.

Amnesty International. (2002). *Unmatched power, unmet principles: the human rights dimensions of US training of foreign military and police forces.* New York.

Amnesty International. (2004). *Helping to break the silence: urgent actions on Iran.* London, UK.

Amnesty International. (2011). *Rape and sexual violence. Human rights law and standard in the International Criminal Court.* London, UK.

Anderson, C., & Carnegey, N. (2004). The social psychology of good and evil. In A. G. Miller (Ed.), *The social psychology of good and evil.* New York: Guilford.

Anonymous. (2006). *Detainee Al Qahtani – Interrogation Log.* Retrieved from http://content.time.com/time/2006/log/log.pdf

Anthony, K. (2008). *Experiments in ethics.* London: Harvard University Press.

Arce, L. (1993). *El infierno [Hell].* Santiago: Editorial Océano.

Arenas, J. G. (2009). The work field of torture and NGOs – the reality and impact. *Psyke & Logos, 30,* 139–52.

Arnoso, M. (2010). Terrorismo de estado en jujuy (Argentina, 1976–1983): trauma sociopolítico y representaciones del pasado y la justicia. *Departamento de Ciencias Politicas.* Universidad del Pais Vasco.

Arrigo, J. M., & Wagner, R. V.(2007). Psychologists and military interrogators rethink the psychology of torture. *Peace and Conflict: Journal of Peace Psychology, 13*(4), 393–98. doi:10.1080/10781910701665550

Arzuaga, J. (2012). *Oso Latza izan da. Tortura Euskal Herrian. [It was very hard. Torture in the Basque Country].* Donostia – San Sebastián: Euskal Memoria.

Assistance Association for Political Prisioners (Burma). (2005). *The darkness we see: torture in Burma's interrogation centers and prisons.* Bangkok.

Association of Chief Police Officers. (2012). *Guidance on the safer detention and handling of persons in custody.* London: National Policing Improvement Agency.

Aussaresses, P. (2010). *The Battle of the Casbah: terrorism and counter-terrorism in Algeria, 1955–1957.*

Baer, H. U., & Vorbrügeen, M. (2007). Humiliation: the lasting effect of torture. *Military Medicine, 172,* 12–29.

Bahbah, B. (1986). *Israel and Latin America: the military connection.* New York: St Martin's Press.

Bandura, A. (1991). Social cognitive theory of self regulation. *Organizational Behaviour and Human Decision Processes, 50,* 248–87.

Bandura, A. (1999). Moral disengagement in the perpetration of inhumanities. *Pers Soc Psychol Rev, 3*(3), 193–209. doi:10.1207/s15327957pspr0303_3

Bandura, A. (2002). Selective moral disengagement in the exercise of moral agency. *Journal of Moral Education., 31*(2), 101–19.

Bandura, A., Barbaranelli, C., Caprara, G. V, & Pastorelli, C. (1996). Mechanisms of moral disengagement in the exercise of moral agency. *Journal of Personality and Social Psychology, 71,* 364–74.

Başoğlu, M. (2009). A multivariate contextual analysis of torture and cruel, inhuman, and degrading treatments: implications for an evidence-based definition of torture. *American Journal of Orthopsychiatry, 79*(2), 135–45. doi:10.1037/a0015681

Başoğlu, M. (1999). *Semi-structured interview for Survivors of War (SISOW).* (mimmeo-personal communication)

Başoğlu, M. (2009). Copia Duplicada – A multivariate contextual analysis of torture and cruel, inhuman, and degrading treatments: implications for an evidence-based definition of torture. *The American Journal of Orthopsychiatry, 79*(2), 135–45. doi:10.1037/a0015681

Başoğlu, M., Jaranson, J., Mollica, R., & Kastrup, M. (2001). Torture and mental health: A research overview. In T. Keane & F. T. E. Garrity (Ed.), *The mental health consequences of torture* (pp. 35–62). New York: Plenum Publishers.

Başoğlu, M., Livanou, M., & Crnobaric, C. (2007). Torture vs other cruel, inhuman, and degrading treatment. *Archives of General Psychiatry, 64,* 277–85.

Başoğlu, M., & Mineka, S. (1992). The role of uncontrollable and impredictable stress in postraumatic stress responses in torture survivors. In M. Basoglu (Ed.), *Torture and its consequences. Current treatment approaches*. New York: Cambridge University Press.

Başoğlu, M., & Paker, M. (1995). Severity of trauma as predictor of long-term psychological status in survivors of torture. *Journal of Anxiety Disorders, 9*(4), 339–350. doi:10.1016/0887-6185(95)00014-F

Başoğlu, M, Paker M., Paker O., Ozmen E., Marks I., Incesu C., Sahin D, and Sarimurat, N. (1994). Psychological effects of torture: a comparison of tortured with nontortured political activists in Turkey. *The American Journal of Psychiatry, 151*, 76–81.

Baum, S. K. (2008). *The psychology of genocide perpetrators, bystanders, and rescuers*. Cambridge, UK: Cambridge University Press.

Baumann, P. (2007). Persons, human beings and respect. *Polish Journal of Phylosophy, 2*, 5–17.

Baykal, T., Schlar, C., & Kapkin, E. (2004). *The Istanbul Project Implementation Protocol. 2003–2005 psychological evidence of torture*. Copenhague: IRCT.

Beck, F., & Godin, W. (1951). *Russian purge and the extraction of confessions*. New York: Hurst and Blackett, Ltd.

Beck, J. G., Coffey, S. F., Palyo, S. A., Gudmundsdottir, B., Miller, L. M., & Colder, C. R. (2004). Psychometric Properties of the Posttraumatic Cognitions Inventory (PTCI): a replication with motor vehicle accident survivors. *Psychological Assessment, 16*(3), 289–98.

Beck, J. G., Palyo, S. A., Canna, M. A., Blanchard, E. B., & Gudmundsdottir, B. (2006). What factors are associated with the maintenance of PTSD after a motor vehicle accident? The role of sex differences in a help-seeking population. *Journal of Behavior Therapy and Experimental Psychiatry, 37*(3), 256–66.

Behan, C. W. (2009). Everybody talks: evaluating the admissibility of coercively obtained evidence in trials by military commission. *Washburn Law Journal, 48*, 563–616.

Beken, T. Vander, & Wu, W. (2010). Police torture in China and its causes: A review of literature. *Australian and New Zealand Journal of Criminology*. doi:10.1375/acri.43.3.557

Bellamy, A. J. (2006). No pain, no gain? Torture and ethics in the war on terror. *International Affairs, 82*, 121–148. doi:10.1111/j.1468-2346.2006.00518.x

Beltran, R. O., Llewellyn, G. M., & Silove, D. (2008). Clinicians' understanding of International Statistical Classification of Diseases and Related Health Problems, 10th Revision diagnostic criteria: F62.0 enduring personality change after catastrophic experience. *Comprehensive Psychiatry, 49*(6), 593–602. doi:10.1016/j.comppsych.2008.04.006

Beltran, R. O., & Silove, D. (1999). Expert opinions about the ICD-10 category of enduring personality change after catastrophic experience. *Comprehensive Psychiatry, 40*(5), 396–403.

Benight, C. C., & Bandura, A. (2004). Social cognitive theory of posttraumatic recovery: the role of perceived self-efficacy. *Behav Res Ther, 42*(10), 1129–48. doi:10.1016/j.brat.2003.08.008 S0005796703002304 [pii]

Berkowitz, L. (1999). Evil is more than banal: situationism and the concept of evil. *Pers Soc Psychol Rev, 3*(3), 246–53. doi:10.1207/s15327957pspr0303_7

Biderman, A. (1957). Communist attempts to elicit false confessions from air force prisoners of war. *Bulletin of the New York Academy of Medicine, 33*, 616–25.

Biderman, A., & Zimmer, H. (1961). *The Manipulation of Human Behaviour*. New York: John Wiley and Sons.

Blagrove, M., & Akehurst, L. (2000). Effects of sleep loss on confidence–accuracy relationships for reasoning and eyewitness memory. *Journal of Experimental Psychology: Applied, 6*(1), 59–73. doi:10.1037/1076-898X.6.1.59

Blasi, A. (1980). Bridging moral cognition and moral action: a critical review of the literature. *Psychological Bulletin, 88*, 1–45.

Blass, T. (1991). Understanding behavior in the Milgram obedience experiment: The role of personality, situations, and their interactions. *Journal of Personality and Social Psychology, 60*(3), 398–413. doi:10.1037//0022-3514.60.3.398

Boire, R. (2000). On cognitive liberty. *Journal of Cognitive Liberties, 1*(1), 1–26.

Boire, R. G. (2005). Searching the brain: the fourth amendment implications of brain-based deception detection devices. *The American Journal of Bioethics: AJOB, 5*(2), 62–3; discussion W5. doi:10.1080/15265160590960933

Borum, R. (2005). Approaching truth: behavioral science lessons on educing information from human sources. In *Educing information interrogation: Science and Art*. Intelligence Science Board.

Borum, R. (2009). Interview and interrogation: a perspective and update from the USA. *Mental Health Law & Policy Faculty Publications. Paper 538*, (January 2009). Retrieved from http://scholarcommons.usf.edu/mhlp_facpub/538

Bradbury, S. G. (2004) Memorandum for John Rizzo (accesed from http://media.luxmedia.com/aclu/olc_05102005_bradbury46pg.pdf).

Breslau, N., Kessler, R. C., Chilcoat, H. D., Schultz, L. R., Davis, G. C., & Andreski, P. (1998). Trauma and posttraumatic stress disorder in the community: the 1996 Detroit Area Survey of Trauma. *Archives of General Psychiatry, 55*(7), 626–32.

Brewin, C., Dalgleish, T., & Joseph, S. (1996). A dual representation theory of posttraumatic stress disorder. *Psychological Review, 103*(4), 670–86.

Brewin, C. R., Lanius, R. A., Novac, A., Schnyder, U., & Galea, S. (2009). Reformulating PTSD for DSM-V: life after Criterion A. *Journal of Traumatic Stress, 22*(5), 366–73. doi:10.1002/jts.20443

Brewin, & Holmes, E. (2003). Psychological theories of post-traumatic stress disorder. *Clinical Psychology Review, 23*(4), 23–56.

Brodsky, S., Griffin, M., & Cramer, R. (2010). The witness credibility scale: an outcome measure for expert witness research. *Behavioral Sciences & the Law, 28*(2), 211–23. doi:10.1002/bsl

Browning, C. R. (1992). *Ordinary men: Reserve Police Battalion 101 and the Final Solution in Poland.* New York: HarperCollins.

Buckley, J. P. (2000). *The Reid Technique of interviewing and interrogation.*

Bushman, B. J., & Baumeister, R. J. (1998). Threatened egotism, narcissism, self-esteem, and direct and displaced aggression: Does self-love or self-hate lead to violence? *Journal of Personality and Social Psychology, 75*(1), 219–229.

Caldas, A. (1981). *Tirando o capuz.* Rio de Janeiro: Garamond Editors.

Cantor, C. (2009). Post-traumatic stress disorder: evolutionary perspectives. *Australian and New Zealand Journal of Psychiatry* (May), 1038–50.

Cantor, C., & Price, J. (2007). Traumatic entrapment, appeasement and complex post-traumatic stress disorder: evolutionary perspectives of hostage reactions, domestic abuse and the Stockholm syndrome. *The Australian and New Zealand Journal of Psychiatry, 41*(5), 377–84. doi:10.1080/00048670701261178

Cardoso, C., & Ellenbogen, M. (2013). Oxytocin and psychotherapy: keeping context and person in mind. *Psychoneuroendocrinology, 38*(12), 3172–3. doi:10.1016/j.psyneuen.2013.08.002

Carinci, A. J., Mehta, P., & Christo, P. J. (2010). Chronic pain in torture victims. *Current Pain and Headache Reports, 14*(2), 73–9. doi:10.1007/s11916-010-0101-2

Carlson, E. B., & Dalenberg, C. (2000). A conceptual framework for the impact of traumatic experiences. *Trauma, Violence & Abuse, 1*(1), 4–28.

Carmena, M., Landa, J. M., Múgica, R., & Uriarte, J. M. (2013). *Informe-base de vulneraciones de derechos humanos en el caso vasco (1960–2013) / Base report on human rights violations in the Basque country case (1960–2013).* Vitoria Gasteiz.

Castaño, C. (2001). *Mi Confesion [My confession].* Bogota: La Oveja Negra.

Castresana, C. (2012). La tortura como mal mayor. *El Viejo Topo, 289*, 17–27.

Catani, C., Adenauer, H., Keil, J., Aichinger, H., & Neuner, F. (2009). Pattern of cortical activation during processing of aversive stimuli in traumatized survivors of war and torture. *European Archives of Psychiatry and Clinical Neuroscience, 259*, 340–51. doi:10.1007/s00406-009-0006-4

Caton, C. L. M., Dominguez, B., Schanzer, B., Hasin, D. S., Shrout, P. E., Felix, A., . . . Hsu, E. (2005). Risk factors for long-term homelessness: Findings from a longitudinal study of first-time homeless single adults. *American Journal of Public Health, 95*(10), 1753–1759. doi:10.2105/ajjph.2005.063321

Center for Bioethics. University of Minnesota. (2014). United States Military Medicine in War on Terror Prisons. Iraq – Operation Iraqi Freedom – OIF Afghanistan – Operation Enduring Freedom – OEF Guantanamo Bay, Cuba – GTMO. Retrieved from www1.umn.edu/humanrts/OathBetrayed/interrogation-index.html

Center for Human Rights & Humanitarian Law. (2006). *Report on torture and cruel, inhuman and degrading treatment of prisoners at Guantanamo Bay, Cuba.* Washington DC: Washington Collegue & Law.

Center for Human Rights & Humanitarian Law. (2009). *Current conditions of confinement at Guantanamo: Still violations of the law.* Washington DC: Washington Collegue & Law.

Center for Human Rights & Humanitarian Law. (2014). *Torture in healthcare settings: reflections on the Special Rapporteur on Torture's 2013 Thematic Repport.* Washington DC: Washington College & Law.

Central Intelligence Agency. (1963). Kubark Counterintelligence Interrogation of Resistance Sources. Washington DC: USA Declassified Document.

Central Intelligence Agency. (1983). Human Resource Exploitation Training Manual. Washington DC: USA Declassified Document.

Chung, M. C., Farmer, S., & Grant, K. (2002). Self-esteem, personality and post traumatic stress symptoms following the dissolution of a dating relationship. *Stress and Health*, *18*(2), 83–90. doi:10.1002/smi.929

Church, D. (2012). Neuroscience in the courtroom: An international concern. *William and Mary Law Review*, *53*(5), 1825–53. Retrieved from http://scholarship.law.wm.edu/cgi/viewcontent .cgi?article=3437&context=wmlr

Cienfuegos, J., & Monelli, C. (1983). The testimony of political repression as a therapeutic instrument. *American Journal of Orthopsychiatry*, *53*, 43–51.

Cobain, I. (2012). Humiliate, strip, threaten: UK military interrogation manuals discovered. *The Guardian*. 25 October.

Cockburn, A., and Cockburn, L. (1991). *Dangerous liaison: the inside story of the U.S.- Israeli covert relationship*. New York: Harper Collins.

Cohen (2001). Democracy and the misrule of law: The Israeli legal system's failure to prevent torture in the occupied territories, 12 *Ind. Int'l and Comp. L. Rev*, 75, 77–8.

Cohrs, J. C., Maes, J., Moschner, B., & Kielmann, S. (2007). Determinants of human rights attitudes and behavior: a comparison and integration of psychological perspectives. *Political Psychology*, *28*(4), 441–69. doi:10.1111/j.1467-9221.2007.00581.x

Cohrs, J., Moschner, B., Maes, J., & Kielman, S. (2010). Personal values and attitudes toward war. *Peace and Conflict*, *11*(3), 293–312.

Colb, S. F. (2009). Why is torture 'different' and how 'different' is it? *Cardozo Law Review*, *30*(4), 1411. doi:10.2139/ssrn.1099061

Collins, A. (1988). *In the sleep room: the story of CIA brainwashing experiments in Canada*. Toronto: Key Porter Books.

Conroy, J. (2000). *Unspeakable acts, ordinary people. The dynamics of torture. An examination of the practice in three democracies*. University of California Press.

Copes, H., Vieraitis, L., & Jochum, J. M. (2007). Bridging the gap between research and practice: how neutralization theory can inform Reid interrogations of identity thieves. *Journal of Criminal Justice Education*, *18*(3), 444–59. doi:10.1080/10511250701705404

Costanzo, M., & Gerrity, E. (2009). The effects and effectiveness of using torture as an interrogation device: using research to inform the policy debate. *Social Issues and Policy Review*, *3*(1), 179–210. doi:10.1111/j.1751-2409.2009.01014.x

Council of Europe. (1973). Standard Minimum Rules for the Treatment of Prisoners. Resolution (73)5. Strasbourg.

Council of Europe. (2006). Recommendation Rec (2006)2 of the Committee of Ministers to member states on the European Prison Rules. Retrieved from http://legislationline.org/documents/action/popup/id/8028

Coyle, A. (2002). *A human rights approach to prison management. Handbook for prison staff*. London: International Center for Prison Studies.

Coyle, A. (2008). The treatment of prisoners: international standards and case law. *Legal and Criminological Psychology*, *13*(2), 219–30. doi:10.1348/135532508X284284

Crampton, D. (2013). *What indicators exist, or may exist, to determine whether a violation of the prohibition of torture, inhuman or degrading treatment or punishment has occurred on the basis of psychological maltreatment, and whether it amounts to psychological torture?* LLM Dissertation. School of Law. University of Essex (personal communication).

Crocker, J., Lee, S., & Park, L. (2004). The pursuit of self-steem: implications for good and evil. In A. G. Miller (Ed.), *The social psychology of good and evil*, pp. 271–302. New York: Guilford Press.

Croissant, K. (1975). *A propos du procès Baader-Meinhof, Fraction Armée Rouge: de la torture dans les prisons de la RFA*. Paris: Christian Bourgeois Éditeur.

CSHRA. (2005). The neurobiology of psychological torture (mimmeo). Retrieved from http://humanrights.ucdavis.edu/projects/the-neurobiology-of-psychological-torture-1/

Culhane, S. E., Hosch, H. M., & Heck, C. (2008). Interrogation technique endorsement by current law enforcement, future law enforcement, and laypersons. *Police Quarterly*, *11*(3), 366–86. doi:10.1177/1098611107309116

Cunniffe, D. (2013). The worst scars are in the mind. Deconstructing psychological torture. *ICL Journal*, 7(1), 1–61.

Cunningham, M., & Cunningham, J. (1997). Patterns of symptomatology and patterns of torture and trauma experiences in resettled refugees. *Australian and New Zealand Journal of Psychiatry, 31*, 555–65.

Cusick, S. G. (2006). Music as torture / Music as weapon. *Trans. Revista Transcultural de Musica.*

Davis, D., & Leo, R. (2012). Acute suggestibility in police interrogation: self-regulation failure as a primary mechanism of vulnerability. In A. M. Ridley, F. Gabert, & D. La Rooy (Eds.), *Suggestibility in legal contexts* (pp. 171–95). John Wiley & Sons. Malden, USA.

de Jong, J., Komproe, I., Spinazzola, J., van der Kolk, B., & Van Ommeren, M. (2005). DESNOS in three postconflict settings: assessing cross-cultural construct equivalence. *Journal of Traumatic Stress, 18*(1), 13–21. doi:10.1002/jts.20005

de Jong, J. T., Komproe, I. H., Van Ommeren, M., El Masri, M., Araya, M., Khaled, N., . . . Somasundaram, D. (2001). Lifetime events and posttraumatic stress disorder in 4 postconflict settings. *JAMA: The Journal of the American Medical Association, 286*(5), 555–62. Retrieved from http://www.ncbi.nlm.nih.gov/pubmed/11476657

Dehn, J. C. (2008). Why Article 5 status determinations are not 'required' at Guantanamo. *J Int Criminal Justice, 6*, 371–383. doi:10.1093/jicj/mqn016

Demarest, G. (2010). Galula or Trinquier? Let's take the French experience in Algeria out of US Counterinsurgency doctrine. *Military Review*, 19–26.

Den Otter, J. (2013). Documentation of torture and cruel, inhuman or degrading treatment of children: A review of existing guidelines and tools. *Forensic Science International, 224*(1–3), 27–32. doi:10.1016/j.forsciint.2012.11.003

Dershowitz, A. M. (2008). *Is there a right to remain silent? Coercive interrogation and the fifth amendment after 9/11*. Oxford Univ Press.

Doris, J. (2010). *The moral psychology handbook*. Oxford: Oxford University Press.

Dotson, T. (2009). Negotiate instead of interrogate – get better results from interrogations through negotiation. Alabama: Maxwell Air Force Base, Alabama.

Drizin, S., & Leo, R. (2004). The problem of false confessions in the post-DNA world. *North Carolina Law Review, 82*, 891–1007.

Dueck, J., Guzman, M., & Verstappen, B. (2009). *HURIDOCS. A Tool for Documenting Human Rights Violations. Micro Thesaurus*. HURIDOCS. Retrieved from www.huridocs.org/

Düwell, M. (2011). Human dignity and human rights. In E. Kaufmann, P., Kuch, H., Neuhäuser, C., & Webster (Eds.), *Humiliation, degradation, dehumanization* (pp. 215–230). Dordrecht: Springer Netherlands.

EATIP, GTNM/RJ, CINTRAS, & SERSOC. (2002). *Paisajes del Dolor, Senderos de esperanza. Salud mental y derechos humanos en el Cono Sur.*

Ebert, A., & Dyck, M. J. (2004). The experience of mental death: the core feature of complex post-traumatic stress disorder. *Clinical Psychology Review, 24*(6), 617–35. doi:10.1016/j.cpr.2004.06.002

ECHR. (1969). *The Greek Case. 12 Yearbook of the European Convention of Human Rights*. Strasbourg.

ECHR. (1978a). *Case of Ireland v. the United Kingdom*. Strasbourg.

ECHR. (1978b). *Case of Ireland v. the United Kingdom*. Separate opinion of Judge O'Donoughe. Strasbourg.

ECHR. (1978c). *Case Tyrer v. United Kingdom*. 5856/72. 15 March 1978. www.refworld.org/docid/402a2cae4.html [accessed 13 June 2016] Strasbourg.

ECHR. (1982). *Case of Campbell and Cosans v. the United Kingdom (Application no. 7511/76; 7743/76)*. 25 February 1982. Strasbourg.

ECHR (1997). *Aydin v. Turkey*, 57/1996/676/866, Council of Europe: European Court of Human Rights, 25 September 1997, available at: http://www.refworld.org/docid/3ae6b7228.html [accessed 13 June 2016].

ECHR. (1999). *Selmouni v. France*, 25803/94, Council of Europe: European Court of Human Rights, 28 July 1999, available at: http://www.refworld.org/docid/3ae6b70210.html [accessed 13 June 2016].

ECHR. (2000a). *Case Akkoç v. Turkey*. 22947/93 and 22948/93. 10 October 2000.

ECHR. (2000b). *Dikme v. Turkey*. 20869/92. 11 July 2000.

ECHR. (2001a). *Case Keenan v. United Kingdom*. 4. March 2001. *(Application no. 27229/95)*.

ECHR (2001b). *Case Peers v. Greece*. 28524/95. 19 April 2001.

ECHR (2002). *Case Kalashnikov v. Russia*. 15 October 2002.

ECHR (2003a). *Case Elci and Others v Turkey*. 23145/93, 25091/94. 24 March 2004. Judgment, 13 November 2003.

ECHR. (2003b). *Case Yankov v. Bulgaria (no. 39084/9711)*. December 2003. Strabourg. Retrieved from http://sim.law.uu.nl/SIM/CaseLaw/hof.nsf/2422ec00f1ace923c1256681002b47f1/2b67e83 6a888f46b41256e1d0038e122?OpenDocument

ECHR 2004. *Case Ilascu and Others v. Moldova and Russia*. 8 July 2004. 48787/99. www.refworld.org/docid/414d9df64.html [accessed 13 June 2016].

Economic and Social Council. (1957). Standard minimum rules for the treatment of prisoners adopted by the First United Nations Congress on the Prevention of Crime and the Treatment of Offenders, held at Geneva in 1955, and approved by the Economic and Social Council by its resolutions 663 C. Retrieved from www.ohchr.org/Documents/ProfessionalInterest/treatmentprisoners.pdf

Ehlers, A., Clark, D., Dunmore, E., Jaycox, L., Meadows, E., & Foa, E. (1998). Predicting response to exposure treatment in PTSD: the role of mental defeat and alienation. *Journal of Traumatic Stress, 11*(3), 457–71. doi:10.1023/A:1024448511504

Ehlers, A., Maercker, A., & Boos, A. (2000). Posttraumatic stress disorder following political imprisonment: The role of mental defeat, alienation, and perceived permanent change. *Journal of Abnormal Psychology, 109*(1), 45–55. doi:10.1037/0021-843X.109.1.45

Ehring, T., Ehlers, A., & Glucksman, E. (2006). Contribution of cognitive factors to the prediction of post-traumatic stress disorder, phobia and depression after motor vehicle accidents. *Behaviour Research And Therapy, 44*(12), 1699–1716.

Elahi, M. (2004). Dual loyalty and human rights in health professional practice: proposed guidelines and institutional mechanisms (review). *Human Rights Quarterly, 26*(3), 781–83. doi:10.1353/hrq.2004.0034

Elsass, P., Carlsson, J., Jespersen, K., & Phuntsok, K. (2009). Questioning western assessment of trauma among Tibetan torture survivors. A quantitative assessment study with comments from Buddhist Lamas. *Torture, 19*(3), 194–203.

Elsea, J. K. (2004). Lawfulness of interrogation techniques under the Geneva Conventions. CRS Report for Congress. Washington DC.

Engler, H., Charlo, P., & Caray, A. (2012). *El Círculo [The Circle]*. Montevideo: Ediciones de la Banda Oriental.

Epstein, O., Schwartz, J., & Schwartz, R. (2011). *Ritual abuse and mind control. The manipulation of attachment needs*. London: Karnac Books.

Erol, F. Ö. (2010). F -Type prisons, isolation and its consequences. In *Proceedings. Situation of political prisoners due to changes in anti-terror legislation and in the law enforcement code. International Expert Meeting*. Bonn.

Evans, J. A. (2012). *Is complex post traumatic stress disorder a valid construct in refugee survivors of torture and war trauma?* Master Thesis. Griffith University.

Evans, J., Meissner, C., Ross, A., Houston, K., Russano, M., & Horgan, A. (2013). Obtaining guilty knowledge in human intelligence interrogations: comparing accusatorial and information-gathering approaches with a novel experimental paradigm. *Journal of Applied Research in Memory and Cognition, 2*(2), 83–8. doi:10.1016/j.jarmac.2013.03.002

Fals-Borda, O., & Rahman, M. (1991). *Action and knowledge: breaking the monopoly with participatory action research*. New York: APEX.

Fanon, F. (1963). *The wretched of the earth*. Trans. C. Farrington. New York: Grove Press.

FBI Review Division. (2008). *A review of the FBI's involvement in and observations of detainee interrogations in Guantanamo Bay, Afghanistan and Iraq*. Washington DC: Office of the Inspector General. Department of Justice.

Fernández Liria, A., & Rodríguez Vega, B. (2001). *La práctica de la psicoterapia: La construcción de narrativas terapéuticas [The practice of psychotherapy: The construction of therapeutic narratives]*. Bilbao: Desclée de Brouwer.

Fields, R. (2008). The neurobiological consequences of psychological torture. In A. E. Ojeda (Ed.), *The trauma of psychological torture* (pp. 139–62). London: Praeger.

Fivecoat, D. G. (2008). Revisiting modern warfare counterinsurgency – following Trinquet. *Military Review* (December), 77–87.

Fletcher, L. E., & Stover, E. (2008). *Guantánamo and its aftermath. US detention and interrogation practices and their impact on former detainees*. Washington DC: Human Rights Center and International Human Rights Law Clinic.

Flynn, M., & Salek, F. (2012). *Screening torture: media representations.* Cambridge, UK: Cambridge University Press.

Foa, E. B., Hearst-Ikeda, D., & Perry, K. J. (1995). Evaluation of a brief cognitive-behavioral program for the prevention of chronic PTSD in recent assault victims. *Journal of Consulting and Clinical Psychology, 63*(6), 948–55.

Foa, E. B., Tolin, D. F., Ehlers, A., Clark, D. M., & Orsillo, S. M.(1999). The Posttraumatic Cognitions Inventory (PTCI): development and validation. *Psychological Assessment, 11,* 303–14.

Forest, E. (2006). Sobre la tortura. [On Torture]. Retrieved from www.sastre-forest.com/forest/pdf/euskalherria.pdf

Forrest, K. D., & Woody, W. D.(2010). Police deception during interrogation and its surprising influence on jurors' perceptions of confession evidence. *The Jury Expert, 22*(6), 9–23.

Frias, M. J. (2011). Gilberto Vázquez justifica tortura. *Ultimas Noticias.*

Galula, D. (1964). *Contrainsurgency warfare: theory and practice.* New York: Frederick A. Prager.

Ganis, G., Rosenfeld, J. P., Meixner, J., Kievit, R. A., & Schendan, H. E.(2011). Lying in the scanner: covert countermeasures disrupt deception detection by functional magnetic resonance imaging. *NeuroImage, 55*(1), 312–9. Retrieved from www.sciencedirect.com/science/article/pii/S1053811910014552

Genefke, I., & Vesti, P. (1998). Diagnosis of governmental torture. In J. Jaranson & M. Popkin (Eds.), *Caring for Victims of Torture* (pp. 43–9). American Psychiatric Press. Washington.

General Counsel of the Department of Defense. (2003). Working group report on detainee interrogations in the global war on terrorism: assessment of legal, historical, policy, and operational considerations.

Geneva Call. (2005). *Armed Non-State Actors and Landmines.* Geneva: PSIO.

Gerrity, E., Keane, T., & Tuma, F. (2001). *Mental health consequences of torture* (1st ed,). Springer: New York.

Gil, D. (1999). *El Capitán Por Su Boca Muere, o, la Piedad de Eros: Ensayo Sobre la Mentalidad de un Torturador* [The Captain by his mouth dies, or Piety of Eros: Essays on the Mentality of a Torturer]. Montevideo: Trilce.

Ginbar, Y. (2009). Celebrating a decade of legalised torture in Israel. *Essex Human Rights Review, 6,* 169–87.

Giridharadas, A. (2008). India's novel use of brain scans in courts is debated. *New York Times. 14 September,* pp. 3–5.

Goffman, E. (1959). *The presentation of self in everyday life.* Edinburgh: University of Edinburgh Social Sciences Research Centre.

Good, A. (2004). Undoubtedly an expert? Anthropologists in British asylum courts. *Journal of The Royal Anthropology Institute, 10,* 113–33. doi:10.1111/j.1467-9655.2004.00182.x

Gorst-Unsworth, C., & Goldenberg, E. (1998). Psychological sequelae of torture and organised violence suffered by refugees from Iraq. Trauma-related factors compared with social factors in exile. *The British Journal of Psychiatry: The Journal of Mental Science, 172,* 90–94. doi:10.1192/bjp.172.1.90

Gourevitch, P. (1998). *We wish to inform you that tomorrow we will be killed with our families: stories from Rwanda.* New York: Farrak Strauss & Giraux.

Grant, M. J. (2013). The illogical logic of music torture. *Torture: Quarterly Journal on Rehabilitation of Torture Victims and Prevention of Torture, 23*(2), 4–13. Retrieved from http://www.ncbi.nlm.nih.gov/pubmed/24480888

Grassian, S. (2006). Psychiatric effects of solitary confinement. *Journal of Law and Policy, 22*(617), 325–83.

Green, D., Rasmussen, A., & Rosenfeld, B. (2010). Defining torture: a review of 40 years of health science research. *Journal of Traumatic Stress, 23,* 528–31. doi:10.1002/jts.20552

Greenberg, K. (2006). *The torture debate in America.* Cambridge University Press. New York.

Grupo de denuncia de la violencia sexual sufrida durante el terrorismo de Estado. (2014). *Vivencias del Horror. Tortura sexual en las cárceles de Uruguay.* Madrid: Irredentos Libros.

Gudjonsson, G. H. (2003). *The psychology of interrogations and confessions. A handbook.* Wiley. London.

Gudjonsson, G. H. (2012). False confessions and correcting injustices. *New England Law Review, 46,* 689–710.

Gudjonsson, G. H., & Pearse, J. (2011). Suspect interviews and false confessions. *Current Directions in Psychological Science, 20*(1), 33–37. doi:10.1177/0963721410396824

Guiora, A. N. (2008). *Constitutional limits on coercive interrogation*. New York: Oxford University Press.

Gutierrez, G. S. (2008). The case of Mohammed Al Qahtani. In A. E. Ojeda (Ed.), *The Trauma of Psychological Torture* (pp. 189–205). Praeger Publisher. Westport, USA.

Guzmán, N. (2000). *Romo, confesiones de un torturador*. Santiago: Editorial Planeta.

Gyulai, G., Kagan, M., Herlihy, J., Turner, S., & Lilli, H. (2013). *Credibility assessment in asylum procedures. A multidisciplinary training manual* (Vol. 1).

Hakun, J. G., Ruparel, K., Seelig, D., Busch, E., Loughead, J. W., Gur, R. C., & Langleben, D. D. (2009). Towards clinical trials of lie detection with fMRI. *Social Neuroscience, 4*(6), 518–27. doi:10.1080/17470910802188370

Haney, C. (2003). Mental health issues in long-term confinement. *Crime and Delinquency, 49*(1), 124–56.

Haney, C., & Lynch, M. (1997). Regulating prisons of the future: psychological analysis of supermax and solitary confinement, XXIII (4):477–570. *New York University Review of Law & Social Change, XXIII*(4), 477–570.

Haritos-Fatouros, M. (2003). *The psychological origins of institutionalized torture*. London: Routledge.

Harman, R., & Lee, D. (2010). The role of shame and self-critical thinking in the development and maintenance of current threat in post-traumatic stress disorder. *Clin Psychol Psychother, 17*(1), 13–24. doi:10.1002/cpp.636

Hartling, L. M., & Luchetta, T. (1999). Humiliation: assessing the impact of derision, degradation and debasement. *The Journal of Primary Prevention, 19*(4), 1–23.

Haslam, S. A., & Reicher, S. (2006). Debating the psychology of tyranny: fundamental issues of theory, perspective and science. *British Journal of Social Psychology, 45*(Pt 1), 55–63. doi:10.1348/014466605X80686

Heckman, K. E., Mark, H. D., & Ballo, J. R. (2005). Mechanical detection of deception: a short review. In D. L. S. Robert Destro, Robert Fein, Pauletta Otis, John Wahlquist, Robert Coulam, Randy Borum, Gary Hazlett, Kristin E. Heckman and Mark D. Happel, Steven M. Kleinman, Ariel Neuman and Daniel Salinas-Serrano (Eds.), *Educing information interrogation: science and art*. National Defence Intelligence College. Washington.

Herlihy, J., & Turner, S. (2006). Should discrepant accounts given by asylum seekers be taken as proof of deceit? *Torture: Quarterly Journal on Rehabilitation of Torture Victims and Prevention of Torture, 16*, 81–92. doi:2006-2.2001-72 [pii]

Herlihy, J., Jobson, L., & Turner, S. (2012). Just tell us what happened to you: Autobiographical memory and seeking asylum. *Applied Cognitive Psychology, 26*(5), 661–76. doi:10.1002/acp.2852

Herman, E., & Chomsky, N. (1979). *The Washington connection and third world fascism*. South End Pr; Edición: First Edition, Highlighting.

Herman, J. (1992a). *Trauma and recovery. The aftermath of violence – from domestic abuse to political terror*. London: Basic Books.

Herman, J. L. (1992b). Complex PTSD: a syndrome in survivors of prolonged and repeated trauma. *J Trauma Stress, 5*(3), 377–89.

Heron, J. (1997). *Co-operative inquiry: research into the human condition*. Thousand Oaks: SAGE.

Hershcovis, M. S. (2011). 'Incivility, social undermining, bullying . . . oh my!': A call to reconcile constructs within workplace aggression research. *Journal of Organizational Behavior, 32*(3), 499–519. doi:10.1002/job.689

Hinkle, L. (1961). The physiological state of the interrogation subject as it affects brain function. In Bierderman A. Biderman, A., & Zimmer, H. (Eds.) (1961). *The Manipulation of Human Behaviour*. New York: John Wiley and Sons.

Hinkle, L., & Wolff, H. (1956). Communist control techniques. An analysis of the methods used by communist state police in the arrest, interrogation, and indoctrination of persons regarded as 'enemies of the state'. Declassified Material.

Hollifield, M., Warner, T. D., Lian, N., Jenkins, J. H., Kesler, J., & Stevenson, J. (2002). Measuring trauma and health status in refugees. *JAMA, 288*(5), 611–21.

Holtz, T. H. (1998). Refugee trauma versus torture trauma: a retrospective controlled cohort study of Tibetan refugees. *The Journal of Nervous and Mental Disease, 186*(1), 24–34.

Honigsberg, P. J. (2013). Lingüistic isolation: a new human rights violation constituting torture and cruel, inhuman and degrading treatment. *University of San Francisco Law Research Paper, 11*, 0–26.

Hooberman, J. B., Rosenfeld, B., Lhewa, D., Rasmussen, A., & Keller, A. (2007). Classifying the torture experiences of refugees living in the United States. *Journal of Interpersonal Violence, 22*(1), 108–23. doi:10.1177/0886260506294999

Hopper, E., & Hidalgo, J. (2006). Invisible chains: psychological coercion of human trafficking victims. *Intercultural Human Rights Law Review, 1,* 185/209.

Hoss, R. (2009). *Yo, comandante de Auschwitz.* Barcelona: Ediciones B.

Hugh, G. M., & Bessler, M. (2006). *Humanitarian negotiations with armed groups: A manual for practitioners.* Retrieved from http://www.eisf.eu/resources/item/?d=3036

Human Rights Committee. (1990). *Miguel Angel Estrella v. Uruguay, Communication No. 74/1980, U.N. Doc. CCPR/C/OP/2 at 93 (1990).*

Human Rights Commitee (1990). *Lucía Arzuaga Gilboa v. Uruguay, Communication No. 147/1983, U.N. Doc. CCPR/C/OP/2 at 176 (1990).*

Human Rights Committee. (1990). *Raúl Cariboni v. Uruguay, Communication No. 159/1983, U.N. Doc. CCPR/C/OP/2 at 189 (1990).*

Human Rights Committee (1994). *Womah Mukong v. Cameroon, Communication No. 458/1991, U.N. Doc. CCPR/C/51/D/458/1991 (1994).*

Hunt, L. (1991). *Secret agenda: the United States Government, Nazi scientists and Project Paperclip 1945–1990.* New York: St. Martin's Press.

Hunter, E. (1951). *Brainwashing in Red China.* New York: Vanguard Press.

Hunter, J. (1987). The Israeli role in Guatemala. *Race & Class, 29*(1), 35–54. doi:10.1177/030639688702900103

Iacopino, V., & Xenakis, S. N. (2011). Neglect of medical evidence of torture in Guantánamo Bay: a case series. *PLoS Medicine, 8*(4), e1001027. doi:10.1371/journal.pmed.1001027

ICTY. (1998). *Prosecutor v. Zdravko Mucic aka "Pavo", Hazim Delic, Esad Landzo aka "Zenga", Zejnil Delalic (Trial Judgement), IT-96-21-T, International Criminal Tribunal for the former Yugoslavia (ICTY),* 16 November 1998, available at: http://www.refworld.org/docid/41482bde4.html [accessed 13 June 2016]

ICTY. (1998a). *Prosecutor v. Anto Furundzija (Trial Judgement), IT-95-17/1-T, International Criminal Tribunal for the former Yugoslavia (ICTY),* 10 December 1998, available at: http://www.refworld.org/docid/40276a8a4.html [accessed 13 June 2016]

ICTY. (1998b). *Prosecutor v. Miroslav Kvocka et al. (Trial Judgement), IT-98-30/1-T, International Criminal Tribunal for the former Yugoslavia (ICTY),* 2 November 2001, available at: http://www.refworld.org/docid/4148117f2.html [accessed 13 June 2016]

ICTY. (2000). *Prosecutor v. Kupreskic et al. (Trial Judgement), IT-95-16-T, International Criminal Tribunal for the former Yugoslavia (ICTY),* 14 January 2000, available at: http://www.refworld.org/docid/40276c634.html [accessed 13 June 2016]

ICTY. (2002). *Prosecutor v. Milorad Krnojelac (Trial Judgement), IT-97-25-T, International Criminal Tribunal for the former Yugoslavia (ICTY),* 15 March 2002, available at: http://www.refworld.org/docid/414806c64.html [accessed 13 June 2016]

Imseis, A. (2001). 'Moderate' torture on trial: the Israeli supreme court judgment concerning the legality of the general security service interrogation methods. *The International Journal of Human Rights, 5*(3), 71–96. doi:10.1080/714003725

Inbau, F. E., Reid, J. E., Buckley, J. P., Jayne, B. C., & Jayne., B. C. (2011). *Criminal interrogation and confessions* (5th ed.). Jones & Bartlett Learning. Burlington, USA.

Inbau, F., & Reid, J. (1963). *Criminal interrogation and confessions.* Washington DC: Williams and Wilkins Co.

Intelligence Science Board. (2006). *Educing information interrogation: science and art.* (D. L. S. Robert Destro, Robert Fein, Pauletta Otis, John Wahlquist, Robert Coulam, Randy Borum, Gary Hazlett, Kristin E. Heckman and Mark D. Happel, Steven M. Kleinman, Ariel Neuman and Daniel Salinas-Serrano, Eds.). Washington DC: National Defense Intelligence College Press.

Intelligence Science Board. (2009). *Intelligence interviewing. Teaching papers and case studies.* Washington DC: National Defense Intelligence College Press.

Inter-American Court of Human Rights. (1996). *Raquel Martí de Mejía v. Perú.* Retrieved from www1.umn.edu/humanrts/cases/1996/peru5-96.htm

Inter-American Court of Human Rights. (1998). *Petruzzi et alt vs Peru (Serie C No. 52). (Vol. 1).*

Inter-American Court of Human Rights. (1999). *Villagran-Morales v. Guatemala.*

Inter-American Court of Human Rights. (2000). *Cantoral Benavides v Perú (Serie C, n° 69)*. Retrieved from www.corteidh.or.cr/docs/casos/articulos/Seriec_69_esp.pdf

Inter-American Court of Human Rights. (2003). *Maritza Urrutia v Guatemala (Series C, N° 103)*.

Inter-American Court of Human Rights. (2004a). *Gómez-Paquiyauri Brothers v Peru (Serie C, N° 110)*. Retrieved from www.corteidh.or.cr/docs/casos/articulos/seriec_110_esp.pdf

Inter-American Court of Human Rights. (2004b). *Tibi v Ecuador (Serie C, N° 114)*.

Inter-American Court of Human Rights. (2004c). *19 Tradesmen v. Colombia*.

Inter-American Court of Human Rights. (2006). *Baldeon Garcia v Perú (Serie C, n° 147)*.

Inter-American Court of Human Rights. (2007). *Rochela Massacre v. Colombia*.

International Forensic Expert Group. (2011). Statement on hooding. *Torture: Quarterly Journal on Rehabilitation of Torture Victims and Prevention of Torture, 21*(3), 186–9.

International Rehabilitation Council for Torture Victims. (2009). *Action against torture. A practical guide to the Istanbul Protocol – for lawyers*. Copenhague.

Iran Human Rights Documentation Center. (2011). *Surviving rape in Iran's prisions*. Teherán.

Jacobs, U. (2008). Documenting the neurobiology of psychological torture: conceptual and neuropsychological observations. In A. E. Ojeda (Ed.), *The trauma of psychological torture* (pp. 163–73). London: Praege.

Jacobs, U., & Iacopino, V. (2001). Torture and its consequences: A challenge to clinical neuropsychology. *Professional Psychology: Research and Practice, 32*(5), 458–464. doi:10.1037//0735-7028.32.5.458

Jaffer, J., & Singh, A. (2006). *Administration of torture. A documentary record from Washington to Abu Ghraib and beyond*. New York: Columbia University Press.

Jamail, M. (1986). *It's no secret: Israel's military involvement in Central America*. Belmont, Mass: Association of Arab-American University Graduates (AAAUG) Press.

Janoff-Bulman, R. (1992). *Shattered assumptions: towards a new psychology of trauma*. New York: Free Press.

Jaranson, J. M., Butcher, J., Halcon, L., Johnson, D. R., Robertson, C., Savik, K., . . . Westermeyer, J. (2004). Somali and Oromo refugees: correlates of torture and trauma history. *American Journal of Public Health, 94*, 591–98. doi:10.2105/AJPH.94.4.591

Jaranson, J. M., & Quiroga, J. (2011). Evaluating the services of torture rehabilitation programmes: history and recommendations. *Torture: Quarterly Journal on Rehabilitation of Torture Victims and Prevention of Torture, 21*(2), 98–140. Retrieved from http://www.ncbi.nlm.nih.gov/pubmed/21715958

Johnson, H., & Thompson, A. (2008). The development and maintenance of post-traumatic stress disorder (PTSD) in civilian adult survivors of war trauma and torture: a review. *Clinical Psychology Review, 28*(1), 36–47. doi:10.1016/j.cpr.2007.01.017

Jongedijk R. A., Carlier, I. V., Schreuder, B. J., & Gersons, B. P.(1996). Complex posttraumatic stress disorder: an exploratory investigation of PTSD and DESNOS among Dutch war veterans. *J Trauma Stress, 9*, 577–86.

Jørgensen, U., Melchiorsen, H., Gottlieb, A. G., Hallas, V., Nielsen, C. V., & Jorgensen, U. (2010). Using the International Classification of Functioning, Disability and Health (ICF) to describe the functioning of traumatised refugees. *Torture: Quarterly Journal on Rehabilitation of Torture Victims and Prevention of Torture, 20*, 57–75. doi:1.2010-10 [pii]

Joseph, S., & Masterson, J. (1999). Posttraumatic stress disorder and traumatic brain injury: are they mutually exclusive? *J Traumatic Stress., 12*(3), 437–53.

Jost, J. T., Krochik, M., Gaucher, D., & Hennes, E. P. (2009). Can a psychological theory of ideological differences explain contextual variability in the contents of political attitudes? *Psychological Inquiry, 20*(2–3), 183–8. doi:10.1080/10478400903088908

Jovic, V., & Opacic, G. (2004). Types of torture. In G. O. Z. Spiric, G. Knezevic, V. Jovic (Eds.), *Torture in war: consequences and rehabilitation of victims*. (pp. 153–70). Belgrade: IAN.

Junghofer, M., Schauer, M., Neuner, F., Odenwald, M., Rockstroh, B., & Elbert, T. (2003). Enhanced fear-network in torture survivors activated by RSVP of aversive material can be monitored by magnetic source imaging. *Psychophysiology, 40 Supplm.*

Kageleiry, P. (2007). Psychological police interrogation methods: pseudoscience in the interrogation room obscures justice in the courtroom. *Military Law Review, 193*(1966), 1–51.

Kaler, M. E., Frazier, P. A., Anders S. L., Tashiro T., Tomich P., Tennen H., & Park, C. (2008). Assessing the psychometric properties of the WAS. *Journal of Traumatic Stress, 21*(3), 326–32.

Karl, A., Schaefer, M., Malta, L., Dorfel, D., Rohleder, N., & Werner, A. (2006). A metanalysis of structural brain abnormalities in PTSD. *Neuroscience and Biobehavioral Reviews, 30*, 1004–31.

Kassin, M., & Kiechel, K. (1996). The social psychology of false confessions: compliance, internalization, and confabulation. *Psychological Science, 7*, 125–28.

Kassin, S. M. (2001). Confessions: psychological and forensic aspects. In N. J. Smelser and P.B. Baltes (Eds.), *International Encyclopedia of the Social and Behavioral Sciences*. Elsevier. Amsterdam.

Kassin, S. M. (2009). Internalized False Confessions. In M. Toglia (Ed.), *Handbook Of Eyewitness Psychology*. Psychology Press. London.

Kassin, S. M., Drizin, S. A., Grisso, T., Gudjonsson, G. H., Leo, R. A., & Redlich, A. D.(2009). Police-induced confessions: Risk factors and recommendations. *Law and Human Behavior, 34*(1), 3–38. doi:10.1007/s10979-009-9188-6

Kassin, S. M., & Fong, C. T. (1999). 'I'm innocent!': Effects of training on judgments of truth and deception in the interrogation room. *Law and Human Behaviour, 23*(5), 499–516.

Kassin, S. M., Gudjonsson, G. H., & Kingdom, U. (2004). The psychology of confessions: a review of the literature and issues. *Psychological Science in the Public Interest, 5*(2), 33–67.

Keller, L. M. (2005). Is truth serum torture? *American University International Law Review, 521*(20), 1–93.

Keller, M. (2012). *Torture Central - E-mails from Abu Ghraib*. Iuniverse.

Kelly, C. E., Miller, J. C., Redlich, A. D., & Kleinman, S. M.(2013). A taxonomy of interrogation methods. *Psychology, Public Policy, and Law, 19*(2), 165–178. doi:10.1037/a0030310

Kerr, I., Binnie, M., & Aoki, C. (2008). Tessling on my brain: the future of lie detection and brain privacy in the criminal justice system. *Canadian Journal of Criminology and Criminal Justice/La Revue Canadienne de Criminologie et de Justice Pénale, 50*(3), 367–87. doi:10.3138/cjccj.50.3.367

King, L., & Snook, B. (2009). Peering inside a canadian interrogation room: an examination of the reid model of interrogation, influence tactics, and coercive strategies. *Criminal Justice and Behavior, 36*(7), 674–694. doi:10.1177/0093854809335142

Kivlahan, C., & Ewigman, N. (2010). Rape as a weapon of war in modern conflicts. *BMJ (Clinical Research Ed.)*. doi:10.1136/bmj.c3270

Klause, I. (2013). Music and 're-education' in the Soviet gulag. *Torture: Quarterly Journal on Rehabilitation of Torture Victims and Prevention of Torture, 23*(2), 24–33. Retrieved from www.ncbi.nlm.nih.gov/pubmed/24480890

Kleinman, S. (1999). The moral, the political and the medical: a sociosomatic view of suffering. In Y. Otsuka, S. Shizu, & S. Kuriyama (Eds.), *Medicine and the History of the Body*. Tokio: Ishiyaku Euroamerica.

Kleinman, S. (2008). *Statement before the House of Representatives Committee on the Judiciary, Subcommittee on Constitution, Civil Rights and Civil Liberties hearing on torture and the cruel, inhuman, and degrading treatment of detainees: the effectiveness and consequences of 'enhanced' interrogation*. Retrieved from http://web.archive.org/web/20080708064007/http://judiciary.house.gov/media/pdfs/Kleinman071108.pdf

Kleinman, S. M. (2006). KUBARK counterintelligence interrogation review: observations of an interrogator lessons learned and avenues for further Research. In D. L. S. Robert Destro, Robert Fein, Pauletta Otis, John Wahlquist, Robert Coulam, Randy Borum, Gary Hazlett, Kristin E. Heckman and Mark D. Happel, Steven M. Kleinman, Ariel Neuman and Daniel Salinas-Serrano (Eds.), *Intelligence Science Board Phase I Report. Educing information*. (pp. 95–140). Washington DC: NIDC Press.

Koenig, K. A. (2013). *The 'worst'. A closer look at cruel, inhuman and degrading treatment*. University of California, Berkeley – School of Law; University of San Francisco. Doctoral Dissertation.

Koenig, K. A., Stover, E., & Fletcher, L. E. (2009). The cumulative effect: A medico-legal approach to United States torture law and policy. *Essex Human Rights Review, 6*(1).

Kohlberg, L., Levine, C., & Hewer, A. (1983). *Moral stages: a current formulation and a response to critics*. Basel: Karger.

Kolassa, I.-T., & Elbert, T. (2007). Structural and functional neuroplasticity in relation to traumatic stress. *Current Directions in Psychological Science, 16*(6), 321–5. doi:10.1111/j.1467-8721.2007.00529.x

Kolber, A. J. (2011). The experiential future of the law. *Emory Law Journal, 60*, 586–654.

Kostelnik, J. O., & Reppucci, N. D.(2009). Reid training and sensitivity to developmental maturity in interrogation: results from a national survey of police. *Behavioral Sciences & the Law, 27*(3), 361–79. doi:10.1002/bsl.871

Kramer, D. (2010). The effects of psychological torture. *Berkeley Law*, (June), 1–9.

Kubzansk, P. E. (1961). The effects of reduced environmental stimulation on human behavior. In A. Biderman & H. Zimmer (Eds.), *The Manipulation of Human Behaviour*. John Wiley and Sons. New York.

Kuch, H. (2011). The rituality of humiliation: exploring symbolic vulnerability. In E. Kaufmann, P., Kuch, H., Neuhäuser, C., & Webster (Ed.), *Humiliation, Degradation, Dehumanization* (pp. 37–56). Dordrecht: Springer Netherlands.

Labkovsky, E., & Rosenfeld, J. P. (2012). The P300-based, complex trial protocol for concealed information detection resists any number of sequential countermeasures against up to five irrelevant stimuli. *Applied Psychophysiology and Biofeedback*, *37*(1), 1–10. doi:10.1007/s10484-011-9171-0

Lacter, E. (2011). Torture-based mind control: psychological mechanisms and. In *Ritual abuse and mind control. The manipulation of attachment needs*. Karnac Books.

Lane, A., Luminet, O., Rimé, B., Gross, J. J., de Timary, P., & Mikolajczak, M. (2013). Oxytocin increases willingness to socially share one's emotions. *International Journal of Psychology: Journal International de Psychologie*, *48*(4), 676–81. doi:10.1080/00207594.2012.677540

Laney, C., & Loftus, E. F. (2013). Recent advances in false memory research. *South African Journal of Psychology*, *43*(2), 137–46. doi:10.1177/0081246313484236

Larreta, J. (1998). Testimonio de un sacerdote vasco [Testimony of a Basque Priest]. In Hiru (Ed.), *Sobre la tortura (on torture)*. Bilbao.

Lassiter, G. D. (2004). *Interrogations, confessions and entrapment*. New York: Springer - USA.

Lazreg, M. (2008). *Torture and the twilight of Empire: from Algiers to Baghdad*.

Leo, R. A. (1996a). Inside the interrogation room. *Journal of Criminal Law and Criminology*, *86*, 266–303.

Leo, R. A. (1996b). Miranda's revenge: Police interrogation as a Confidence game. *Law and Society Review*, *30*(2).

Leo, R. A. (2008). *Police Interrogation and American Justice*. Cambridge, MA: Harvard University Press.

Lerner, M. (1980). *The belief in a just world: a fundamental delusion*. New York: Plenum Press.

Levinson, S. (2006). *Torture: a collection*. Oxford: Oxford University Press.

Lewis, J., & Cuppari, M. (2009). The polygraph: the truth lies within. *Journal of Psychiatry & Law*, *37*(1), 85–92.

Lewis, M. W. (2010). A dark descent into reality: making the case for an objective definition of torture. *Wash & Lee Law Review*, *77*, 77–136.

Lifton, R. (1987). *The future of inmortality and other essays for a nuclear age*. New Tork: Basic Books.

Lifton, R. J. (1961). *Thought reform and the psychology of totalism. A study of 'brainwashing' in China*. New York, London: Norton and Co.

Liscano, C. (2004). *El furgón de los locos [Truck of fools: a testimonio of torture and recovery]*. Nashville: Vanderbilt University Press.

Littleton, H. (2007). An evaluation of the coping patterns of rape victims: integration with a schema-based information-processing model. *Violence against Women*, *13*(8), 789–801.

Luban, D. (2009). Human dignity, humiliation, and torture. *Kennedy Institute of Ethics Journal*, *19*, 211–30.

Luban, D., & Shue, H. (2012). Mental torture: A critique of erasures in U.S. law. *The Georgetown Law Journal*, *100*, 823–63.

Luber, B., Fisher, C., Appelbaum, P., Ploesser, M., & Lisanby, S. H. (2009). Non-invasive brain stimulation in the detection of deception: scientific challenges and ethical consequences. *Behavioral Science and the Law*, *208*(March), 191–208.

Macdonald, K., & Macdonald, T. M. (2010). The peptide that binds: a systematic review of oxytocin and its prosocial effects in humans. *Harvard Review of Psychiatry*, *18*(1), 1–21. doi:10.3109/10673220903523615

Mackey, A., & Barnes, J. (2013). *Assessment of credibility in refugee and subsidiary protection claims under the EU Qualification Directive Judicial criteria and standards*. Prepared by Allan Mackey and John Barnes for the International Association of Refugees.

Maercker, A., Brewin, C. R., Bryant, R. a, Cloitre, M., van Ommeren, M., Jones, L. M., . . . Reed, G. M. (2013). Diagnosis and classification of disorders specifically associated with stress: proposals for ICD-11. *World Psychiatry*, *12*(3), 198–206. doi:10.1002/wps.20057

Magid, L. (2001). Deceptive police interrogation practices: How far is too far? *Michigan Law Review*, *99*, 1168–1210.

Magwaza, A. S. (1999). Assumptive world of traumatized South African adults. *The Journal of Social Psychology*, *139*(5), 622–30.

Maier, A. (2011). Torture. How denying moral standing violates human dignity. In E. Kaufmann, P., Kuch, H., Neuhäuser, C., & Webster (Eds.), *Humiliation, degradation, dehumanization* (pp. 101–18). Dordrecht: Springer Netherlands.

Maiter, S., Simich, L., Jacobson, N., & Wise, J. (2008). Reciprocity: an ethic for community-based participatory action research. *Action Research, 6*(3), 305–25. doi:10.1177/1476750307083720

Marks, J. H. (2007). Interrogational neuroimaging in counterterrorism: a 'no-brainer' or a human rights hazard? *American Journal of Law & Medicine, 33*(2-3), 483–500. Retrieved from www.ncbi .nlm.nih.gov/pubmed/17910168

Marks, J. H. (2010). A neuroskeptic's guide to neuroethics and national security. *American Journal of Bioethics: Neuroscience, 1*(2), 4–12.

Marlowe, A. (2010). *David Galula: his life and intellectual context.* Carlisle, PA (USA): Strategic Studies Institute. US Army War College.

Martin-Baró, I. (1990). *Psicología social de la guerra. Trauma y terapia [Social psychology of war. Trauma and therapy].* San Salvador: Ediciones Universidad Centroamericana de El Salvador (UCA).

Masmas, T. N., Møller, E., Buhmannr, C., Bunch, V., Jensen, J. H., Hansen, T. N., . . . Ekstrøm, M. (2008). Asylum seekers in Denmark – a study of health status and grade of traumatization of newly arrived asylum seekers. *Torture: Quarterly Journal on Rehabilitation of Torture Victims and Prevention of Torture, 18*(2), 77–86. doi:2008-2.2008-28 [pii]

Mason, O. J., & Brady, F. (2009). The psychotomimetic effects of short-term sensory deprivation. *The Journal of Nervous and Mental Disease, 197*(10), 783–5. doi:10.1097/NMD.0b013e3181b9760b

Matthews, L. T., & Marwit, S. J.(2004). Examining the assumptive world views of parents bereaved by accident, murder, and illness. *OMEGA: The Journal of Death and Dying, 48*(2), 115–36. doi:10.2190/KCB0-NNVB-UGY6-NPYR

Mausfeld, R. (2009). Psychology, 'white torture' and the responsibility of scientists. *Psychologische Rundschau, 60*, 229–40.

McClelland, R. T. (2011). A naturalistic view of human dignity. *Journal of Mind and Behavior, 32*, 5–48. Retrieved from http://search.proquest.com/docview/888752880?accountid=4485

McColl, H., Higson-Smith, C., Gjerding, S., Omar, M. H., Rahman, B., Hamed, M., . . . Awad, Z. (2010). Rehabilitation of torture survivors in five countries: common themes and challenges. *International Journal of Mental Health Systems, 4*(1), 16. doi:10.1186/1752-4458-4-16

McCoy, A. (2009). Confronting the CIA's mind maze. Retrieved September 5, 2014, from www .thepeoplesvoice.org

McCoy, A. W. (2006). *A short history of psychological torture: its discovery, propagation, perfection, and legalization.* University of California, Los Angeles.

McCoy, A. W. (2008). Legacy of a dark decade: CIA mind control, classified behavioral research and the origins of modern medical ethics. In A. Ojeda (Ed.), *The trauma of psychological torture.* Praeger Publisher, pp.40–69.

McCoy, A. W. (2012). *Torture and impunity: The U.S. doctrine of coercive interrogation.* University of Wisconsin Press.

Mcdonnell, M.-H. M., Nordgren, L. F., & Loewenstein, G. (2011). Torture in the eyes of the beholder: the psychological difficulty of defining torture in law and policy. *Vanderbilt Journal of Transnational Law, 44*, 87–122.

McGlynn, C. (2009). Rape, torture and the European Convention on Human Rights. *International and Comparative Law Quarterly, 58*(03), 565. doi:10.1017/S0020589309001195

McHenry, J. R. (2002). The prosecution of rape under international law. *Vanderbilt Journal of Transnational Law, 35*, 1278.

McKenna, B. S., Dickinson, D. L., & Orff, H. J.(2007). The effects of one night of sleep deprivation on known-risk and ambiguous-risk decisions. *J Sleep Research, 16*, 245–52.

Mcnally, R. J. (2010). Can we salvage the concept of psychological trauma? *The Psychologist, 23*(5), 386–90.

Medical Foundation for the Care of Victims of Torture. (2013). *'We will make you regret everything'. Torture in Iran since the 2009 elections.* London.

Meissner, C. (2012). *Interview and interrogation methods and their effects on investigative outcomes.* Campbell Systematic Reviews (Vol. 13). doi:10.4073/csr.2012.13

Meissner, C. A., Redlich, A. D., Michael, S. W., Evans, J. R., Camilletti, C. R., Bhatt, S., & Brandon, S. (2014). Accusatorial and information-gathering interrogation methods and their effects on true and false confessions: a meta-analytic review. *Journal of Experimental Criminology, 10*(4), 459–86. doi:10.1007/s11292-014-9207-6

Meissner, C. A., & Russano, M. B.(2003). The psychology of interrogations and false confessions. *The Canadian Journal of Police & Security Services*, *1*(1), 53–64.

Mendez, J. (2010). *Report of the Special Rapporteur on torture and other cruel, inhuman or degrading treatment or punishment*. UN Report. Retrieved from www2.ohchr.org/english/bodies/hrcouncil/docs/13session/A.HRC.13.39.Add.5_en.pdf

Mendez, J. (2011). UUNN Special Reporteur Statement on solitary confinement. (A/66/268). Vol. 44570.

Mendez, J. (2013). *Thematic Report - Exclusionary rule and its fundamental role in upholding the prohibition of torture and other cruel, inhuman or degrading treatment*.

Mendez, J. (2014). *Thematic report – standard minimum rules for the treatment of prisoners needs updating* (Vol. 42285). Washington: United Nations.

Merino, M. A. (1993). *Mi verdad: mas alla del horror,yo acuso [My truth: beyond the horror, I accuse]*. Santiago de Chile: Merino Vega.

Metzner, J. L., & Fellner, J. (2010). Solitary confinement and mental illness in U.S. prisons: a challenge for medical ethics. *The Journal of the American Academy of Psychiatry and the Law*, *38*(1), 104–8. Retrieved from www.ncbi.nlm.nih.gov/pubmed/20305083

Miles, S. H. (2009). *Oath betrayed. America's torture doctors*. (2nd ed.). Los Angeles: University of California Press.

Miller, A. G. (Ed.) (2004). *The social psychology of good and evil*. New York: The Guilford Press.

Miller, H., & Young, G. (1997). Prison segregation: administrative detention remedy of mental health problem? *Criminal Behaviour and Mental Health*, 7, 85–94.

Mind. (2010). *Achieving justice for victims and witnesses with mental distress. A mental health toolkit for prosecutors and advocates*. London: Mind-For better health.

Mirzaei, S., Knoll, P., Keck, A., Preitler, B., Gutierrez, E., Umek, H., . . . Pecherstorfer, M. (2001). Regional cerebral blood flow in patients suffering from post-traumatic stress disorder. *Neuropsychobiology*, *43*(4), 260–64. doi:10.1159/000054900

Mollica, R., Donelan, K., Tor, S., Lavelle, J., Elias, C., Frankel, M., & Blendon, R. J. (1993). The effect of trauma and confinement on functional health and mental health status of Cambodians living in Thailand-Cambodia border camps. *JAMA: The Journal of the American Medical Association*, *270*, 581–6. doi:10.1001/jama.270.5.581

Mollica, R. F., Lyoo, I. K., Chernoff, M. C., Bui, H. X., Lavelle, J., Yoon, S. J., . . . Renshaw, P. F. (2009). Brain structural abnormalities and mental health sequelae in South Vietnamese ex-political detainees who survived traumatic head injury and torture. *Archives of General Psychiatry*, *66*(11), 1221. doi:10.1001/archgenpsychiatry.2009.127

Mollica, R., Gaspi-Yavin, Y., Bollini, P., & Truongp, T. (1992). Validating a cross-cultural instrument for measuring torture, trauma, and posttraumatic stress disorder in Indochinese refugees. *The Journal of Nervous and Mental Disease*, *180*, 111–6.

Montagut, M. (2012). *Les possibilités d'être après la torture. Sociologie clinique du système torturant*. Université Paris-Diderot. Paris.

Monteleone, G. T., Phan, K. L., Nusbaum, H. C., Fitzgerald, D., Irick, J.-S., Fienberg, S. E., & Cacioppo, J. T. (2009). Detection of deception using fMRI: better than chance, but well below perfection. *Social Neuroscience*, *4*(6), 528–38.

Moore-King, B. (1998). *White man, black war*. Zimbabwe: Baobab Books.

Morgan, R., & Evans, M. (1999). *Protecting prisoners. The standards of the European Commitee for the Prevention of Torture in context*. Oxford: Oxford University Press.

Morgan, R., & Evans, M. (2001). *CPT standards regarding prisoners*. Geneva: Association for The Prevention of Torture.

Morris, D. J. (2009). Empires of the mind: SERE, Guantanamo and the legacies of torture. *Virginia Quarterly Review*, (Winter), 211–21.

Mortensen, L.-T. B. (2012). *Social deprivation as torture: a bibliography research about adult animals in social isolation*. Tromso: University of Tromso.

Mosteller, R. P. (2007). Confessions and police disclosure: Police deception before Miranda warning: The case for per se prohibition of an entirely unjustified practice at the most critical moment. *Texas Tech Law Review*, *39*, 1240–1273.

Mueller, P. (1946). *Japanese methods of prisioner of war interrogation*.

Mukamana, D., & Brysiewicz, P. (2008). The lived experience of genocide rape survivors in Rwanda. *Journal of Nursing Scholarship: An Official Publication of Sigma Theta Tau International Honor Society of Nursing / Sigma Theta Tau*, *40*, 379–84. doi:10.1111/j.1547-5069.2008.00253.x

Mullenix, P. A. (2007). Interrogation strategies for an unconventional extremist enemy. *Journal of the American Polygraph, 36*(3), 121–32.

Muller, R. (2010). *Trauma and the avoidant client*. New York: W.W. Norton & Company.

Muncey, T. (2010). *Creating autoethnographies*. Bangalore. India: SAGE.

Myjer, E. (2004). *Prison security and human rights. The Strasbourg case law*. Strasbourg: European Court of Human Rights. Interim Reports.

Nath, V. (1998). *A Cambodian prison portrait. One year in the Khmer Rouge's S-21*. Bangkok: White Lotus Lmtd.

National Research Council. (2009). *Opportunities in neuroscience for future army applications*. Washington, D.C.: National Academies Press.

Navarro, M. A., Pérez-Sales, P., Lopez, G., Arnoso, M., & Morentin, B. (2016). Psychological and psychiatric consequences of ill-treatment and torture in incommunicado detention in Spain: trauma and human worldviews. Torture Journal (2016). In press.

NDS. (1940). Gestapo interrogation methods. Retrieved from http://www.americantorture.com/documents/torture_memos/TM0.pdf

Nederveen, J. (1984). *Israel's role in the third world*. Amsterdam: Emancipation Research.

Neequaye, D. A. (2011). *Making them talk! Educing information through schema priming and inquisitorial interviewing*. University of Ghana. Degree Thesis.

Neuman, A., & Salinas-Serrano, D. (2006). Custodial interrogations: what we know, what we do, and what we can learn from law enforcement experiences. In Robert Destro, Robert Fein, Pauletta Otis, John Wahlquist, Robert Coulam, Randy Borum, Gary Hazlett, Kristin E. Heckman and Mark D. Happel, Steven M. Kleinman, Ariel Neuman and Daniel Salinas-Serrano (Eds.), *Educing information interrogation: science and art*. Washington DC: National Defense Intelligence College.

Neumeister, A., Shannan, H., & Krystal, J. (2007). Neurocircuitry and neuroplasticity in PTSD. In M. Friedman, T. Keane, & P. Resick (Eds.), *Handbook of PTSD*. New York: Guilford Press.

Neuner, F., Kurreck, S., Ruf, M., Odenwald, M., Elbert, T., & Schauer, M. (2010). Can asylum-seekers with posttraumatic stress disorder be successfully treated? A randomized controlled pilot study. *Cognitive Behaviour Therapy, 39*(2), 81–91. doi:10.1080/16506070903121042

Newbery, S. (2009). Intelligence and controversial British interrogation techniques: the Northern Ireland Case, 1971–2. *Irish Studies in International Affairs, 20*(-1), 103–19. doi:10.3318/ISIA.2009.20.103

Neziroglu, I. (2007). A comparative analysis of mental and psychological suffering as torture, inhuman or degrading treatment or punishment under international human rights treaty law prohibition and definition of torture, inhuman and degrading treatment or punishment under International Human Rights Treaty Law. *Essex Human Rights Review, 4*(1), 1–16.

Nordgren, L. F., McDonnell, M.-H. M., & Loewenstein, G. (2011). What constitutes torture? psychological impediments to an objective evaluation of enhanced interrogation tactics. *Psychological Science: A Journal of the American Psychological Society / APS, 22*, 689–94. doi:10.1177/0956797611405679

Nowak, M. (2006). What practices constitute torture? US and UN standards. *Human Rights Quarterly, 28*(4), 809–41. doi:10.1353/hrq.2006.0050

Nowak, M. (2009). Torture and enforced disappearance. In C. Krause & M. Scheinin (Eds.), *International protection of human rights: a textbook*. (pp. 151–82). Turku: Institute for Human Rights, Åbo Akademi University.

Nowak, M. (2011). Introduction. In E. Kaufmann, P., Kuch, H., Neuhäuser, C., & Webster (Eds.), *Humiliation, degradation, dehumanization* (pp. 1–3). Dordrecht: Springer Netherlands.

Nowak, M., & McArthur, E. (2006). The distinction between torture and cruel, inhuman or degrading treatment. *Torture: Quarterly Journal on Rehabilitation of Torture Victims and Prevention of Torture, 16*(3), 147–51. Retrieved from http://www.ncbi.nlm.nih.gov/pubmed/17251647

Nowak, M., & McArthur, E. (2008). *The United Nations Convention Against Torture. A commentary*. Cambridge University Press.

O'Mara, S. (2015). *Why torture doesn't work. The neuroscience of interrogation*. Cambridge, MA: Harvard University Press.

O'Mara, S., & O'Mara, S. (2009). Torturing the brain: on the folk psychology and folk neurobiology motivating 'enhanced and coercive interrogation techniques'. *Trends in Cognitive Sciences, 13*, 497–500. doi:10.1016/j.tics.2009.09.001

Office of Professional Responsability. (2009). Investigation into the Office of Legal Counsel's Memoranda concerning issues relating to the Central Intelligence Agency's use of 'Enhanced Interrogation Techniques' on suspected terrorists. Department of Justice. Desclassified Document.

Office of the High Commisioner for Human Rights. (2010). *The prosecution of sexual violence in conflict: The importance of human rights as means of interpretation.*

Ojeda, A. E. (2008). What is psychological torture? In A. E. Ojeda (Ed.), *The trauma of psychological torture* (pp. 1–22). London: Praeger.

Open Society. (2012). *Written comments in the case of Etxebarria Caballero versus Spain (ECHR – Application 74016/12).* Washington DC: Open Society Justice Initiative.

Organisation for the Prohibition of Chemical Weapons. (1997). Convention on the prohibition of the development, production, stockpiling and use of chemical weapons and on their destruction.

Organization of African Unity. African Charter on Human and Peoples' Rights. (1981). Nairobi: Organization of African Unity.

Otterman, M. (2007). *American torture: from the cold war to Abu Ghraib and beyond.* Melbourne: Melbourne University Press.

PACE. (1984). Police and Criminal Evidence Act. Chapter 60.

Packer, D. J. (2008). Identifying systematic disobedience in Milgram's obedience experiments: a meta-analytic review. *Perspectives on Psychological Science, 3*(4), 301–4. doi:10.1111/j.1745-6924.2008.00080.x

Panayiotou, A., Jackson, M., & Crowe, S. F. (2010). A meta-analytic review of the emotional symptoms associated with mild traumatic brain injury. *Journal of Clinical and Experimental Neuropsychology, 32*(5), 463–73. doi:10.1080/13803390903164371

Panh, R. (2003). *La machine Khmère Rouge.* Paris: Flammarion.

Papaeti, A. (2013). Music and 're-education' in Greek prison camps: from Makronisos (1947–1955) to Giaros (1967–1968). *Torture: Quarterly Journal on Rehabilitation of Torture Victims and Prevention of Torture, 23*(2), 34–43. Retrieved from www.ncbi.nlm.nih.gov/pubmed/24480891

Pardo, P. (2014). *El Monstruo. Memorias de un interrogador.* Madrid, España: Libros del KO.

Paris, M. L. (1997). Lying to ourselves. *Oregon Law Review, 76,* 817–832.

Parry, J. T. (2003). What is torture, are we doing it, and what if we are. *Pitt. Law Review, 64,* 237–49.

Patel, N., Williams, A. C. D. C., & Kellezi, B. (2016). Reviewing outcomes of psychological interventions with torture survivors : Conceptual, methodological and ethical Issues. *Torture Journal, 26*(1), 2–16.

Payne, L. (2009). *Testimonios perturbadores. Ni verdad ni reconciliacion en las confesiones de violencia de Estado.* Bogota: Universidad de los Andes – Fundación Ideas para la Paz.

Pearse, J., & Gudjonsson, G. H. (2003). The identification and measurement of 'oppressive' police interviewing tactics in britain. In G. H. Gudjonsson (Ed.), *The psychology of interrogations and confessions* (pp. 75–114). Chichester, UK: John Wiley & Sons, Ltd. doi:10.1002/9780470713297.ch4

Peel, M. (Ed.) (2004). *Rape as a method of torture.* London: Medical Foundation for the Care of Victims of Torture.

Pelcovitz, D., Van der Kolk, B., Roth, S., Mandel, F., Kaplan, S., & Resick, P. (1997). Development of a criteria set and a Structured Interview for Disorders of Extreme Stress (SIDES). *Journal of Traumatic Stress, 10*(1), 3–16.

Pérez-Sales, P. (Ed.) (2006). *Trauma, culpa y duelo: hacia una psicoterapia integradora.* Bilbao: Desclée de Brouwer.

Pérez-Sales, P. (2009). *Peritación psicológica y psiquiátrica de maltrato y tortura en solicitantes de asilo. Uso del Protocolo de Estambul.* In I. Márquez, F.-L. A, & P. Pérez-Sales, (Eds.), *Violencia y salud mental.* Madrid, España: AEN.

Pérez-Sales, P., Eiroa-Orosa, F. J., Olivos, P., Barbero-Val, E., Fernández-Liria, A., & Vergara, M. (2012). Vivo Questionnaire: A measure of human worldviews and identity in trauma, crisis, and loss—validation and preliminary findings. *Journal of Loss and Trauma, 17*(3), 236–59. doi:10.1080/15325024.2011.616828

Pérez-Sales, P., Morentin, B., Barrenetxea, O., & Navarro, M. A. (2015). Incommunicado detention and torture in Spain. Enhanced credibility assessment based on the Istanbul Protocol. *In Press.*

Pérez-Sales, P., Navarro, M., Lopez, G., & Barrios, O. (2014). *Incommunicado detention and torture. Assessments using the Istanbul Protocol.* Bilbao: Marra. Retrieved from http://ome-aen.org/files/2014/09/inf_incomunicacion_y_tortura_en.pdf

Pfeiffer, A., & Elbert, T. (2011). PTSD, depression and anxiety among former abductees in Northern Uganda. *Conflict and Health, 5*(1), 14. doi:10.1186/1752-1505-5-14

Phillips, E. M. (2011). Pain, suffering, and humiliation: the systemization of violence in kidnapping for ransom. *Journal of Aggression, Maltreatment & Trauma, 20*(8), 845–69. doi:10.1080/10926771 .2011.626512

Physicians for Human Rights. (2005). *Break them down. Systematic use of psychological torture by US Forces.* PHR.

Physicians for Human Rights. (2010). *Experiments in torture: Evidence of human subject research and experimentation in the 'Enhanced' Interrogation Program.* Washington: Physicians for Human Rights.

Phythian, M. (2000). *The politics of British arms sales since 1964.* Manchester: Manchester University Press.

Pollmann, A. (2011). Embodied self-respect and the fragility of human dignity: a human rights approach. In E. Kaufmann, P., Kuch, H., Neuhäuser, C., & Webster (Eds.), *Humiliation, degradation, dehumanization* (pp. 243–63). Dordrecht: Springer Netherlands.

Porter, S., & Brinke, L. (2010). The truth about lies: what works in detecting high-stakes deception? *Legal and Criminological Psychology, 15*, 57–75. doi:10.1348/135532509X4331SI

Pottie, K., Greenaway, C., Feightner, J., Welch, V., Swinkels, H., Rashid, M., . . . Tugwell, P. (2010). Evidence-based clinical guidelines for immigrants and refugees. *Canadian Medical Association Journal, 183*(12), E824–E925. doi:10.1503/cmaj.090313

Pratto, F., Sidanius, J., Stallworth, L., & Malle, B. (1994). Social dominance orientation: a personality variable predicting social and political attitudes. *Journal of Personality and Social Psychology, 67*, 741–763.

Priebe, S., & Bauer, M. (1995). Inclusion of psychological torture in PTSD Criterion A. *American Journal of Psychiatry, 152*(11), 1691–2.

Punamäki, R., Quota, S., & Sarraj, E. El. (2010). Nature of torture, PTSD, and somatic symptoms among political ex-prisoners. *Journal of Traumatic Stress, 23*(4), 532–6. doi:10.1002/jts.

Pustilnik, A. C. (2012). Pain as a fact and heuristic: how pain neuroimaging illuminates moral dimensions of law. *Cornell Law Review, 97*, 801–48. Retrieved from www.ncbi.nlm.nih.gov/pubmed/22754972

Quiroga, J., & Jaranson, J. (2008). Torture. In *Encyclopedia of Psychological Trauma.* Wiley. London.

Rasumussen, A. (2016). Personal communication.

Rasmussen, A., Crager, M., Keatley, E., Keller, A. S, & Rosenfeld, B. (2011). Screening for torture: A narrative checklist comparing legal definitions in a torture treatment clinic. *Zeitschrift Fur Psychologie / Journal of Psychology, 219*(3), 143–9. doi:10.1027/2151-2604/a000061

Ray, W. J., Odenwald, M., Neuner, F., Schauer, M., Ruf, M., Wienbruch, C., . . . Elbert, T. (2006). Decoupling neural networks from reality: dissociative experiences in torture victims are reflected in abnormal brain waves in left frontal cortex. *Psychological Science, 17*(10), 825–9. doi:10.1111/j.1467-9280.2006.01788.x

Redlich, A. D., Kelly, C. E., & Miller, J. C.(2014). The who, what, and why of human intelligence gathering: self-reported measures of interrogation methods. *Applied Cognitive Psychology, 28*(6), 817–28. doi:10.1002/acp.3040

Redress. (2004). *Actions against torture. A practical guide to the Istanbul Protocol for lawyers in Uganda.* Copenhague.

Redress. (2007). *UK Army in Iraq: time to come clean on civilian torture.* London.

Reicher, S., & Haslam, A. (2006). Rethinking the psychology of tyranny: the BBC prison study. *British Journal of Social Psychology, 45*(1), 1–40. doi:10.1348/014466605x48998

Rejali, D. (2007). *Torture and democracy.* Princeton: Princeton University Press.

Resick, P. A., & Miller, M. W.(2009). Posttraumatic stress disorder: anxiety or traumatic stress disorder? *Journal of Traumatic Stress, 22*(5), 384–90. doi:10.1002/jts.20437

Ressler, K. J., Mercer, K. B., Bradley, B., Jovanovic, T., Mahan, A., Kerley, K., . . . May, V. (2011). Post-traumatic stress disorder is associated with PACAP and the PAC1 receptor. *Nature, 470*(7335), 492–7. doi:10.1038/nature09856

Reyes, H. (2008). The worst scars are in the mind: psychological torture. *International Review of the Red Cross, 89*(867), 591–617. doi:10.1017/S1816383107001300

Reynolds, J. L. (1997). Post-traumatic stress disorder after childbirth: the phenomenon of traumatic birth. *Canadian Medical Association Journal, 156*(6), 831–5.

Rizvi, S., Kaysen, D., Gutner, C., Griffin, M., & Resick, P. (2008). Beyond fear: the role of peritraumatic responses in posttraumatic stress and depressive symptoms among female crime victims. *Journal of Interpersonal Violence, 23*, 853–68.

Rizzolatti, G., & Craighero, L. (2004). The mirror-neuron system. *Annual Review of Neuroscience, 27,* 169–192. doi:1146/annurev.neuro.27.070203.144230

Robin, M.-M. (2004). *Escadrons de la mort, l'école française [Death squads, the French school].* Paris: Ed La Découverte.

Roccato, M. (2008). Right-wing authoritarianism, social dominance orientation, and attachment: An Italian study. *Swiss Journal of Psychology, 67*(4), 219–229.

Rochat, F., & Modigliani A. (1995). The ordinary quality of resistance: from Milgram's laboratory to the Milage of Le Chambon. *Journal of Social Issues, 51*(3), 195–210.

Rodley, N. S., & Pollard, M. (2009). *The treatment of prisoners under international law* (3rd ed.). Oxford: Clarendon Press.

Rodriguez, S. (2011). *Fact sheet: psychological effects of solitary confinement.* Retrieved from www.solitarywatch.com

Rodriguez, S. A. (2007). The impotence of being earnest: 1. status of the United Nations standard minimum rules for the treatment of prisoners in Europe and the United States. *New England Journal on Criminal and Civil Confinement, 611,* 61–122.

Rosenfeld, J. P., Soskins, M., Bosh, G., & Ryan, A. (2004). Simple, effective countermeasures to P300-based tests of detection of concealed information. *Psychophysiology, 41*(2), 205–19. doi:10.1111/j.1469-8986.2004.00158.x.

Roth, S., Newman, E., Pelcovitz, D., van der Kolk, B., & Mandel, F. (1997). Complex PTSD in victims exposed to sexual and physical abuse: results from the DSM-IV field trial for posttraumatic stress disorder. *J Trauma Stress, 10,* 539–55.

Rousseau, C., Pottie, K., Greenaway, C., Feightner, J., Welch, V., Swinkels, H., … Tugwell, P. (2011). Evidence-based clinical guidelines for immigrants and refugees. *Canadian Medical Association Journal, 183*(12), E824–E925. doi:10.1503/cmaj.090313

Ruiz, F. (2011). No hay zonas grises, uno sabe si esta torturando [No gray areas, you know if this is torturing]. *El Mundo,* p. 15–16. Madrid. Retrieved from http://elmundo.orbyt.es/2011/09/07/orbyt_en_elmundo/1315374532.html

Rumsfeld, D. (2003). Memorandum for the General Counsel of the Department of Defense. Working Group Report on detainee interrogations in the global war on terrorism: assessment of legal, historical, policy and operational considerations. Washington, DC.

Russano, M. B., Meissner, C. A., Narchet, F. M., & Kassin, S. M.(2005). Investigating true and false confessions within a novel experimental paradigm. *Psychological Science: A Journal of the American Psychological Society / APS, 16*(6), 481–6. doi:10.1111/j.0956-7976.2005.01560.x

Sagarin, B. J., Cialdini, R. B., Rice, W. E., & Serna, S. B. (2002). Dispelling the illusion of invulnerability: The motivations and mechanisms of resistance to persuasion. *Journal of Personality and Social Psychology, 83*(3), 526–541. doi:10.1037//0022-3514.83.3.526

Saks, M. J. (1992). Obedience versus disobedience to legitimate versus ilegitimate authorities issuing good versus evil directives. *Psychological Science, 3*(4), 221–3.

Saporta, J., & Kolk, B. van der. (1992). Psychobiological consequences of severe trauma. In M. Basoglu (Ed.), *Torture and its consequences. Current treatment approaches.* (pp. 151–81). New York: Cambridge University Press.

Sar, V. (2011). Developmental trauma, complex PTSD, and the current proposal of DSM-5. *European Journal of Psychotraumatology, 2,* 1–9. doi:10.3402/ejpt.v2i0.5622

Scarry, E. (1985). *The body in pain.* London: Oxford University Press.

Schafer, J. R., & Navarro, J. (2010). *Advanced interviewing techniques. Proven strategies for law enforcement, military and security personnel.* Springfield. Ill.: Charles C. Thomas Publisher.

Schauer, F. (2010). Neuroscience, lie-detection, and the law: contrary to the prevailing view, the suitability of brain-based lie-detection for courtroom or forensic use should be determined according to legal and not scientific standards. *Trends in Cognitive Sciences, 14*(3), 101–3. doi:10.1016/j.tics.2009.12.004

Schein, E. H. (1960). *Brainwashing.* Center for International Studies. Massachusetts Institute of Technology.

Schwartz, S. (1994). Rape as a weapon of war in the former Yugoslavia. *Hastings Women Law Journal, 5,* 69–74. Retrieved from www.islamicpluralism.org/documents/1068.pdf\nhttp://www.webcitation.org/6H987OdEK

Semel, M. D. (2013). Military interrogations: best practices and beliefs. *Perspectives on Terrorism, 7*(2), 39–62.

Senese, L. C. (2014). *Anatomy of Interrogation Themes.* Washington: John E. Reid and Associates.

Shalev, S. (2008). *A sourcebook on solitary confinement.* London: Mannheim Centre for Criminology. London School of Economics and Political Science.

Shalev, S. (2011). Solitary confinement and supermax prisons: a human rights and ethical analysis. *Journal of Forensic Psychology Practice*, *11*(2-3), 151–83. doi:10.1080/15228932.2011.537582

Shane, B. S., Johnston, D., & Risen, J. (2007). Secret US endorsement of severe interrogations. *New York Times*. Retrieved from www.spiegel.de/international/0,1518,509355,00.html

Shoeb, M., Weinstein, H., & Mollica, R. (2007). The Harvard Trauma Questionnaire: Adapting a cross-cultural instrument for measuring torture, trauma and posttraumatic stress disorder in Iraqi refugees. *International Journal of Social Psychiatry*. doi:10.1177/0020764007078362

Shrestha N. M., Sharma B, Van Ommeren (1998). Impact of torture on refugees displaced within the developing world: symptomatology among Bhutanese refugees in Nepal. *JAMA.*, *280*, 443–8.

Shue, H. (1978). Torture. *Philosophy and Public Affairs*, *1*, 124–43.

Silove, D. (1998). Is posttraumatic stress disorder an overlearned survival response? An evolutionary-learning hypothesis. *Psychiatry*, *61*, 181–90.

Silove, D., Steel, Z., McGorry, P., Miles, V., & Drobny, J. (2002). The impact of torture on post-traumatic stress symptoms in war-affected Tamil refugees and immigrants. *Comprehensive Psychiatry*, *43*(1), 49–55. Retrieved from http://www.ncbi.nlm.nih.gov/pubmed/11788919

Simcoe, R. (2006). The effects of training on the creation of a memory schema for Reid method deception cues. Retrieved from www.researchgate.net/publication/242422400_The_Effects_of_Training_on_the_Creation_of_a_Memory_Schema_for_Reid_Method_Deception_Cues

Simmons, S. (2008). Joint Task Force Guantanamo. BSCT operation integral to JTF mission success. Retrieved September 9, 2014, from www.jtfgtmo.southcom.mil/storyarchive/2008/January/012808-1-BSCT.html

Singh, S. P. (2008). *Fundamentals of the interrogation techniques*. Delhi: Kalpaz Publications.

Sip, K. E., Roepstorff, A., McGregor, W., & Frith, C. D. (2008). Detecting deception: the scope and limits. *Trends in Cognitive Sciences*, *12*(2), 48–53. doi:10.1016/j.tics.2007.11.008

Skylv, G. (1992). The physical sequelae of torture. In M. Başoğlu (Ed.), *Torture and its consequences. Current treatment approaches* (pp. 38–55). Cambridge University Press.

Slobogin, C. (1997). Deceit, pretext, and trickery: Investigative lies by the police. *Oregon Law Review*, *76*, 775–816.

Slobogin, C. (2007). Confession and police disclosure: Lying and confessing. *Texas Tech Law Review*, *39*, 1275–1292.

Smith, P. S. (2008a). Solitary confinement. an introduction to the Istanbul Statement on the Use and Effects of Solitary Confinement. *Torture: Quarterly Journal on Rehabilitation of Torture Victims and Prevention of Torture*, *18*(1), 56–62.

Smith, P. S. (2008b). The Istanbul Statement on the Use and Effects of Solitary Confinement. *Torture: Quarterly Journal on Rehabilitation of Torture Victims and Prevention of Torture*, *18*(1), 63–6.

Soldz, S., Raymond, N., & Reisner, S. (2015). *All the president's psychologists: The American Psychological Association's secret complicity with the White House and US intelligence community in support of the CIA's 'enhanced' interrogation program*. American Psychological Association. Washington, DC.

Solzhenitsyn, A. (1975). *The Gulag Archipelago (1918–1956)* (1st ed.) London: Harper & Row.

Southwick, S., Davis, L., Aikins, D., Rasmusson, A., Barron, J., & Morgan ChA. (2007). Neurobiologiocal alterations associated with PTSD. In M. Friedman, T. Keane (Eds.), *Handbook of PTSD*. New York: Guilford Press.

Spjut, R. (1979). Torture under the European Convention on Human Rights. *AJIL*, *73*, 267–71.

Startup, M., Makgekgenene, L., & Webster, R. (2007). The role of self-blame for trauma as assessed by the Posttraumatic Cognitions Inventory (PTCI): a self-protective cognition? *Behaviour Research and Therapy*, *45*(2), 395–403. doi:S0005-7967(06)00045-3 [pii]10.1016/j.brat.2006.02.003

Staub, E. (1999). The roots of evil: social conditions, culture, personality, and basic human needs. *Pers Soc Psychol Rev*, *3*(3), 179–92. doi:10.1207/s15327957pspr0303_2

Staub, E. (2003). *The psychology of good and evil. Why children, adults and other groups help and harm others.* Cambridge University Press.

Steel, Z., Chey, T., Silove, D, Marnane, C, Bryant, R. A., van Ommeran, M. (2009). Association of torture and other potentially traumatic events with mental health outcomes among populations exposed to mass conflict and displacement: A systematic review and meta-analysis. *JAMA.*, *302*(5), 537–49.

Stoecker, R. (2011). Three crucial turns on the road to an adequate understanding of human dignity. In E. Kaufmann, P., Kuch, H., Neuhäuser, C., & Webster (Eds.), *Humiliation, degradation, dehumanization* (pp. 7–20). Dordrecht: Springer Netherlands.

Suedfeld, P. (1990). *Psychology and torture*. Washington DC: Hemisphere Publishing Corp.

Sussman, D. (2005). What's wrong with torture? *Philosophy and Public Affairs, 33*(1), 1–32. doi:10.1111/j.1088-4963.2005.00023.x

Sussman, D. (2006). Defining torture. *Case Western Reserve Journal of International Law, 37,* 225.

Sutker, P., Vasterling, J., Brailey, K., & Allain, A. (1995). Memory, attention, and executive deficits in POW survivors: contributing biological and psychological factors. *Neuropsychology., 9,* 118–25.

Syed, H. R., Dalgard, O. S., Dalen, I., Claussen, B., Hussain, A., Selmer, R., & Ahlberg, N. (2006). Psychosocial factors and distress: a comparison between ethnic Norwegians and ethnic Pakistanis in Oslo, Norway. *Bmc Public Health, 6.* doi:10.1186/1471-2458-6-182

Task Group on Solitary Confinement. (2008). The Istanbul Statement on the use and effects of solitary confinement. *Torture Journal, 18*(1), 63–6.

Taylor, K. (2004). *Brainwashing: the science of thought control.* Oxford: Oxford University Press.

Theidon, K. (2004). *Entre prójimos: El conflicto armado interno y la política de la reconciliación en el Perú.* Lima, Perú: IEP Ediciones.

Theidon, K. (2010). Histories of innocence: post-war stories in Peru. In R. Shaw, L. Waldorf, & P. Hazan (Eds.), *Beyond the toolkit: rethinking the paradigm of transitional justice.* Palo Alto: Stanford University Press.

Thomas, G. (2001). *Mindfield.* Dublin: Mentor Books.

Thomas, G. C., III (2007). Confessions and police disclosure: Regulating police deception during interrogation. *Texas Tech Law Review, 39,* 1293–1319.

Thompson, S. K. (2005). The legality of the use of psychiatric neuroimaging in intelligence interrogation. *Cornell Law Review, 90,* 1601–38.

Toch, H. (1992). *Mosaic of despair: human breakdown in prison.* Washington DC: American Psychological Association.

Tringer, E. (2007). *Action research.* Thousand Oaks. California,: SAGE.

Trinquier, R. (1961). *La guerre moderne.* Paris: La Table ronde.

Trinquier, R., Duchemin, J., & Bailley, J. Le. (1963). *Notre guerre au Katanga [Our war in Katanga].* Paris: La Pensée Moderne.

Troccoli, J. N. (1996). *La ira de Leviatán. Del método de la furia a la búsqueda de la paz.* (Centro de Informaciones e Investigaciones del Uruguay, Ed.). Montevideo.

Tunning, W. (1978). Torture and philosophy. *Proceedings of the Aristotelian Society, 52,* 143–94.

UNESCO. Universal Declaration on Bioethics and Human Rights (adopted by UNESCO's General Conference on 19 October 2005) (2005). Retrieved from www.unesco.org/new/en/social-and-human-sciences/themes/bioethics/bioethics-and-human-rights/

United Nations High Commissioner for Human Rights. (2004). *Istanbul Protocol. Manual on the effective investigation and documentation of torture and other cruel, inhuman or degrading treatment or punishment.* (PROFESSION.). Geneva.

United Nations High Commissioner for Human Rights. (2005). *Human rights and prisons. Manual on human rights training for prison officials.*

US Army. (1992). *FM 34–52. Intelligence interrogation.* Washington DC.

US Army. (2006). *FM 2-22.3. Human intelligence collector operations.* (Vol. 3). Washington DC.

Van der Hart, O., Nijenhuis, E., & Steele, K. (2005). Dissociation: an insufficiently recognized major feature of complex posttraumatic stress disorder. *Journal of Traumatic Stress, 18*(5), 413–23.

van der Kolk, B., Roth, S., Pelcovitz, D., Sunday, S., & Spinazzola, J. (2005). Disorders of extreme stress: the empirical foundation of a complex adaptation to trauma. *Journal of Traumatic Stress, 18*(5), 389–99.

van Ommeren, M., de Jong, J. T. V. M., Sharma, B., Komproe, I., Thapa, S. B., & Cardeña, E. (2001). Psychiatric disorders among tortured Bhutanese refugees in Nepal. *Archives of General Psychiatry, 58*(5), 475. doi:10.1001/archpsyc.58.5.475

Vasiliades, E. (2004). Solitary confinement and international human rights: why the U.S. prison system fails global standards. *American Journal of International Law Review, 21,* 71–100.

Vecchio, N. Del, Elwy, A. R., Smith, E., Bottonari, K. A., & Eisen, S. V.(2011). Enhancing self-report assessment of PTSD: development of an item bank, *24*(2), 191–9. doi:10.1002/jts.

Victor., J. (1980). *Hugo Garcia Rivas: memorias de un ex-torturador.* Cordoba. Argentina: Ed CiD.

Vidal-Naquet, P. (1975). *Les Crimes de l'Armée Française en Algérie [Crimes of the French Army in Algeria].* Paris: Editions Le Decouverte.

Villani, M. (2011). *Desaparecido. Memorias de un cautiverio. Club Atlético. El Banco, El Olimpo, Pozo de Quilmes y ESMA.* Buenos Aires: Biblos.

Viñar, M., & Ulriksen, M. (1990). *Fracturas de la Memoria. Cronicas de una memoria por venir.* [Memory fractures. Chronicles of a memory to come]. Montevideo: Trilce.

Vorbrüggen, M., & Baer, H. U. (2007). Humiliation: the lasting effect of torture. *Military Medicine*, *172*, 29–33.

Vos, C. M. De. (2007). Mind the gap: purpose, pain, and the difference between torture and inhuman treatment. *Human Rights Brief*, *14*(2), 4–10.

Waldron, J. (2008). *Cruel, inhuman, and degrading treatment: the words themselves. New York University Public Law and Legal Theory Working Papers #98.* New York.

Wang, S.-J., Haque, M. A., Masum, S.-U.-D., Biswas, S., & Modvig, J. (2009). Household exposure to violence and human rights violations in western Bangladesh (II): history of torture and other traumatic experience of violence and functional assessment of victims. *BMC International Health and Human Rights*, *9*, 31. doi:10.1186/1472-698X-9-31

Wasco, S. M. (2003). Conceptualizing the harm done by rape. *Trauma, Violence and Abuse*, *4*(4), 309–22.

Weathers, F. W., & Keane, T. M.(2007). The criterion a problem revisited: controversies and challenges in defining and measuring psychological trauma. *Journal of Traumatic Stress*, *20*(2), 107–21.

Webster, E. (2011). Degradation: a human rights law perspective. In E. Kaufmann, P., Kuch, H., Neuhäuser, C., & Webster (Eds.), *Humiliation, degradation, dehumanization* (pp. 67–84). Dordrecht: Springer Netherlands.

Weierstall, R., Junghöfer, M., Ruf, M., Schauer, M., Neuner, F., Rockstroh, B., & Elbert, T. (2011). The tortured brain. *Zeitschrift Für Psychologie.* doi:10.1027/2151-2604/a000064

Weinstein, C. S., Fucetola, R., & Mollica, R. (2001). Neuropsychological issues in the assessment of refugees and victims of mass violence. *Neuropsychology Review*, *11*, 131–41. doi:10.1023/A: 1016650623996

Weissbrodt, D., Aolain, F., Fitzpatrick, J., & Newman, F. (2009). *International human rights: law, policy, and process* (4th ed.). LEXISNEXIS.

Welch, M. (2009). American 'pain-ology' in the war on terror: a critique of 'scientific' torture. *Theoretical Criminology*, *13*(4), 451–74. doi:10.1177/1362480609340394

Wessells, M. (2009). *Child soldiers: from violence to protection.* New York: Harvard University Press.

WHO-EU. (2007). *Health in prisons. A WHO guide to the essentials in prison health.* Copenhague: WHO.

Williams, A., & van der Merwe, J. (2013). The psychological impact of torture. *British Journal of Pain*, *7*(2), 101–6. doi:10.1177/2049463713483596

World Health Organization. (2010). *International Classification of Diseases 10th Revision.* Geneva.

World Medical Association (1975). *Declaration of Tokyo (1975).* Adopted by the World Medical Association, Tokyo, Japan. October 1975.

Yehuda, R., Flory, J. D., Pratchett, L. C., Buxbaum, J., Ising, M., & Holsboer, F. (2010). Putative biological mechanisms for the association between early life adversity and the subsequent development of PTSD. *Psychopharmacology*, *212*(3), 405–17. doi:10.1007/s00213-010-1969-6

Zawati, H. M. (2007). Impunity or immunity: wartime male rape and sexual torture as a crime against humanity. *Torture: Quarterly Journal on Rehabilitation of Torture Victims and Prevention of Torture*, *17*, 27–47. doi:2007-1.2006-0032 [pii]

Zimbardo, P. G. (2004). A situationist perspective on the psychology of evil: understanding how good people are trsformed into eprpetrators. In A. Miller (Ed.), *The social psycology of good and evil*, pp. 21–50. New York: Guilford Press.

Zimbardo, P. G. (2007). Thoughts on psychologists, ethics, and the use of torture in interrogations: don't ignore varying roles and complexities. *Analyses of Social Issues and Public Policy*, *7*(1):1–9, 070606100408001–??? doi:10.1111/j.1530-2415.2007.00122.x

Zimbardo, P. G. (2008). *The Lucifer effect.* Random House Inc. New York · London.

INDEX

because I know that
you will go further than me

'Si arribeu' © Lluís Llach 1977

Antoni i Trini, Mireia, Marc i Pol, Santi, Rosa, Roseta i Guillem, María Vergara, Jesús Antona, Inma Albí, Gabriela López, Marta Moya, Teresa González, Oihana Barrios, Miguel Ángel Navarro, Saioa Magunazelaia, Sara "Nodo" López, Eva y Guille, Elena y Finn, Valeria y Ale, Myriam Rivera, Susana Navarro, Martha Nubia Bello, Alfonso Rodriguez, Jose Antonio y Pili, Pepa, Antonio, Carla, Cesar y Sofia, Manuel, Verónica, Chris, Nico y Daniela, Mariángeles y Bernardo, Monika, María Luisa y Carlos, Bernardo, Reyes, Irene y Dani, Ángeles Plaza, Salva Lacruz, Pablo Olivos, Irina Kohan, Lidia y Lourdes, Itziar y Amos, Jorge y Marta (siempre Arizcun), Susana y Jorge, Ángela Palau, Beatriz Rodriguez, Blanca Amador, Marifé Bravo, Arancha García, Iñaki Márkez, Benito Morentin, Olatz Barrenechea, Nagore Lopez, Itziar Gandarias, SiRa Manrique y sus secuaces, Cristina y Dani, Maitane Arnoso, Roberta Bacic, Maren y Marcelo Viñar, Víctor Maturana, Jose Quidel y los araucanos, Vicente Amado, Maricel Robaina, Graciela Loarche y todos los que una quinquagesima noche de febrero regalaron sus sonrisas para que todo volviera a empezar.